W0050576

Principles of Microsurgical Techniques in Infertility

Principles of Microsurgical Techniques in Infertility

Edited by

J. Victor Reyniak

and

Niels H. Lauersen

Mount Sinai School of Medicine
New York, New York

Plenum Medical Book Company
New York and London

Library of Congress Cataloging in Publication Data

Main entry under title:

Principles of microsurgical techniques in infertility.

Bibliography: p.
Includes index.
1. Sterility, Female—Surgery. 2. Fallopian tubes—Surgery. 3. Microsurgery. 4. Vasovasostomy. I. Reyniak, J. Victor. II. Lauersen, Niels. [DNLM: 1. Microsurgery—Methods. 2. Sterility—Surgery. WP 570 P957]
RG201.P74   618.1′78059   81-3045
ISBN-13: 978-1-4684-4012-6   e-ISBN-13: 978-1-4684-4010-2 ACR2
DOI: 10.1007/978-1-4684-4010-2

Contributors

Richard D. Amelar, M.D.
Professor of Clinical Urology
New York University School of Medicine
New York, New York 10016

Ancel Blaustein, M.D.
Clinical Professor of Pathology
New York University School of Medicine
New York, New York 10016

Sami S. David, M.D.
Clinical Instructor
Department of Obstetrics and Gynecology
Mount Sinai School of Medicine
New York, New York 10029

W. P. Dmowski, M.D., Ph.D.
Professor of Obstetrics and Gynecology
Director, Division of Reproductive
  Endocrinology and Infertility
Department of Obstetrics and Gynecology
University of Arkansas for Medical
  Sciences
Little Rock, Arkansas 72205

Lawrence Dubin, M.D.
Professor of Clinical Urology
New York University School of Medicine
New York, New York 10016

Carlton A. Eddy, Ph.D.
Associate Professor
Department of Obstetrics and Gynecology
The University of Texas Health Science
  Center
San Antonio, Texas 78284

Martin S. Goldstein, M.D.
Assistant Clinical Professor
Department of Obstetrics and Gynecology
Mount Sinai School of Medicine
New York, New York 10029

Martin Greenberg, M.D.
Fellow, Reproductive Endocrinology
Department of Obstetrics and Gynecology
Mount Sinai School of Medicine
New York, New York 10029

Saul B. Gusberg, M.D.
Professor and Chairman
Department of Obstetrics and Gynecology
Mount Sinai School of Medicine
New York, New York 10029

Niels H. Lauersen, M.D.
Associate Professor
Department of Obstetrics and Gynecology
Mount Sinai School of Medicine
New York, New York 10029

J. Victor Reyniak, M.D.
Clinical Professor of Gynecology
   and Obstetrics
Director, Division of Reproductive
   Endocrinology
Mount Sinai School of Medicine
New York, New York 10029

John A. Rock, M.D.
Assistant Professor
Department of Obstetrics and Gynecology
Director, Division of Reproductive
   Endocrinology
Head, Reproductive Surgery
The Johns Hopkins Hospital
Baltimore, Maryland 21205

Alexander Sedlis, M.D.
Professor of Obstetrics and Gynecology
State University of New York
Downstate Medical Center
Brooklyn, New York 11203

John J. Stangel, M.D.
Associate Clinical Professor of Obstetrics
   and Gynecology
Director, Section of Reproductive
   Endocrinology and Infertility
New York Medical College
Westchester County Medical Center
Valhalla, New York 10595

Foreword

While this world eagerly awaits the ideal contraceptive technique that could efficiently, safely, and esthetically save this planet from the starvation and squalor of overcrowding and offer women control over their reproductive capacity, the individual faced with the frustration, even desperation, induced by infertility begs for help in achieving the desired conception.

The discipline of gynecology and obstetrics, recognizing the importance of these problems and the need for special expertise in reproductive endocrinology and its attendant clinical challenges in fertility and infertility, has now formalized the training of specialists in this area of scientific knowledge in a further effort to advance the skills of diagnosis and treatment attendant on these complex problems.

Slowly but steadily, as befits the complexity of the endocrine and metabolic pathways involved, the scientific basis of reproductive physiology has been revealed by the research of physicians, biochemists, and physiologists. It is clear that no significant clinical advance can be made without the foundation of such new knowledge. Indeed, the successful treatment of infertility resulting from failure of ovulation was based on just such a scientific advance.

At the same time, caring gynecologists have been frustrated by their meager success in dealing with organic causes of infertility, especially those causing impairment of the transport mechanisms of ovum and sperm. The introduction of microsurgical techniques for the resolution of the problem of organic tubal obstruction suggests a strategy that enables the gynecologic surgeon to deal gently and effectively with these problems and bring the diseased Fallopian tube as close as possible to its normal physiological transport capacity. There is little doubt of its effectiveness, and it may, in fact, be revolutionary.

This volume offers the clinician an expert view of the microsurgical method by seasoned gynecologic surgeons and teachers in addition to describing the pre- and postoperative clinical and psychoemotional preparation so important in problems of reproductive disorders.

S. B. Gusberg, M.D., D.Sc., FACS, FACOG, FRCOG

Preface

The purpose of this book is to present guidelines for the application of microsurgical principles to the management of infertility. The endpoint to be utilized in judging the success of microsurgery for infertility is the delivery of a term infant. This ultimate goal cannot be achieved by the bare knowledge of microsurgical techniques isolated from the knowledge of the reproductive system. Microsurgery can statistically improve the success rate as compared to standard infertility surgery, and this volume provides a detailed description of the microsurgical principles, tools, and instrumentation and the most current techniques. In addition, it offers important information to enhance the reader's understanding of the physiology and the pathophysiology of the reproductive structures that are the subjects of the microsurgery. The most skillful surgery performed by the most knowledgeable physician, however, is doomed to failure in an inappropriate candidate. Patient selection and preoperative counseling are, therefore, emphasized. Finally, the present availability of microsurgery offers a physician the ability to maintain or restore fertility in patients in whom such maintainence or restoration previously would have been very difficult if not impossible. Therefore, the management of certain conditions, such as ectopic pregnancy, is considered in the light of microsurgery.

This book has been designed for the full range of physicians concerned with infertility, from the surgeon who will utilize these instruments and techniques to the clinician who will counsel the infertile couple as to the appropriateness of microsurgery for their particular problem. The editors and contributing authors hope that this book will add to the knowledge of and the ability to correct a rapidly increasing clinical problem, infertility.

J. Victor Reyniak, M.D.
Niels H. Lauersen, M.D.

Acknowledgments

The editors wish to thank all the contributing authors, whose knowledge, enthusiasm, and effort made this book a reality. A special acknowledgment is owed to Kathleen H. Wilson for her skillful editing and organization of this textbook.

We are grateful to our secretary, Lori Leeds, for her dedication and professionalism. We also wish to thank Carol Mercado for her efforts in the typing and preparation of the manuscripts. Our thanks also go to Connie DeGrazia for her typing assistance. Our appreciation also goes to Dr. Zoë R. Graves for her assistance on the final proof of this volume.

We are indebted to Laurel Purington and Leonard Dank for their excellent medical illustrations and artwork. We finally wish to thank the staff at Plenum Publishing Corporation for their valuable assistance in the preparation of this book.

J. V. R.
N. H. L.

Contents

Principles of Microsurgical Techniques in Infertility

1 Principles of Microsurgery in Infertility

J. Victor Reyniak

Department of Obstetrics and Gynecology
Division of Reproductive Endocrinology
Mount Sinai School of Medicine
New York, New York 10029

Microsurgical techniques have become an integral part of those surgical subspecialties that deal with small anatomical structures. Application of microsurgical techniques often results in an improved clinical outcome as compared with conventional methods.

Infertility surgeons have been relatively tardy in utilizing these techniques in their surgery, for the components of the reproductive tract in both male and female are essentially "macro" structures. Furthermore, many aspects of the physiology and function of the Fallopian tubes and the vas deferens are still not fully understood. In the past, conventional infertility surgeons frequently considered these structures as mere conduits and attempted to restore patency alone at all costs. For this reason, the functional potential of these structures could even have been jeopardized by the use of large-caliber, reactive suture materials and application of various mechanical devices to assure patency.

The first use of an operating microscope in Fallopian tube surgery is credited to Wolfgang Waltz in 1959.[1] Subsequently, Swolin introduced microsurgical techniques to reconstructive tubal surgery.[2,3] Instrumentaion, magnification, and techniques were adapted from other surgical specialties that dealt with true microstructures—ophthalmology, otology, vascular, and neurosurgery.[4] Microsurgical anastomosis of previously ligated Fallopian tubes was first reported in the United States by Garcia,[5] and Silber[6] utilized microsurgical techniques in vasovasotomy for reversal of operative male sterilization. Subsequently, a period of animal microsurgical experimentation ensued.[7-9] The application of microsurgical techniques in human infertility surgery eventually gained wider acceptance in the late 1960s and early 1970s.[10,11] The final result of those innovative techniques has been a change in the overall approach to infertility surgery that has evolved within the past 10 years. A cluster of techniques and principles referred to as microsurgery has been adopted by most infertility surgeons. The obvious reason for such acceptance was the reported improvement in the outcome of infertility surgery as measured by the number of live births and low rate of ectopic gestations (see Chapter 5).

Microsurgery represents an additional skill that can be added to the armamentarium of the infertility surgeon if that person has sufficient time, motivation and patience to undergo both the new training and the retraining required by the microsurgical approach. Most infertility surgeons have been trained in conventional surgical techniques, and the learning of the new skills demanded by microsurgery implies a considerable change in both mental and physical attitude toward the surgical procedure. The technical challenge of operating on reproductive structures under optic magnification cannot, however, be met by a surgeon who does not possess an in-depth knowledge and understanding of both physiology and pathophysiology of these organs (see Chapters 2 and 3).

Furthermore, microsurgical techniques, even in the most skilled hands, may not be the answer in a variety of pathological conditions, such as when the damage to the oviduct has been too extensive or in conditions with obscure deleterious effect on fertility potential, e.g., endometriosis in the female and absence of testicular spermatogenesis in the male. Thus, the surgeon's responsibility is patient preselection, which involves careful preoperative evaluation of all factors affecting fertility of the couple, followed by indepth counseling (see Chapters 5 and 6). Only then may the application of the mechanical skill of microsurgery be reasonable and beneficial to the clinical outcome.

MICROSURGICAL TRAINING

In contrast to conventional infertility surgery, microsurgical techniques cannot be learned by assisting in the operating room. The basic skills must be learned in the laboratory, and the number of hours necessary to acquire these skills varies from individual to individual. Initially, the surgeon may practice "operating" under the microscope on rubber or nylon tubing or gauze sponges. Thereafter, ideally, laboratory animals should be used, although excised human Fallopian tubes or even segments of umbilical cord are suitable *in vitro* laboratory specimens. The prospective microsurgeon must learn hand–eye coordination under various magnifications and develop the ability to place suture so as to minimize tissue trauma.

The proper position of the needle in the spring-loaded needle holder and the needle holder in the surgeon's hand is very important (Fig. 1). In the course of a microsurgical procedure, multiple sutures must be tied, and the technique of tying an instrument-tied square knot under magnification must be learned (Fig. 2). It is essential to master these skills in the laboratory, for clumsy technique in the operating

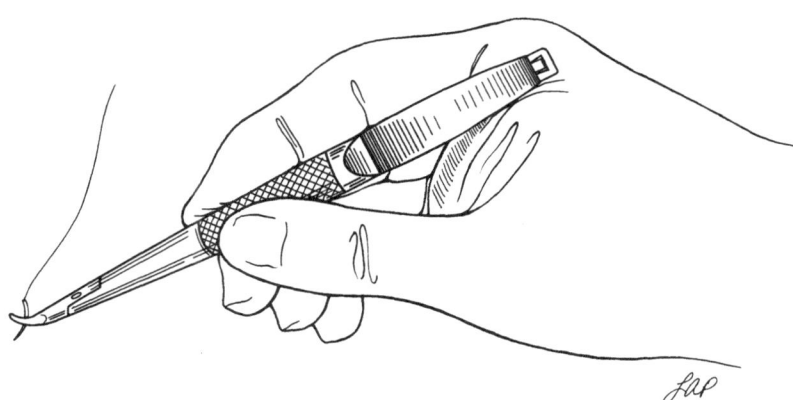

Figure 1. Proper position of the needle in the needle holder and of the needle holder in the hand. Note that with this positioning the placement of the suture in the tissue would require minimal rotation of the needle holder.

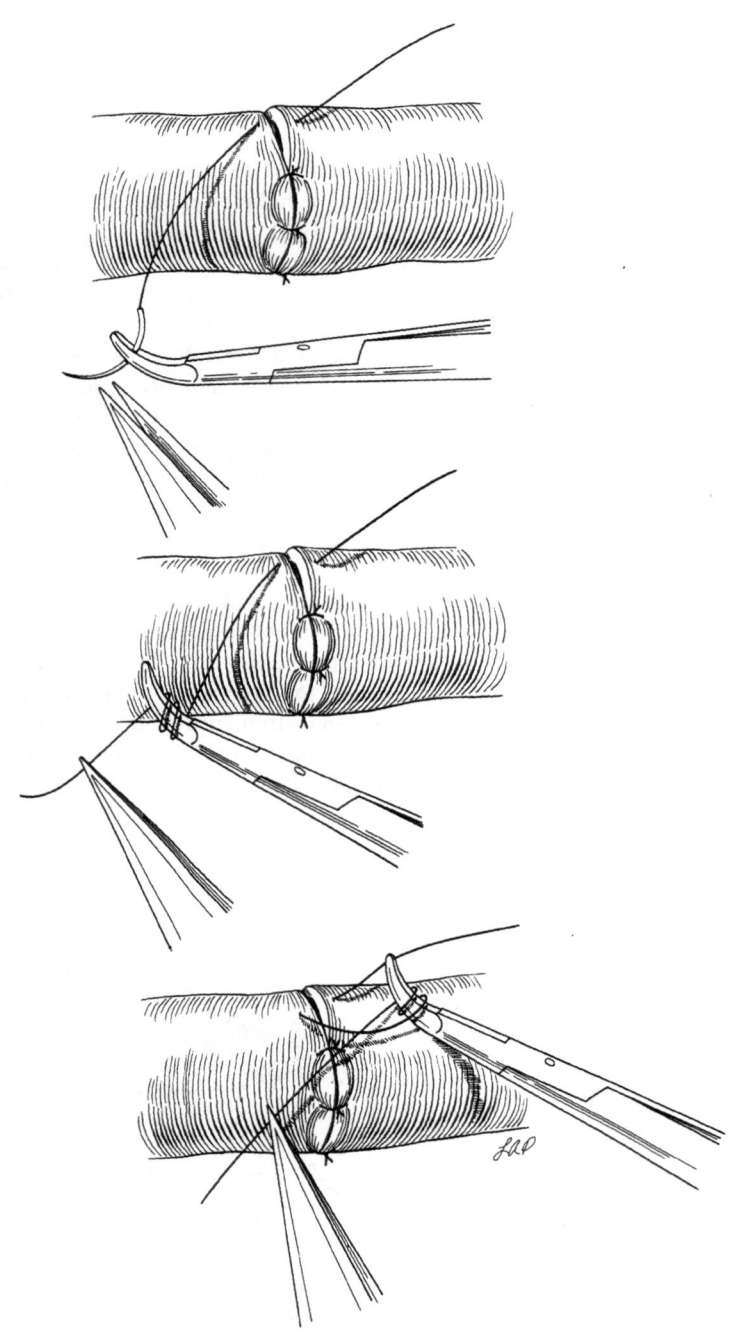

room results in prolonged operating time with the deleterious effects of inadvertant atmospheric drying of exposed pelvic structures by the heat of the operating room lights. The technical aspects of microsurgical procedures will be discussed in detail in subsequent chapters of this volume (Chapters 4, 7, 8, 10, and 13). It is essential, however, to understand that although not all cases of infertility surgery lend themselves to the use of high optic magnification, the microsurgical principles can be beneficially applied every time a procedure designed to promote or restore fertility potential is performed (Chapters 9, 11, and 12).

MICROSURGICAL PRINCIPLES

The following principles must therefore be followed in infertility surgery:

1. Reconstructive surgery is an elective procedure and, as such, in the female, it should be scheduled preferably during the proliferative phase of the cycle, which is considered the anabolic generative interval.[12] In addition, operating on the adnexa during the preovulatory phase eliminates the risk of inadvertant damage to the recent corpus luteum.

2. *Meticulous hemostasis* must be observed regardless of the type of incision. During laparotomy in the female, a low transverse incision is usually adequate for exposure; the edges of the incision should be covered with moistened laparotomy pads before the placement of self-retaining retractors.[13]

3. *Adequate elevation and immobilization of structures* to be operated on are essential to allow ap-

Figure 2. Technique of instrument tying under magnification. Following placement of the suture, its long end with needle attached is grasped 2-3 cm from the suture emergence from the tissue by tying forceps, which are held in the left hand. The needle is then released from the needle holder. The long end of the suture is looped twice around the point of the needle holder with the tying forceps. The short (distal) end of the suture is then grasped with the needle holder. Traction allows for tying of the first knot. The identical steps are repeated for the second and third throws of the knot.

plication of optic magnification with its shallow depth of field. In female infertility surgery, this may be accomplished by packing the vagina prior to laparotomy with moist laparotomy pads or gauze rolls to elevate the uterus and adnexa. After division and excision of adhesions, moistened packs can be placed both in the cul-de-sac and anteriorly under the pubis to further improve the exposure and immobilization. A pediatric Foley catheter can be placed transcervically into the uterine cavity and brought into the sterile field with extension tubing for tubal perfusion. When transfundal perfusion is necessary, Hellman–Siegler or Buxton clamps are used to occlude the uterocervical junction and to permit elevation of the uterus. The use of Babcock clamps or traction sutures on the fundus must be avoided to minimize tissue trauma and adhesion formation.

4. *Versatility in the use of optic magnification is necessary.* The main purpose of magnification is to allow identification and excision of pathological tissues while following the physiological tissue planes and, subsequently, to permit precise and accurate approximation of tissues and placement of sutures. Low magnifications are required for lysis of adhesions. *Loupes,* with magnification of $\times 2$ to $\times 6$, provide a comfortable focal length, a fairly wide field of view, and a greater depth of field as compared with the microscope. Their use usually requires an additional light source such as a fiberoptic cable or a headlamp.

The *operating microscope* is the preferred instrument for anastomosis procedures. Microscopes provide a selection of magnification from $\times 4$ to $\times 40$. Optical combinations for operating microscopes set up for infertility surgery include: eye pieces of $\times 10$, $\times 12.5$, or $\times 16$ magnification with an objective lens of 250, 275, or 300 mm. Therefore, the range of magnification can vary from $\times 2$ to $\times 20$. The most useful combination entails eyepieces of $\times 12.5$ and an objective lens of 275-mm focal length and provides a range of magnification from $\times 3$ to $\times 15$.[13] Magnifications above $\times 10$ are rarely used in infertility surgery (see Chapter 4 for a detailed discussion of optic magnification).

5. *Maximally atraumatic operating technique must be used.* Tissue handling should be avoided whenever possible. Fingers, plastic, or glass rods are less traumatic than abrasive metal instruments for manipulation or traction. When excising adhesions, the surgeon must avoid disturbing the peritoneal surface. Inadvertent peritoneal trauma should be repaired using fine sutures that are to be placed without traction. Division of adhesions is best accomplished with a monopolar needle microelectrode. The cutting should be performed along the axis of a plastic or glass rod placed under the adhesive bands; this allows the adhesions to be placed under tension to delineate tissue planes. The use of plastic or glass avoids possible damage to adjacent tissues by current spread. The use of $\times 4$ loupes provides the best delineation of tissue planes and permits precise division of adhesions. The use of microscopes for lysis is less advantageous because the size of the operating area would necessitate constant lens readjustment. Excessive magnification can actually impede the progress of the procedure and increase the operating time.[12]

6. *An understanding of the principles in electrosurgery is essential.* Microbipolar forceps are optimal for pinpoint hemostasis. Electrodissection with hemostasis is best accomplished by the use of a monopolar needle microelectrode connected to a low cutting current. Overzealous coagulation must be avoided. Magnification and tissue irrigation allow for precise identification and coagulation of bleeding points.

7. *All exposed serosal surfaces must be kept moist at all times.* Physiological saline, with or without added heparin,[12] or Ringer's lactate have been recommended. We prefer 6% dextran 70 solution (see Chapters 7 and 12). A syringe with attached 18-guage plastic cannula can be used to constantly moisten tissues and help in the identification of bleeding points by providing a fine stream of fluid. This "wet" technique, developed for

neurosurgery, not only reduces tissue drag and shrinkage but prevents the coagulated tissue from adhering to the forceps.[14,15] Sponging of tissues should be avoided at all costs.

8. *Approximation of tissues should be delicate, precise, and follow actual anatomical tissue planes.* Hemostasis must be meticulous, and both bipolar microforceps and fine ligature ties are superior to unipolar, one-point coagulation. In the latter method, the current spreads in conical area beneath the surface, and this results in desiccation of tissue with the increased possibility for fibrosis and adhesion.

9. *All available measures must be utilized to prevent formation of postoperative adhesions* (see Chapter 12). Adhesions formed on the tissue of the Fallopian tube may cause kinking, impairment of mobility, or even total blockage of the lumen.[16–18]

10. *Atraumatic microneedles and fine inert or nonreactive sutures must be used.* The most versatile suture material is 7-0 to 8-0 polyglactin suture, although nylon sutures of this or finer caliber may be utilized. A 6-0 material is sufficient for re-peritonealization when necessary. Sutures of larger caliber should be avoided.[12] (For detailed discussion of sutures and needles, see Chapter 6.)

11. *Fine delicate instruments must be used.* The number of instruments should be kept to a minimum to avoid cluttering the operative field. A spring-loaded microneedle holder is superior to the locking type for totally atraumatic placement of the needle through the tissues. The only other instruments necessary for most cases are microscissors, iris scissors, toothed microforceps, and tying forceps.

In conclusion, the cluster of technical principles termed microsurgery should be applied to every operation aimed at restoration of fertility, for the approach is advantageous to the surgical outcome. The use of an operating microscope is not always necessary, because not all cases lend themselves to the use of high magnification. Specifically, in lysing of adhesions, fimbrial lysis, and most cases of pelvic endometriosis, operating loupes may offer sufficient magnification and versatility. The application of the basic principles and techniques delineated in this chapter aims at the attainment of the optimal clinical outcome.

REFERENCES

1. Waltz W: Sterilitatsoperationen an der Tube mit hilfe eines Operationmikroskupe. *Z Geburtshilfe Gynaekol* 153:49, 1959.
2. Swolin K: Fertilitatsoperationen. I. Literatur und Methodik. *Acta Obstet Gynecol Scand* 46:234, 1967.
3. Swolin K: Fifty fertility operations. I: Literature and methods. *Obstet Gynecol Surg* 23:382, 1968.
4. Kraus H: Foreword: Microsurgery, in Koos WT, Bock FW, Spetzler RT (eds): *Clinical Microsurgery*. Stuttgart, Georg Thieme, 1976, p 18.
5. Garcia C-R: Oviductal anastomosis procedures, in: Richard RM, Prager DJ (eds): *Human Sterilization*. Springfield, Ill., Charles C Thomas, 1972, p 116.
6. Silber SJ: Microsurgery of the male genitalia: nonvascular, in Silber SJ (ed), *Microsurgery*. Baltimore, Williams & Wilkins, 1979, p 332.
7. David A, Brackett BG, Garcia C-R: Effects of microsurgical removal of the rabbit uterotubal junction. *Fertil Steril* 20:250, 1969.
8. Paterson P, Wood C: The use of microsurgery in the reanastomosis of the rabbit Fallopian tube. *Fertil Steril* 25:757, 1974.
9. Winston RML: Microsurgical reanastomosis of the rabbit oviduct and its functional and pathological sequelae. *Br J Obstet Gynaecol* 82:513, 1975.
10. Gomel V: Tubal renanastomosis by microsurgery. *Fertil Steril* 28:58, 1977.
11. Diamond E: Microsurgery in infertility: Instrumentation and technique, in: Phillips DM (ed): *Microsurgery in Gynecology*. Downey, Calif., American Association of Gynecologic Laparoscopists, 1977, p 20.
12. Garcia C-R, Mastroianni L: Microsurgery for treatment of adnexal disease. *Fertil Steril* 34:413, 1980.
13. Gomel V: Recent advances in surgical correction of tubal disease producing infertility. *Curr Probl Obstet Gynecol* 1(10):1, 1978.
14. Greenwood J Jr: Two points coagulation: A follow-up report on a new technique and instrument for electrocoagulation in neurosurgery. *Arch Phys Ther* 23:552, 1942.
15. Greenwood J Jr: Two-point or interpolar coagulation: Review after a twelve-year period with notes on addition of a sucker tip. *J Neurosurg* 12:196, 1955.
16. Diamond E: Lysis of postoperative pelvic adhesions in infertility. *Fertil Steril* 31:287, 1979.
17. Gomel V: Causes of failed reconstructive tubal microsurgery. *J Reprod Med* 24:239, 1980.
18. Holtz G: Prevention of postoperative adhesions. *J Reprod Med* 24:141, 1980.

2 Physiology of the Fallopian Tube

Carlton A. Eddy

Department of Obstetrics and Gynecology
The University of Texas Health Science Center
San Antonio, Texas 78284

Tubal infertility surgery is a heterogeneous collection of techniques performed by surgeons of widely differing capabilities, insights, and motivations on patients with a variety of conditions, the successful treatment of which is defined by an elusive event temporally remote from the original surgery—the term delivery of a normal infant.

Macrosurgery, at least historically, has been guided by the simplistic impression of the oviduct as a hollow viscus prone to losing its patency but amenable to surgical reopening and, failing that, to being replaced by an appropriately hollow substitute such as the appendix or a section of fetal umbilical blood vessel. This attitude has largely relegated tubal surgery to a procedure without special technique, instruments, or suture. Until recently, most tubal macrosurgery had as its goal the reestablishment of patency—assured through the use of assorted probes, stents, hoods, and spirals over which the oviduct was sewn and allowed to heal, in some cases for up to 6 months, using suture and techniques common to general gynecologic and abdominal surgery. Tubal macrosurgery tended not to be undertaken specifically to conserve or restore complex tubal anatomy and its associated physiological function because the naked eye could not perceive such structure.

In contrast, it has become almost axiomatic that the practitioner of gynecologic microsurgery regards the oviduct as an anatomically and physiologically complex structure and seeks to preserve and restore functional anatomy. With the resolution of the operating microscope in concert with specialized instruments, nonreactive microsutures, and a high level of surgical competence, very precise reconstruction of internal genital anatomy is possible, thereby maximizing the potential for the restoration of complex physiological function. Only when such function has been restored, either macrosurgically or microsurgically, can a return to fertility be realistically anticipated. This chapter will describe some of those functions.

TUBAL ANATOMY

The historical and continuing clinical preoccupation with the diagnosis and the restoration of tubal patency reflects the fact that the oviduct is basically a tubular structure. The oviducts are paired pelvic organs that furnish a functional communication between the ovaries and the uterus. Anatomically, they arise from the superior lateral aspect of the uterine fundus and extend to the ovaries. Each oviduct is supported throughout its length by a mesenteric peritoneal fold, the mesosalpinx. The oviducts are directed laterally to the ovaries, over which they arch, and terminate in an abdominal ostium, an opening surrounded by fimbriated mucosal projections collectively referred to as the fimbria (Fig. 1).

The oviduct is a seromuscular organ composed of an outer serous coat, the serosa, a middle smooth muscle coat, the myosalpinx, with outer longitudinal and inner circular layers, and an internal mucous coat, the endosalpinx, composed of ciliated and secretory cells. The oviduct averages 10–12 cm in length and may be divided into four segments based on characteristic morphological differences: (1) the intramural segment contained within the wall of the uterus; (2) the isthmus, proximal to the uterus, constituting approximately one-third of the extrauterine oviduct; (3) the ampulla, distal to the uterus, constituting the virtual remaining two-thirds of the oviduct; and (4) the infundibulum, the short (1–2 cm) terminal segment, the most prominent feature of which is the fimbriated abdominal ostium (Fig. 2).

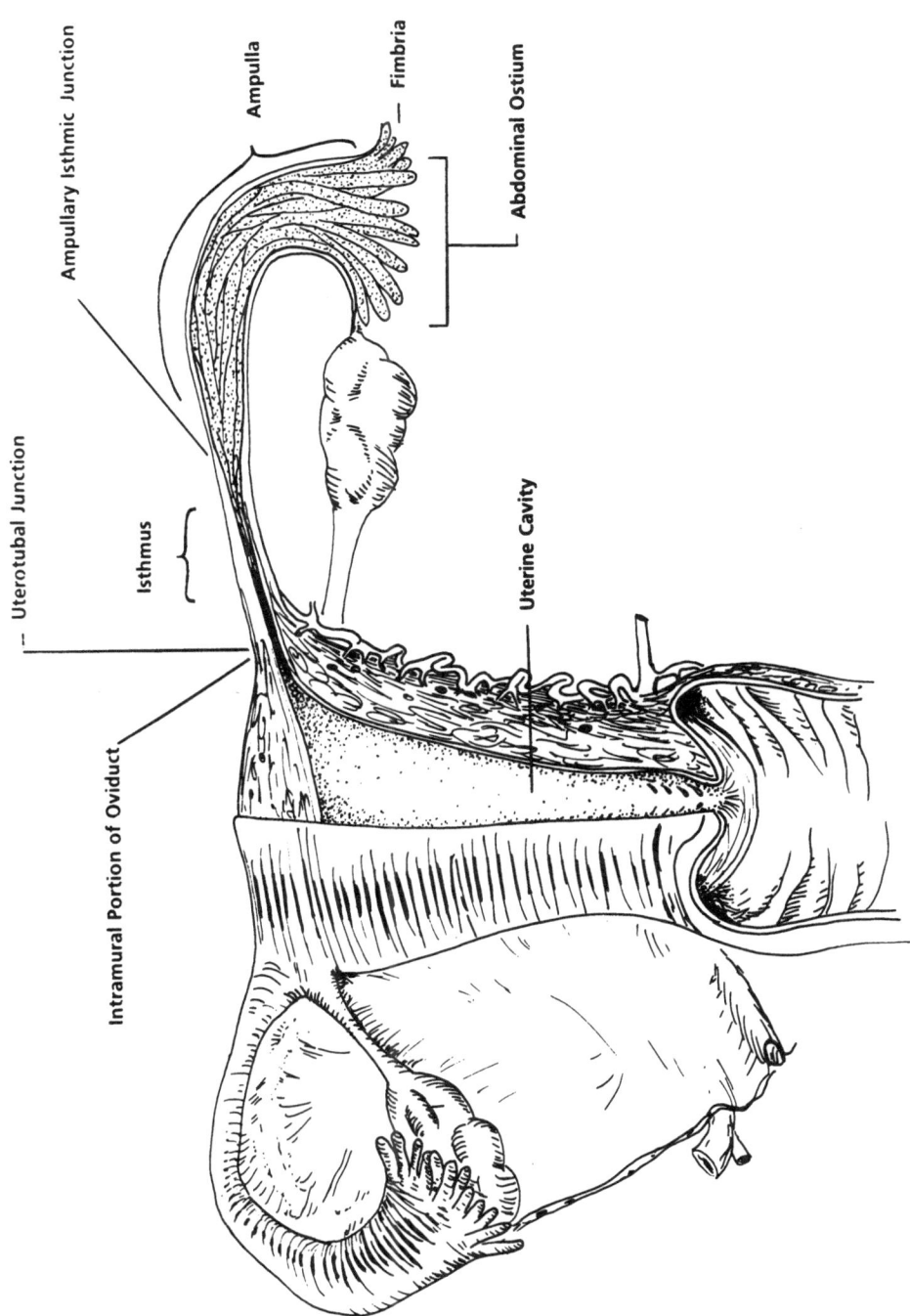

Figure 1. The human female reproductive tract. The relationship of the oviduct to the uterus, ovary, and supporting mesenteries is shown. On the right side, the uterus and oviduct are depicted in section to reveal internal structure and blood supply.

Labels: Uterotubal Junction, Ampullary Isthmic Junction, Ampulla, Fimbria, Abdominal Ostium, Isthmus, Uterine Cavity, Intramural Portion of Oviduct

PHYSIOLOGY OF THE FALLOPIAN TUBE | **13**

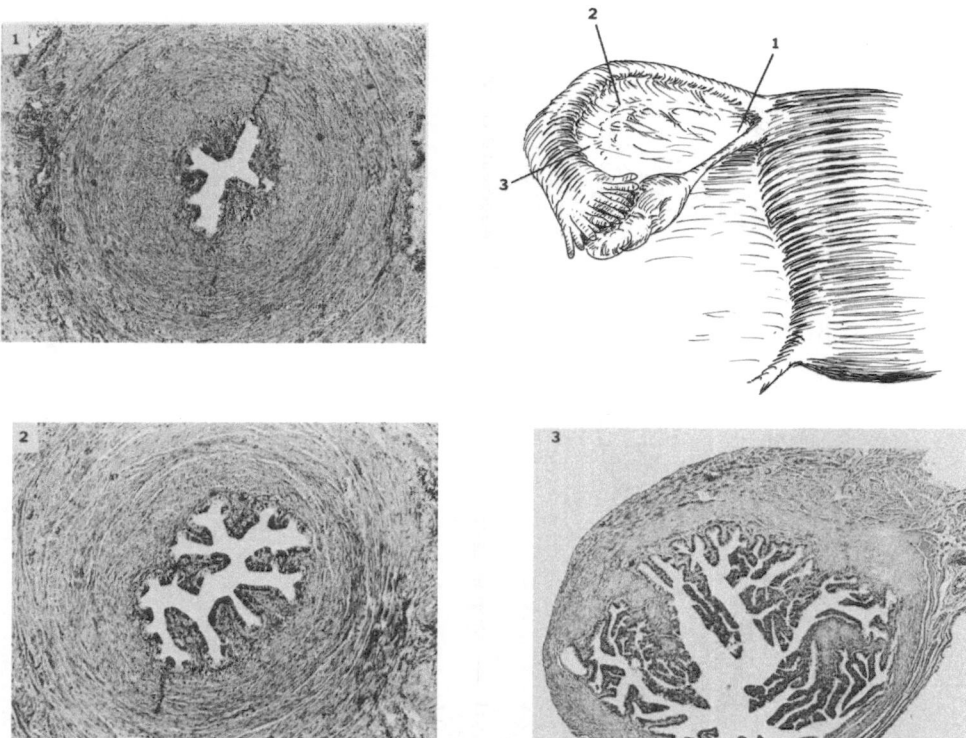

Figure 2. Cross-sectional morphology of the oviduct at the level of (1) the proximal isthmus near the uterotubal junction, (2) the distal isthmus near the ampullary isthmic junction, and (3) the ampulla. The cross sections correspond to the areas indicated in the accompanying drawing (4). Note the progressive increase in luminal diameter and endosalpinx complexity from proximal isthmus to distal ampulla and the corresponding decrease in myosalpinx thickness.

Interstitial Segment

The interstitial segment of the oviduct transverses the uterine wall and, hence, is surrounded by a substantial myometrium thickness. The myosalpinx comprises an external uterine layer of longitudinally arranged smooth muscle bundles, an intermediate, circularly arranged layer, and an inner longitudinal layer.[1,2] Ciliated mucosa of intermediate type, between that of the endometrium and that of the oviduct, line the lumen, which is approximately 400 μm in diameter and may describe a variety of paths to the endometrial cavity.[3] The transition from extrauterine to interstitial oviduct, the uterotubal junction (UTJ), has long been considered to function as a physiological sphincter that regulates passage of ova into the uterus and of spermatozoa into the oviduct. The existence of such a sphincter, however, has not been demonstrated convincingly. A recent report of successful pregnancies in approximately 50% of patients treated for proximal tubal obstruction with bilateral uterotubal implantation at the posterior uterine fundus[4] suggests that the UTJ is not critical to normal reproduction.

Isthmus

The isthmus is the most densely muscular segment of extrauterine oviduct. The myosalpinx contains well-developed outer longitudinal and inner circular muscle layers with an additional inner longitudinal layer that extends proximally to the uterus and distally to the ampulla. The endosalpinx is moderately folded into three to five primary folds that describe a cruciform shape in cross-section in the area adjacent to the UTJ. Toward the ampulla, the folds become more numerous and complex. Secretory cells predominate over ciliated, although the latter are also abundant. The isthmic lumen is narrow, averaging 400 μm (range 100 μm-1 mm).

The thick myosalpinx, narrow lumen, and dense adrenergic innervation strongly suggest that the isthmus is a physiological sphincter that, in concert with UTJ, regulates the passage of gametes, thereby insuring normal fertilization and proper timing of the embryo's entrance into the endometrial cavity. Clinical studies[5] and animal experiments[6,7] in which major portions or the entire isthmus have been removed indicate that the isthmus may not be critical to normal fertility because pregnancy can occur in its absence. Certainly, subtotal resection of the isthmus is consistent with normal fertility.

Winston and Margara[8] reported on microsurgical reversal of previous elective tubal sterilization in 95 patients who underwent anastomosis at various anatomic locations. The most successful of the reversal procedures was isthmo-isthmic anastomosis, which produced a 78% pregnancy rate. This success rate may have been the result of several factors: the relative technical ease of suturing the thick-walled isthmus with its relatively uncomplicated endosalpinx; the inability of minor postoperative isthmic adhesions to cause distortion and kinking of the isthmus; and the possible physiological dispensability of major proportions of the isthmus.

Ampulla   The ampulla is the largest portion of the oviduct. Unlike the isthmus and intramural segments, the ampulla is thin walled with a large lumen, measuring 1–2 cm at the ampullary–isthmic junction (AIJ). The myosalpinx consists of outer longitudinal and inner circular muscle layers. A discontinuous inner longitudinal arrangement of fibers may be observed in portions of the proximal ampulla. The endosalpinx is extensively folded, rendering the lumen a virtual space. In contrast to the isthmus, ciliated cells predominate in the distal ampulla and gradually decrease in numbers toward the isthmus. Cilia throughout the tube beat toward the uterus and are thought to be important in ovum and embryo transport to the uterus.

In contrast to the isthmus, the ampulla appears to be more important for normal fertility. Resection of a segment of ampulla followed by ampullary anastomosis tends to be among the least successful sterilization reversal procedures with the exception of salpingostomy. Because of its thin-walled anatomy, the ampulla is easily collapsed. The inevitable peritubal adhesions that follow tuboplastic surgery, even if mild by subjective appraisal, may be sufficient to place tension on the ampulla, resulting in functional occlusion of the lumen. Similarly, the difficulty of placing anastomosis sutures accurately to avoid the endosalpinx may interfere with the complex system of mucosal folds and lead to partial or complete occlusion of the lumen or to the formation of blind passages. This architectural damage to the tube may be an important determinant in the occurrence of ectopic pregnancy. The post-tubal-surgery patient is always at an increased risk of ectopic pregnancy. The majority of tubal ectopic implants occur in the ampulla,[1] a logical occurrence since fertilization and early embryo development occur at this location. Derangement of the ovum transport mechanism or occlusion of the ampullary lumen may allow fertilization but deny passage of the developing embryo, with subsequent implantation in the ampulla.

Infundibulum   The infundibulum is the trumpet-shaped distal portion of the oviduct that terminates in the fimbriated tubal abdominal ostium. It is thin walled with outer longitudinal and inner circular muscle layers surrounding a lumen that often exceeds 1 cm in diameter. The tubal epithelium is extensively plicated. The majority of cells are ciliated. Surrounding the tubal ostium is the extensively fringed fimbria, which is thrown into numerous lanciform folds that surround and cover the ostium. The fimbrial epithelium is densely ciliated; the distribution of such cells approaches 70% in normal, fertile women. The direction of ciliary beat is toward the uterus, as it is throughout the oviduct.

As the functional connection between ovary and oviduct, the infundibulum and fimbria lie in close apposition to the ovary. The anatomic approximation is maintained by the mesenteries and ligaments that support the ovaries and oviducts. These structures contain smooth muscle fibers that contract vigorously at the time of ovulation, thereby drawing the ovary and fimbria closer together, a result that may facilitate ovum pickup. Because of the highly specialized nature of the fimbria and its role in the ovum pickup mechanism, pathologically or iatrogenically induced loss of the fimbria is consistent with infertility and remains one of the most difficult conditions to correct surgically.

TUBAL PHYSIOLOGY

The anatomic complexity of the oviduct is mirrored in its muscular, secretory, and ciliary activity, which vary with the endocrine status. Through integration of such activity, the oviduct supports a number of diverse and complex processes including sperm transport, capacitation, ovum pickup, fertilization, early embryo development, and ovum and embryo transport. The efficiency and regularity of these processes, particularly when considered within the context of rather precise temporal requirements for gamete survival, union, and initial embryo development, attest to the oviduct's complexity and account for the present incompleteness of our understanding of these processes and of their integration.

Tubal Contractility

A great deal of descriptive information has been acquired about patterns of contractility in the human oviduct throughout the menstrual cycle. The oviduct exhibits a continuous, complex pattern of spontaneous activity. Complete quiescence never occurs. Even during pregnancy, when the uterus has been rendered quiescent by high levels of circulating progesterone, the oviducts remain spontaneously active, although at a reduced rate similar to that of the late luteal or early proliferative phase of the menstrual cycle.[9] Two peaks of contractility occur: one at menstruation, when estrogen levels are lowest; the other around the time of ovulation, when estrogen levels are highest. The relative refractoriness of the oviduct to the uterine inhibitory influence of progesterone, which is rising during the period of ovum transport, may be important to insure that gamete transport can proceed despite uterine quiescence. Although the relationship between tubal contractility and gamete transport remains undefined, contractility is generally thought to be a major component.

As in other muscular tissues, contractile activity of the smooth muscle of the oviduct is preceeded and triggered by action potentials arising within and propagated through the oviductal muscular syncytium.[10] Because of the arrangement of muscle fibers in layers oriented in circular and longitudinal fashion, the oviduct is capable of generating a variety of contractile patterns including peristaltic, antiperistaltic, and segmental contractions. Unlike the gut, which is adapted for continuous transport of luminal contents over great distances and to which the oviduct is often but erroneously compared, the oviduct does not appear to experience regular peristaltic contractions. It instead undergoes segmental contractions that propagate simultaneously in opposite directions over short distances. Ovum transport therefore assumes a discontinuous pattern of reciprocal movements in which the ovum is forced out of areas of contraction into inactive regions. Thus, ovum transport appears to be a series of random movements that, over a period of several days, acquire a gradual net bias toward the uterus.

Laboratory studies[11,12] using the rabbit, in which propagation of action potentials and the effect of the resultant contractile activity of the oviduct on ovum transport were measured, have allowed the following hypothesis to be evolved. Shortly after ovulation, contractile activity predominates in the distal oviduct while the major portion of the isthmus is quiescent. This inactive region acts as a passive "absorbing barrier" into which the ovum tends to collect because there are no contractions to push the ovum back to the active region. The gradual movement of this inactive region toward the uterus during the 3-day period of ovum

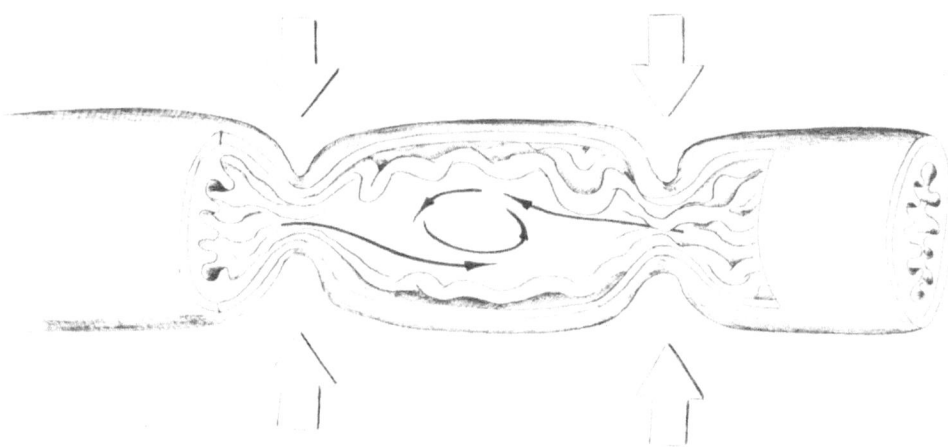

Figure 3. Semidiagrammatic representation of segmental tubal contractility. Wide, light arrows depict points of spontaneous segmental contraction. Narrow solid arrows depict transient, turbulent flow within the short segment of oviduct momentarily created by two adjacent segmental contractions. Such a flow pattern may be of importance in transporting gametes.

transport combined with the prouterine beat of cilia lining the fimbria, infundibulum, and ampulla, which actively impedes net movement of the ovum toward the ovary, ultimately result in entrance of the ovum into the uterus.

The role of tubal contractility in sperm transport is less clear. Unlike the ovum, which has no innate mechanism of locomotion, spermatozoa are capable of movement and thus may actively participate in their own transport through the female reproductive tract. The segmental contraction of the endosalpinx, myosalpinx, and mesosalpinx may compartmentalize the oviduct, randomly moving its contents throughout the tube (Fig. 3). This mechanism, in concert with the sperm's innate motility, may result in spermatozoa being transported to the vicinity of the newly ovulated ovum.

Secretory Activity   The oviduct is the site of and furnishes the environment for tubal gamete transport and survival, fertilization, and early embryo development. Tubal secretions constitute the medium in which these processes take place. It is therefore not unreasonable to assume that tubal secretions are of functional importance in reproduction.

Tubal fluid is a complex product derived primarily from hormone-dependent secretory activity of the tubal epithelium and selective transudation from the blood with varying contributions from the uterus, peritoneal cavity, and, in the postovulatory interval, the ovarian follicle. Tubal secretion, a predominantly estrogen-dependent phenomenon, is antagonized by progesterone. Estrogen alone, when given exogenously, is capable of maintaining normal tubal secretory rates in the ovariectomized rabbit.[13] In the rabbit,[13] ewe,[14] and rhesus monkey,[15] tubal secretion is maximal at the time of maximum estrogen production. A similar increase in ampullary[16,17] and interstitial[18] secretion at the time of ovulation in the human has been described.

Tubal secretory cells undergo definite morphological changes during the ovarian cycle. During the early proliferative stage, under low-estrogen conditions, the tubal mucosa is thin, exhibiting a low cuboidal profile. Secretory activity is absent at this time. Ultrastructurally, the cells display a compact Golgi apparatus, a limited and poorly developed endoplasmic reticulum, and decreased size and numbers of mitochondria. As the cycle progresses, rising estrogen levels result in progressive mucosal thickening. Secretory cells increase in height and become domed. The Golgi apparatus, endoplasmic reticulum, and mitochondria become more prominent. Following the preovulatory estrogen peak, the mucosal epithelium attains maximal thickness. The domed, microvilli-covered apices of secretory cells protrude into the lumen above the tips of ciliated cells, rendering their cilia inconspicuous. The subcellular synthetic apparatus is maximally developed. The large cell nucleus assumes a basal position to accommodate the extensively developed supranuclear Golgi with its numerous dilated cisternae. The remaining cytoplasmic space is densely populated with well-developed endoplasmic reticulum and abundant secretory granules, the latter appearing in greater numbers beneath the cell membrane facing the lumen.

At ovulation, the granules discharge their contents into the oviductal lumen by exocytosis. The secretory granule membrane fuses with the cell membrane, thereby releasing material directly into the lumen. Granule aggregation may also occur prior to release of secretory material into the lumen, giving rise to greatly expanded cell surface membrane area.[19] Apocrine secretion, consisting of secretory granules extruded along with cytoplasm and ribosomes, occurs following diminished exocrine secretion several days after ovulation and may be a means of clearing the cell of extrasynthetic subcellular organelles in anticipation of the next cycle. During the late luteal and menstrual phases of the cycle, the mucosa again thins out, and secretory activity is halted.

Secretory function is more prominent in the isthmus than in the ampulla. The number of secretory cells increases from the ampulla to the isthmus. Quantitative differences[20] in secretion therefore exist in different segments of the oviduct, the major volume being produced by the isthmus. Qualitative differences[21] have also been demonstrated. Histochemical studies[22,23] indicate that regionalization of secretory glycoproteins occurs, the isthmus being the primary site of production of mucin, a tubal secretory product that may be of importance in sperm and ovum transport.

Biochemical evidence exists that indicates the presence of nonserum, possibly unique proteins in the tubal secretions of the human oviduct. Endogenous protease inhibitors have been detected in the tubal fluid of women[24,25] and other species.[26] Since fertilization *in vivo* and *in vitro* can be blocked by exogenous trypsin inhibitors, presumably by inhibition of sperm penetrability through the ovum zona pellucida, the role of these inhibitory proteins may be to regulate fertility. These inhibitory substances are present in tubal fluid throughout the cycle except for the short period following ovulation when their concentration is significantly depressed. Thus, a putative role could be that of inhibiting fertilization of aged ova.

Tubal fluid may also contain inhibitors of embryonic growth. In the rabbit, there appears to be an estrogen-modulated protein produced by the ampulla that inhibits embryo development during the first postovulatory day.[19,27] Its subsequent removal allows the fertilized ovum to undergo cleavage and normal development. A similar substance has been detected in estrogen-dominated tubal fluids in the mouse.[28]

It is possible that an interaction between the developing embryo and tubal epithelium may occur, giving rise to secretory changes necessary for embryo survival and growth.

Such a dynamic interaction could insure optimum quantitative and qualitative secretory activity to accommodate the constantly changing demands of the embryo during its sojourn in the oviduct prior to its entrance into the uterus.

The degree to which such an interaction exists in the human oviduct has not been determined. It is clear, however, that the oviduct does supply an appropriate milieu for fertilization and early embryo development. The effects of elective sterilization or tubal pathology in diminishing that function and the potential for its restoration are central to infertility surgery.

Ciliary Activity   Ciliated cells constitute the second of the two major cell types that compose the tubal mucosal epithelium. The ciliated cell is characterized by the presence of 250–300 elongated, regularly arranged kinocilia at the cell apex.[29] Each individual cilium originates from a basal body complex just below the cell surface and displays the typical microtubule arrangement of two central filaments and nine double lateral filaments. The cytoplasm contains numerous ribosomes, endoplasmic reticula, and mitrochondria. The pattern of distribution of ciliated and secretory cells is somewhat random throughout the oviduct. It is possible to find highly localized areas in which one particular cell type predominates. In general, ciliated cells tend to be found in greatest numbers on the apex and sides of mucosal folds, whereas secretory cells occupy a more basal position. At the level of the fimbria, up to 70% of the cells are ciliated (Fig. 4). This number diminishes minimally in the ampulla and significantly declines in the isthmus. As the tube enters the uterus, there is an increase in the number of ciliated cells.[18]

In the newborn, ciliated and secretory cells are well developed and appear functional.[16] This advanced differentiation seen at birth suggests that the tubal epithelium is responsive to the high levels of circulating maternal ovarian estrogen prior to birth. Following delivery and the removal of maternal hormonal support, both ciliated and secretory cells regress. At the same time, changes are occurring in the maternal epithelium. Deciliation of the tubal isthmus in the third trimester has been described[30,31] and is thought to be the result of prolonged exposure to a sustained elevation in progesterone. Such deciliation is variable during pregnancy

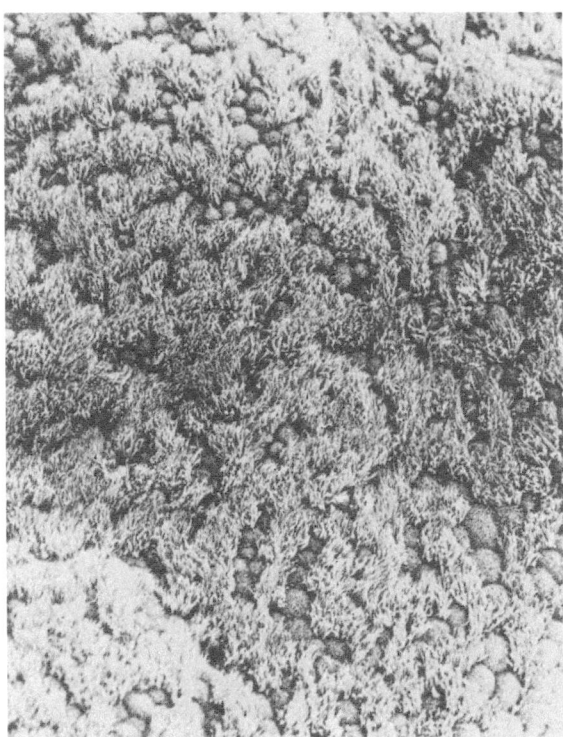

Figure 4. Scanning electron photomicrograph of tubal fimbria. Note the predominance of ciliated epithelial cells interspersed with microvilli-covered secretory cells ($\times 1200$).

but is fairly extensive later in the puerperium when the full effects of estrogen and progesterone withdrawal are realized.[30,32]

In the nonhuman primate, tubal epithelium undergoes well-defined morphological changes during the ovarian cycle. Ciliated cells increase in height during the estrogen-dominated follicular phase and shrink during the progesterone-dominated luteal phase. The cilia are shed and regenerated in cyclic fashion during the menstrual cycle. This process varies with the region of the oviduct. In the fimbria, over 95% of the ciliated cells shed and regenerate their cilia each cycle. In the ampulla, only a small number of cells show complete loss and renewal of their cilia; instead, cyclic changes are restricted to changes in cell height.[33]

In the human, there is disagreement concerning specific changes in the detailed morphology and distribution of ciliated cells during the cycle.[1] It appears that human tubal epithelium does not undergo cyclic, estrogen-driven ciliogenesis. Some changes, such as increase in cell size, number of cytoplasmic granules, and mitochondria may occur as the cycle progresses. Some renewal of ciliated cells does occur, but there is no evidence for either transformation of ciliated into secretory cells or widespread deciliation. Thus, little is known concerning the ability of the epithelium to undergo functional regeneration following surgical trauma or destructive pathological changes.

The cilia are kinetic organelles exhibiting a highly organized synchronized pattern of contractility in which a propulsive power stroke is followed by a nonpropulsive retracting stroke. Ciliary activity in the human is directed toward the uterus[31] as it is in most mammalian species. In the rabbit, there is a progressive increase in the rate of ciliary beat following ovulation.[34] The increase peaks at 20% and is maintained for 3–4 days after ovulation. The occurrence of a similar increase in ciliary beat in the human has been reported[31] and denied.[35]

The importance of ciliary activity in ovum transport through the ampulla has been demonstrated in two experiments. Complete paralysis of the rabbit ampullary musculature with pharmacological agents that allow ciliary beating to continue does not alter ovum transport time.[36] Additionally, segmental reversal of the rabbit ampulla does not allow passage of ova across the reversed segment because of the ovarian direction of ciliary beat within the reversed segment which actively prevents passage of ova.[37]

The importance of ciliary activity in human reproduction has recently been questioned by reports of normal fertility in women suffering from the so called "immobile cilia syndrome." This syndrome is characterized by a congenital absence of ciliary motility.[38] This cilia defect has been demonstrated morphologically in the endocervical cells[39] and tubal ciliated cells of fertile women.[40] However, direct motility studies on tubal cilia have not been performed in these patients. Recent observations that indicate that dynein-defective cilia retain some motility but lack coordination cast some doubt on the existence of the immotile cilia syndrome in the oviduct.[41]

Ovum Pickup

Ovum pickup is the process in which ovulated ova are transported from the surface of the ovary to the interior of the oviduct. Although ovum pickup has been studied extensively in experimental animals and humans, the exact role and degree of interaction of the mechanical, cilial, and suction mechanisms invoked to define the process are not well known, particularly in women and nonhuman primates. In the rabbit, it has been determined that as ovulation approaches, the fimbria and oviductal ostium are brought into contact with the ipsilateral ovary through integrated contractions of the oviduct, mesotubarium superius, mesosalpinx, and fimbria ovarica.[42] Studies in monkeys[46] and anecdotal laparoscopic observations in women are consistent with this scenario (Fig. 5).

In response to continuing contractions, the fimbria constantly sweep across the ovarian surface. At ovulation, the densely ciliated fimbrial mucosa, the cilia of which beat toward the ostium, is positioned over the ovulatory stigmata and their adherent, viscous, ovum-containing cumulus masses. Direct ciliary contact with the cumulus mass has been shown to be important in its detachment from the ovarian surface and in the subsequent passage of ova into the tubal lumen.[43] If the mesenteries responsible for positioning the fimbria in close proximity to the ovary are resected, ovum pickup is significantly reduced. Resection of the mesotubarium superius has been shown to reduce ovum pickup from a mean of 91% in control rabbits to 65% following resection.[47] If the entire fimbria is surgically removed in the rabbit, the cumulus masses remain adherent to the ovary for an extended period.[43] Following fimbriectomy, ovum pickup is reduced to between 7% and 14%.

Clinically, the ability of the fimbria to be positioned over the site of ovulation may similarly be important to normal ovum pickup. Cohen[48] has reported on seven patients with "idiopathic infertility," whose only clinical finding appeared to be derangement of the fimbrial–ovarian

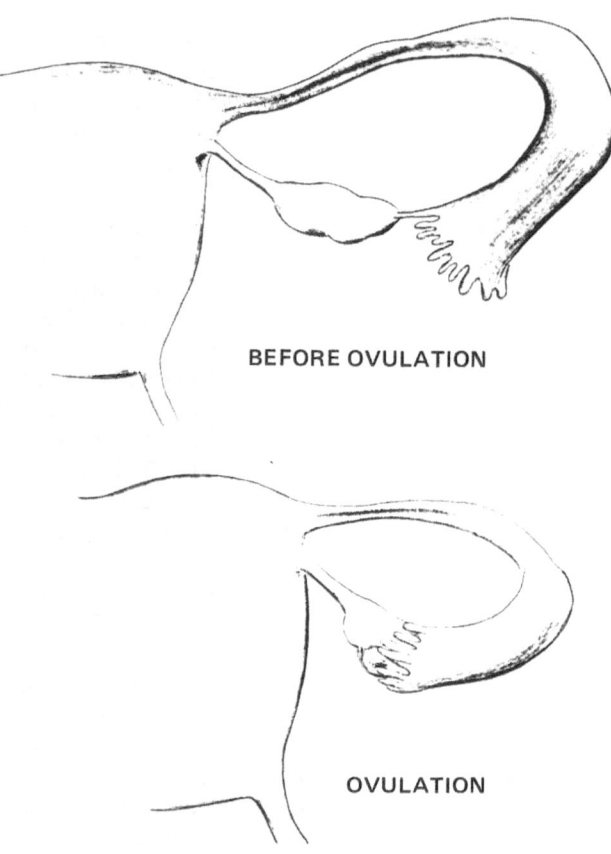

BEFORE OVULATION

OVULATION

Figure 5. Diagrammatic representation of ovum pickup in the human. Before ovulation, the fimbria and ovary exhibit a normal separation. At ovulation, the fimbria and ovary become functionally juxtaposed.

relationship because of elongation of the fimbria ovarica to greater than 4 cm and associated uterine retroversion noted at laparoscopy. During a 12-month period of exposure to conception under optimal conditions prior to surgery, one patient conceived. The remainder underwent surgical plication of the fimbria ovarica and round ligaments to bring the fimbria into normal proximity to the ovaries. Five became pregnant. Three delivered at term, and two aborted.

Pregnancy can occur in women with one ovary and only the contralateral oviduct,[49] suggesting that ovum pickup from the cul-de-sac can occur. In this situation, the existence of a negative pressure, as demonstrated by Maia and Coutinho[50] using intraluminal catheters in the human oviduct, could play an important role complementing that of tubal cilia and mobility of the fimbria.

Reversal of fimbriectomy sterilization has recently been reported with a pregnancy rate of 44% after transverse salpingostomy and cuff eversion using microsurgical technique.[51] This marked improvement over results of salpingostomy in patients with hydrosalpinges probably reflects the absence of pathologically induced changes in the oviducts that underwent fimbriectomy but remained otherwise healthy. It was noted[51] that the ideal candidate for fimbriectomy reversal has an oviduct at least 8 cm long, an ampulla at least 1 cm in diameter, rugal patterns discernable on hysterosalpingography, and minimal peritubal adhesions. Most notably, successful reversal was associated with spontaneous eversion of the endosalpinx at the time of surgery which tended to form a neofimbrialike structure. All of these factors favor ovum pickup and are usually absent or severely compromised in the post-pelvic inflammatory disease patient with hydrosalpinges.

Sperm Transport

The oviduct has the unique and paradoxical task of bringing the ovum and sperm into close proximity from opposite directions so that fertilization can occur. To date, the anatomic and physiological basis for this complex transport capability is incompletely understood. Many important observations, however, concerning gamete transport have been documented and allow the formulation of a tentative description of the process.

The average normal human ejaculate deposited at the cervix contains in excess of 100 million spermatozoa, a low but significant percentage of which are morphologically and possibly functionally abnormal. Of this large and heterogenous population of spermatozoa, most, including many abnormal forms, remain in the vagina or lower reproductive tract to be later expelled or phagocytized. The remaining small percentage undergo a selective filtering process as they sequentially ascend the female reproductive tract to insure that an optimum number of normal, highly fertile spermatozoa reach the ovum.

Two phases of sperm transport appear to occur, an initial short phase[52] in which spermatozoa are rapidly transported to the ampulla and a subsequent sustained phase[53] in which spermatozoa are less rapidly transported to the site of fertilization. The rapid phase of transport which requires only minutes is an acute phenomenon that appears to be effected primarily through contractile activity of the reproductive tract. Interestingly, spermatozoa transported during this phase survive poorly and probably do not participate in fertilization. The average number of spermatozoa in the oviduct increases during the first 15 min after insemination and thereafter appears to remain somewhat constant as the second phase of sustained transport begins.

It has been determined that spermatozoa are cleared to the peritoneal cavity. Ahlgren[54] found a maximum of several hundred spermatozoa per tube in women with patent tubes, but up to 23,000 per tube in women with hydrosalpinges. This observation suggests that spermatozoa are prevented from leaving the ampulla through the fimbriated end to enter the abdominal cavity. This results in a progressive accumulation of spermatozoa and the attainment of high numbers characteristic of a hydrosalpinx. In the patent tube, a normal complement of spermatozoa is maintained via continuous replacement of those lost in the peritoneal cavity by others from reservoirs below during the sustained phase of transport.

Both the cervix and the tubal isthmus appear to act as selective filters and as reservoirs of spermatozoa. In the human, the population of spermatozoa that reach the ampulla contains a higher proportion of normal forms than does the ejaculate.[54] Furthermore, in rabbits, the fertilizing ability and motility of spermatozoa are greater in those recovered from the ampulla than in sperm recovered from the isthmus.[55,56] The mechanism of sustained transport of spermatozoa following colonization of the isthmus has not been defined but may include intrinsic motility of the spermatozoa, chemotactic attraction of the ovum, or tubal muscular, ciliary, or secretory activity.

While residing in the isthmus, sperm exhibit reduced intrinsic motility. The flagellar activity of isthmic sperm increases with the passage of time after coitus in the rabbit, so that ascent to the site of fertilization is functionally associated with increased motility and temporally coincident with ovulation. The importance of sperm motility in their passage through the isthmus has been demonstrated in the estrous rat. Only motile sperm are capable of reaching the ampulla. Dead sperm or inert particles of India ink are not transported.[57]

Because of the large volume of the ampulla compared to the small size of the ovum and the relative sparseness of spermatozoa present, the concept of chemotactic attraction of sperm by the egg is of interest. However, there is no good evidence that the ovum produces a chemical signal capable of attracting sperm. Such a signal would be highly diluted by the tubal fluid. In addition, sperm reach the site of fertilization in the absence of an ovum. If a chemotactic attraction does exist, it probably is restricted to the immediate vicinity of the ovum. The constant presence and transport of fertile sperm, their intrinsic motility, and the 12- to 24-hr fertilizable life-span of the ovum are probably sufficient for a successful chance encounter of the ovum and the fertilizing spermatozoon.

The role of contractility of the myosalpinx and tubal mesenteries in sperm transport has not been defined experimentally. The segmental contraction of the oviduct may compartmentalize the lumen and cause a turbulent movement of tubal fluid which would tend to cause a reflux of suspended spermatozoa throughout the segment. Successive segmental contractions could result in continuous random transport of spermatozoa throughout the oviduct.

Sperm transport proceeds counter to the direction of ciliary beating. Although narrow paths of cilia beating toward the ovary occur in the isthmus of some species,[58] all tubal cilia in the human oviduct beat toward the uterus. If sperm are deposited on the tubal mucosa of a freshly opened oviduct *in vitro,* the strong ciliary currents rapidly transport spermatozoa toward the uterus, completely independent of their own flagellar activity.[43] It would therefore appear that spermatozoa would have to be protected from this directionally inappropriate ciliary beating in order to be transported to the site of fertilization. Contraction-induced compartmentalization of the tubes may integrate with ciliary activity to create the countercurrent pattern of fluid flow previously described. Alternatively, secretory activity into the tube may play an important role in sperm transport. According to Koester,[59] oviductal secretory activity is greatest in the isthmus. Within the isthmus, secretory rates are high at ovulation but decline following ovulation. Flow is in the ovarian direction, rapid through the isthmus and relatively slow through the ampulla, thus favoring transport toward the ovary. In addition, the protuberant secretory cells tend to obscure the cilia, rendering them relatively ineffective. Most recently, it has been proposed[23] that the tubal isthmus at the time of ovulation contains viscous mucus that masks the cilia and promotes the passage of spermatozoa in similar fashion to cervical mucus. After ovulation, isthmic luminal contents lose viscosity and disappear as secretory cell dominance is lost, and cilia once again become prominent.

Capacitation   Freshly ejaculated spermatozoa or those removed from the epididymis are not capable of penetrating the ovum and fertilizing it. Spermatozoa must first undergo a physiological change called capacitation[60,61] that renders them capable of fertilizing the ovum. The ability of spermatozoa to exist in two forms may be of functional importance. Since capacitated spermatozoa are very active metabolically, their lifespan in both male and female tract would be enhanced by the noncapacitated state. Further, since capacitated spermatozoa are highly penetrable of tissue, noncapacitated spermatozoa remain noninvasive in both the male and female, a characteristic of great importance, particularly in the male.

During its development in the ovarian follicle, the ovum is surrounded by an acellular mucopolysaccharide layer, the zona pellucida, and by numerous layers of follicular granulosa cells, collectively termed the cumulus oophorus. Those cells adjacent to the zona pellucida and densely adherent to each other and to the zona are termed the corona radiata. These cellular investments persist around the ovum after ovulation and must be penetrated by the spermatozoa before fertilization can occur.

The head of the spermatozoon contains several enzymes located on the outer and inner acrosomal membranes that may be important in this penetration. Among these are hyaluronidase, acrosin, and a corona-dispersing enzyme. Hyaluronidase is thought to be located on the outer acrosomal membrane and, together with biocarbonate ion present in oviduct fluid,[62] is responsible for dispersing the loose aggregate of cumulus cells. Acrosin and the corona-dispersing enzyme may be located on the inner acrosomal membrane. These enzymes assist in the removal of corona cells and in sperm penetration through the zona pellucida.[63] Capacitation involves a destabilization of the plasma membrane of the spermatozoon head that renders these enzymes accessible. The process, however, is poorly understood. The oviduct appears capable of furnishing all of the appropriate conditions for capacitation. Because fertilization of human ova has been achieved *in vitro*[63-65] in defined media, the necessity or occurrence of capacitation of human spermaotozoa has not been demonstrated.

Fertilization

Fertilization is the process by which chromosomes of the male and female gametes unite to form a new and genetically unique individual. The process entails penetration of the ovum by a spermatozoon, formation and development of male and female pronuclei, and subsequent union of their chromosomes. Fertilization occurs in the oviduct, most probably in the distal ampulla.

Sperm await the arrival of the ovum in the oviduct. The fertile life of sperm within the female genital tract is shorter than the motile life and has been estimated at 24–48 hr in women.[66-68] Recent estimates place the figure as high as 120 hr.[69] Possible inaccuracies in timing the occurrence of ovulation, however, invite caution in interpreting this figure. It is generally accepted that the fertilizable life-span of the human ovum is less than 24 hr.[70] Pre- or postovulatory aging of ova or of spermatozoa may result in chromosomal abnormalities.

Although fertilization normally occurs in the oviduct, it is doubtful that the tubal lumen contains unique substances that are essential for fertilization. Successful *in vitro* fertilization in defined media and term delivery have been accomplished.[71,72] It is, therefore, likely that considerable alterations of tubal functions may be consistent with normal fertilization.

Early Embryo Development

The fertilized ovum begins to cleave while still in the oviduct. Between ovulation and implantation, a period of approximately a week, the developing embryo exists suspended in the fluids of the genital tract in a free-living state and must obtain its metabolic support from the tubal and uterine surroundings.

In order to develop and undergo cleavage, the fertilized ovum requires a source of both energy and biosynthetic precursors. At ovulation, the ovum contains a wide variety of enzymes capable of catalyzing the necessary metabolic reactions in support of embryonic development. The types, amounts, and activities of these enzymes reflect the progressive changes in metabolic activities of the developing embryo. Early embryos are much more fastidious in their requirements than embryos in later stages of development. The two-celled mouse embryo, for example, is capable of utilizing a limited number of growth factors.[73]

Unlike the embryos of lower forms, such as invertebrates or amphibians, which rely on stored nutrients in an otherwise hostile environment, the mammalian embryo is dependent on continuing support from the maternal environment. The oviduct, therefore, provides ideal conditions for early embryo development. Although the oviductal lumen does supply this environment, the necessity of normal tubal epithelial function for embryo development remains to be established. The human embryo is capable of implanting and developing to advanced stages in the oviduct. Because ectopic implantation often occurs in tubes that have been damaged by infection or previous elective sterilization and subsequent surgical repair, it is unlikely that functional tubal mucosa is indispensible for survival of the early human embryo. In contrast, it is very likely that a normal and functional tubal mucosa is necessary for proper embryo transport, particularly through the ampulla.

Ovum Transport

Ovum transport is remarkably similar in most mammalian species with regard to its duration, an average of 3–4 days being required for the ovum or embryo to transit the length of the oviduct and enter the uterus.[74] By far, the greatest amount of knowledge concerning ovum transport has been gained using laboratory species, particularly the rabbit. The rabbit is an ideal species for ovum transport studies for several reasons. Rabbits are induced or reflex ovulators. Ovulation occurs 10–14 hr after coitus or following the administration of exogenous luteinizing hormone or human chorionic gonadotropin.[75] Therefore, the time of ovulation can be accurately and consistently determined. Rabbits are also polytocous, releasing several ova from each ovary. A large number of ova are therefore available for transport studies.

The detailed pattern of ovum transport in the rabbit has been determined, Ova move rapidly from the infundibulum to the AIJ. Transampullary times of less than 10 min have been observed.[76,77] Ova are then retained at the AIJ for 12–36 hr. At this time, they begin entering the distal isthmus and are gradually transported to the UTJ over a period of approximately 24–36 hr. Ova then enter the uterus.[78]

Similar detailed information for primate species, including man, has only recently begun to be obtained. Primates ovulate spontaneously and generally release only a single egg. In the absence of overt external signs of ovulation, the accurate determination of the occurrence of ovulation is difficult. Similarly, should failure to recover the single ovum and determine its location occur, the results obtained would be of minimal use. Using daily determination of periovulatory estrogen levels and serial diagnostic laparoscopy to accurately establish the time of ovulation, the detailed time course of ovum transport has been determined in two species of primates, the Rhesus monkey[79] and the baboon.[80] In each species, ovum transport requires 3 days and is characterized by prolonged retention within the ampulla and fairly rapid transit through the isthmus into the uterus.

Using estrogen and LH determinations to approximate the time of ovulation in women, Croxatto and his colleagues in Santiago, Chile, have recovered ova from the tubes and uteri of women operated on at various intervals after ovulation. Transport of ova in women is characterized by retention in the ampulla for approximately 72 hr followed by rapid transit through the isthmus. Ova are delivered to the endometrial cavity approximately 80 hr after release from the follicles.[81–83] Thus, the detailed time course of ovum transport in women and monkeys is virtually identical, but both differ dramatically from the rabbit.

Ovum transport is thought to be the result of the interaction of tubal contractility, ciliary activity, fluid dynamics, and changes in mucosal fold arrangement and topography. The degree to which each of these functional components contributes to or is necessary for successful transport of the developing embryo to the uterus is unknown. Mechanical obstruction of the tubal lumen through intra- or peritubal adhesions, alteration in epithelial and myosalpingeal function, or anatomically imperfect tuboplastic procedures may be expected to alter tubal function. In general, the degree of functional impairment and its capacity for regeneration are inversely proportional to surgical salvageability.

REFERENCES

1. Woodruf JD, Pauerstein CJ: *The Fallopian Tube: Structure, Function, Pathology and Management*. Baltimore, Williams & Wilkins Co, 1969.
2. Wilhelmsson L, Lindblom B, Wiqvist N: The human uterotubal junction: Contractile patterns of different smooth muscle layers and the influence of prostaglandin E_2, prostaglandin $F_2\alpha$, and prostaglandin I_2 *in vitro*. *Fertil Steril* 32:303, 1979.
3. Sweeney WJ: The interstitial portion of the uterine tube: Its gross anatomy, course and length. *Obstet Gynecol* 19:3, 1962.
4. Peterson EP, Musich JR, Behrman SJ: Uterotubal implanation and obstetric outcome after previous sterilization. *Am J Obstet Gynecol* 128:662, 1977.
5. Winston RML: Microsurgical tubocornual anastomosis for reversal of sterilization. *Lancet* 1:284, 1977.
6. Eddy CA: Tuboplastic microsurgery: Appropriate sites for tubal repair, in Brosens I, Winston RML (eds): *Reversibility of Female Sterilization*. London, Academic Press, 1978, p 47.
7. Winston RML: The future of microsurgery in infertility. *Clin Obstet Gynecol* 5:607, 1978.
8. Winston RML, Margara RA: Techniques for the improvement of microsurgical tubal anastomosis, in Crossignani PG, Rubin BL (eds): *Microsurgery in Female Infertility*. London, Academic Press, 1980, p 31.
9. Coutinho EM, Maia H Jr, Mattos CER: Contractility of the fallopian tube. *Gynecol Invest* 6:146, 1975.
10. Daniels EE: A functional analysis of the myogenic control systems of the human fallopian tube. *Am J Obstet Gynecol* 121:1046, 1975.
11. Hodgson BJ, Talo A, Pauerstein CJ: Oviductal ovum surrogate movement: Interrelation with muscular activity. *Biol Reprod* 16:394, 1977.
12. Portnow J, Talo A, Hodgson BJ: A random walk model of ovum transport. *Bull Math Biol* 39:349, 1977.
13. Mastroianni L Jr, Beer F, Shah U, et al: Endocrine regulation of oviduct secretions in the rabbit. *Endocrinology* 68:92, 1961.

14. Perkins JL: Fluid flow of the oviduct, in Johnson AD, Foley CW (eds): *The Oviduct and its Functions*. New York, Academic Press, 1974, p 119.

15. Mastroianni L Jr, Shah U, Abdul-Karim R: Prolonged volumetric collection of oviduct fluid in the rhesus monkey. *Fertil Steril* 12:417, 1961.

16. Patek E, Nilsson L, Johannisson E: Scanning electron microscopic study of the human fallopian tube, report ii. Fetal life, reproductive life and post menopause. *Fertil Steril* 23:719, 1972.

17. Ludwig H, Metzger H: *The Human Female Reproductive Tract. A Scanning Electron Microscopic Atlas*. New York, Springer-Verlag, 1976.

18. Fadel HE, Berns D, Zaneveld LJD, et al: The human uterotubal junction: A scanning electron microscope study during different phases of the menstrual cycle. *Fertil Steril* 27:1176, 1976.

19. Stone SL, Hamner CE: Biochemistry and physiology of oviductal secretions. *Gynecol Invest* 6:234, 1975.

20. Bajpai VK, Shipstone AC, Gupta DN, et al: Differential response of the ampullary and isthmic cells to oviductomy and estrogen treatment: An Ultrastructural study. *Endokrinologie* 69:11, 1977.

21. Bajpai VK, Shipstone AC, Gupta, DN, et al: Studies on the ultrastructure of the fallopian tube: Part 2, changes in the secretory cells of the rabbit fallopian tube during ovum transport. *Indian J Exp Biol* 12:123, 1974.

22. Fredricsson B: Histochemistry of the oviduct, in Hafez ESE, Blandau RJ (eds): *The Mammalian Oviduct*. Chicago, University of Chicago Press, 1969, p 311.

23. Jansen RPS: Cyclic changes in the human fallopian tube isthmus and their functional importance. *Am J Obstet Gynecol* 136:292, 1980.

24. Moghissi KS: Human fallopian tube fluid. 1. Protein composition. *Fertil Steril* 21:821, 1970.

25. Hirschhauser C, Kionke V, Daume E: Trypsin inhibitors in the human female genital tract. *Acta Endocrinol (Kbh)* 68:413, 1971.

26. Stambaugh R, Seitz HM Jr, Mastroianni L Jr: Acrosomal proteinase inhibition in rhesus monkey oviduct fluid. *Fertil Steril* 25:352, 1974.

27. Kille JW, Hamner CE: The influence of oviductal fluid on the development of one-cell rabbit embryos *in vitro*. *J Reprod Fertil* 35:415, 1973.

28. Cline EM, Randall PA, Oliphant G: Hormone mediated oviductal influence on mouse embryo development. *Fertil Steril* 28:766, 1977.

29. Borell U, Nilsson O, Wersall J, et al: Electron-microscope studies of the epithelium of the rabbit fallopian tube under different hormonal influences *Acta Obstet Gynecol Scand* 35:35, 1956.

30. Andrews MC: Epithelial changes in the puerperal fallopian tube. *Am J Obstet Gynecol* 62:28, 1951.

31. Cristoph FN, Dennis KJ: The cellular composition of the human oviduct epithelium. *Br J Obstet Gynaecol* 84:219, 1977.

32. Seki K, Rawson J, Eddy CA, et al: Deciliation in the puerperal fallopian tube. *Fertil Steril* 29:75, 1978.

33. Brenner RM: Renewal of oviduct cilia during the menstrual cycle of the rhesus monkey. *Fertil Steril* 20:599, 1969.

34. Borell U, Nilsson O, Westman A: Ciliary activity in the rabbit fallo-

pian tube during oestrus and after copulation. *Acta Obstet Gynecol Scand* 36:22, 1957.

35. Westrom L, Mardh PA, von Mecklenburg C, et al: Studies on ciliated epithelia of the human genital tract. II. The mucociliary wave pattern of fallopian tube epithelium. *Fertil Steril* 28:955, 1977.

36. Halbert SA, Tam PY, Blandau RJ: Egg transport in the rabbit oviduct: The roles of cilia and muscle. *Science* 191:1052, 1976.

37. Eddy CA, Flores JJ, Archer DR, et al: The role of cilia in fertility: An evaluation by selective microsurgical modification of the rabbit oviduct. *Am J Obstet Gynecol* 132:814, 1978.

38. Afzelius BA, Camner P, Mossberg B: On the function of cilia in the female reproductive tract. *Fertil Steril* 29:72, 1978.

39. Bleau G, Richer CL, Bosquet D: Absence of dynein arms in cilia of endocervical cells in a fertile woman. *Fertil Steril* 30:362, 1978.

40. Jean Y, Langlais J, Roberts KD, et al: Fertility of a woman with nonfunctional ciliated cells in the fallopian tubes. *Fertil Steril* 31:349, 1979.

41. Sturgess JM, Chao J, Turner JAP: Transposition of ciliary microtubules, another cause of impaired ciliary motility. *N Engl J Med* 303:318, 1980.

42. Westman AA: A contribution to the question of the transit of the ovum from ovary to uterus in rabbits. *Acta Obstet Gynecol Scand* 5:1, 1926.

43. Blandau RJ: Gamete transport comparative aspects, in Hafez ESE, Blandau RJ (eds): *The Mammalian Oviduct.* Chicago, University of Chicago Press, 1969, p 129.

44. Halbert SA, Conrad JT: *In vitro* contractile activity of the mesotubarium superius from the rabbit oviduct in various endocrine states. *Fertil Steril* 26:248, 1975.

45. Doteuchi M, Takeda H: Adrenergic innervation and contractile activity of the mesotubarium superius of the rabbit oviduct. *J Reprod Fertil* 52:213, 1978.

46. Dukelow WR: The morphology of follicular development and ovulation in nonhuman primates. *J Reprod Fertil [Suppl]* 22:23, 1975.

47. Metz KGP, Mastroianni J Jr: Dispensibility of fimbria: Ovum pickup by tubal fistulas in the rabbit. *Fertil Steril* 32:329, 1979.

48. Cohen BM: Surgical repair of abnormal fimbrial gonadal relationships in the human female. *J Reprod Med* 25:33, 1980.

49. First A: Transperitoneal migration of ovum or spermatozoon. *Obstet Gynecol* 4:431, 1954.

50. Maia H, Coutinho EM: Peristalsis and antiperistalsis of the human fallopian tube during the menstrual cycle. *Biol Reprod* 2:305, 1970.

51. Novy MJ: Reversal of Kroener fimbriectomy sterilization. *Am J Obstet Gynecol* 137: 198, 1980.

52. Overstreet JW, Cooper GW: Sperm transport in the reproductive tract of the female rabbit. I. The rapid transit phase of transport. *Biol. Reprod* 19:101, 1978.

53. Overstreet JW, Cooper GW, Katz DF: Sperm transport in the reproductive tract of the female rabbit. II. The sustained phase of transport. *Biol Reprod* 19:115, 1978.

54. Ahlgren M: Sperm transport to and survival in the human fallopian tube. *Gynecol Invest* 6:206, 1975.

55. Cohen J, McNaughton DC: Spermatozoa: The probable selection of a

small population by the genital tract of the female rabbit. *J Reprod Fertil* 39:297, 1974.

56. Overstreet JW, Cooper GW: Reduced sperm motility in the isthmus of the rabbit oviduct. *Nature* 258:718, 1975.

57. Leonard SL, Perlman PL: Conditions effecting the passage of spermatozoa through the utero–tubal junction of the rat. *Anat Rec* 104:89, 1949.

58. Gaddum-Rosse P, Blandau RJ: Comparative observations on ciliary currents in mammalian oviducts. *Biol Reprod* 14:605, 1976.

59. Koester H: Ovum transport, in Gibian H, Platz EJ (eds): *Mammalian Reproduction*. New York, Springer, 1970, p 189.

60. Austin CR: Observations on the penetration of the sperm into the mammalian egg. *Aust J Sci Res* B4:581, 1951.

61. Chang MC: Fertilizing capacity of spermatozoa deposited into the fallopian tubes. *Nature* 168:697, 1951.

62. Stambaugh R, Noreiga C, Mastroianni L Jr: Bicarbonate ion: The corona cell dispersing factor of rabbit tubal fluid. *J Reprod Fertil* 18:51, 1969.

63. Brackett BG, Seitz HM Jr, Rocha G, et al: The mammalian fertilization process, in Moghissi KS, Hafez ESE (eds): *Biology of Mammalian Fertilization and Implantation*. Springfield, Illinois, Charles C Thomas, 1973, p 165.

64. Edwards RG, Bavister BD, Steptoe PC: Early stages of fertilization *in vitro* of human oocytes matured *in vitro*. *Nature* 221:632, 1969.

65. Edwards RG, Steptoe PC, Purdy JM: Fertilization and cleavage *in vitro* of preovulatory human oocytes. *Nature* 227:1307, 1970.

66. Bedford JM: The saga of mammalian sperm from ejaculation to syngamy, in Gibian H, Plotz EJ (eds): *Mammalian Reproduction*. New York, Springer-Verlag, 1970, p 124.

67. Cohen MR, Stein IF: Sperm survival at the estimated ovulation time. *Fertil Steril* 2:20, 1950.

68. Tietze C: Probability of pregnancy resulting from a single unprotected coitus. *Fertil Steril* 11:485, 1960.

69. Ferin J, Thomas K, Johansson ED: Ovulation detection, in Hafez ESE, Evans T (eds): *Human Reproduction: Conception and Contraception*. New York, Harper & Row, 1973, p 261.

70. Hartman CG: *Science and the Safe Period*. Baltimore, Williams and Wilkins, 1962.

71. Steptoe PC, Edwards RG: Birth after the reimplantation of a human embryo. *Lancet* 2:366, 1978.

72. Lopata A, Brown JB, Leeton JF, et al: *In vitro* fertilization of preovulatory oocytes and embryo transfer in infertile patients treated with clomiphene and human chorionic gonadotropin. *Fertil Steril* 30:27, 1978.

73. Whitten WK: Culture of tubal ova. *Nature* 179:1081, 1957.

74. Croxatto HB, Ortiz MES: Egg transport in the fallopian tube. *Gynecol Invest* 6:215, 1975.

75. Harper MJK: The time of ovulation in the rabbit following the injection of luteinizing hormone. *J Endocrinol* 22:147, 1961.

76. Boling JL, Blandau RJ: Egg transport through the ampulla of the oviducts of rabbits under various experimental conditions. *Biol Reprod* 4:174, 1971.

77. Harper MJK: The mechanisms involved in the movement of newly ovulated eggs through the ampulla of the rabbit fallopian tube. *J Reprod Fertil* 2:522, 1961.
78. Pauerstein CJ, Anderson V, Chatkoff ML, et al: Effect of estrogen and progesterone on the time course of tubal ovum transport in rabbits. *Am J Obstet Gynecol* 120:299, 1974.
79. Eddy CA, Garcia RG, Kraemer DC, et al: Detailed time course of ovum transport in the rhesus monkey (*Macaca mulatta*). *Biol Reprod* 13:363, 1975.
80. Eddy CA, Turner T, Kraemer D, et al: Pattern and duration of ovum transport in the baboon (*Papio anubis*). *Obstet Gynecol* 47:658, 1976.
81. Cheviakoff S, Diaz S, Carril M, et al: Ovum transport in women, in Harper MJK, Pauerstein CJ, Adams CE, et al (eds): *Ovum Transport and Fertility Regulation*. Copenhagen, Scriptor, 1976, p 416.
82. Avendano S, Croxatto HD, Pereda J, et al: A seven cell human egg recovered from the oviduct. *Fertil Steril* 26:1167, 1975.
83. Croxatto HB, Ortiz ME, Diaz S, et al: Studies on the duration of egg transport by the human oviduct. II. Ovum location at various intervals following luteinization hormone peak. *Am J Obstet Gynecol* 132:629, 1978.

3 Pathophysiology of the Fallopian Tube in Infertility

Alexander Sedlis

Department of Obstetrics and Gynecology
State University of New York
Downstate Medical Center
Brooklyn, New York 11203

and

Ancel Blaustein

Department of Pathology
New York University School of Medicine
New York, New York 10016

Diseases of the Fallopian tube are usually bilateral, and, therefore, they adversely affect reproductive function. Moreover, the pathological changes often extend throughout the entire length of the tube, making it difficult to correct the damage by surgery. Tubal disease may cause mechanical obstruction or disturb the interaction between cilliary and secretory activity and muscular contractility. The result of such dysfunction is loss or impairment of ovum pickup, sperm transport, and transport of fertilized ova to the uterus.

A severe degree of tubal damage causes total sterility by preventing fertilization. The less severe dysfunction may only retard the transport of the fertilized ovum and favor ectopic implantation. Paradoxically, treatment of tubal disease may increase risk of ectopic pregnancy. Delayed or inadequate antibiotic therapy of salpingitis, for example, will leave the tube partially patent, allowing fertilization but at the same time favoring tubal implantation. Similarly, the hazard of ectopic pregnancy is increased after reconstructive surgery aimed at restoring tubal patency.

In the overwhelming majority, diseases of the Fallopian tube result from inflammation. Tubal neoplasms, both benign and malignant, are rare and usually affect women past the reproductive age and therefore play an insignificant role in infertility.

INFLAMMATORY DISEASES

Salpingitis and Its Sequelae

Salpingitis is caused in most instances by microorganisms reaching the Fallopian tube by an ascending route from the vagina and cervix via the endometrial cavity. The alternate route of infection is either by continuity from the adjacent organs in the abdominal cavity or through the lymphatic channels.

Bacteriology of salpingitis has not been investigated adequately because of inaccessibility of the tube for routine bacterial sampling and difficulty in growing the fastidious pathogenic organisms such as gonococci, *Chlamydia, Mycoplasma,* and the anaerobes.

According to the prevalent view, sexually transmitted microorganisms are responsible for the majority of cases of salpingitis.[1] Until recently, the gonococcus was considered to be the main offender in pelvic infections, but during the last few years evidence has begun to accumulate that other sexually transmitted organisms such as *Chlamydia* and *Mycoplasma* are also involved in the etiology of salpingitis.[1-3] Much of objective evidence of bacteriological flora in pelvic inflammation was obtained by Westrom using routine laparoscopy or laparotomy and direct bacterial cultures for "objectivized" diagnosis of acute pelvic inflammatory disease.[4] According to this study, *Chlamydia trachomatis* were found in 30% of women with acute salpingitis, and gonococcus was isolated in 4% of the cases.

Acute Salpingitis

An acute primary infection of the Fallopian tube affects mainly the mucosa of the endosalpinx. On gross examination at laparotomy or laparoscopy, purulent exudate is seen exuding from tubal ostium, the diameter of the tube is only slightly enlarged by edema, and the serosal coat is congested and sometimes covered with fibrous exudate. Microscopic examination reveals the columnar epithelium and the subepithelial layers of tubal mucosa to be infiltrated with inflammatory cells, mostly polymorphonuclear leukocytes. The tubal lumen is filled with inflammatory exudate composed of pus cells, desquamated epithelial cells, proteinaceous material, and necrotic debris (Fig. 1). Patches of necrosis of surface epithelium with fibrinous exudate may be seen on light microscopy and in improved detail on scanning electron microscopy.[5]

Although initial acute episodes of salpingitis respond to treatment with prompt disappearance of symptoms, they may lead to permanent changes in tubal structure and function in a high percentage of cases. At present, the exact percentage of permanent damage is not known.

These residual changes are responsible for the chronic inactive phase of pelvic inflammatory disease, for subsequent acute exacerbations, and for impaired fertility. According to Westrom,[4] tubal occlusion occurs in 15% of women after a single infection, in 35% after two infections, and in 75% after three or more infections. The rate of ectopic pregnancy increases after tubal infection from one in 100 to one in 29 intrauterine pregnancies.

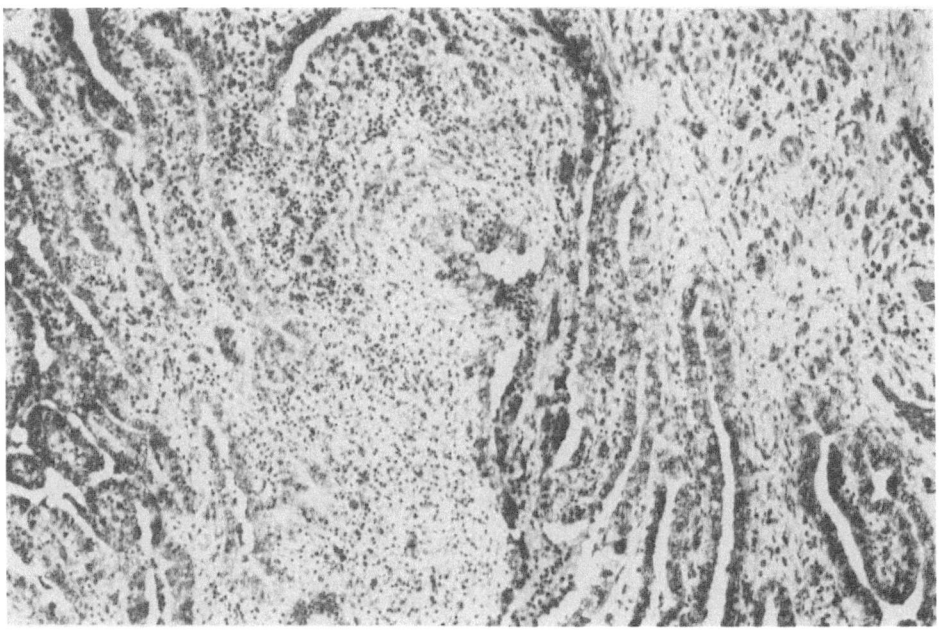

Figure 1. Acute salpingitis. Purulent exudate in the tubal lumen and inflammatory infiltration of the mucosa.

Chronic Inactive Inflammatory Disease

Follicular Salpingitis. Follicular salpingitis is the result of adhesions developing between the adjacent surfaces of tubal mucosal folds at multiple sites of epithelial damage produced by acute infection. During the healing process the fibroblasts penetrate the fibrinous exudate over the focal epithelial necrosis and cross over to the necrotic areas of the neighboring mucosal folds, causing fusion between the folds. Follicular salpingitis in its quiescent stage is totally asymptomatic, and the gross appearance of the Fallopian tube is unremarkable. On microscopic examination, the cross section of the tube with follicular salpingitis has a loculated, "sievelike" appearance with thin septa dividing the tubal lumen into multiple compartments, each completely surrounded by tubal epithelium (Fig. 2). During the silent phase, no inflammatory cell infiltration is observed, nor is there any other evidence of active inflammation. Complete or partial obstruction of the tubal lumen in follicular salpingitis is the key factor in future complications, acute exacerbation of infection, infertility, and ectopic pregnancy.

Hydrosalpinx. Hydrosalpinx, an accumulation of clear liquid in the distended tubal lumen, develops when the

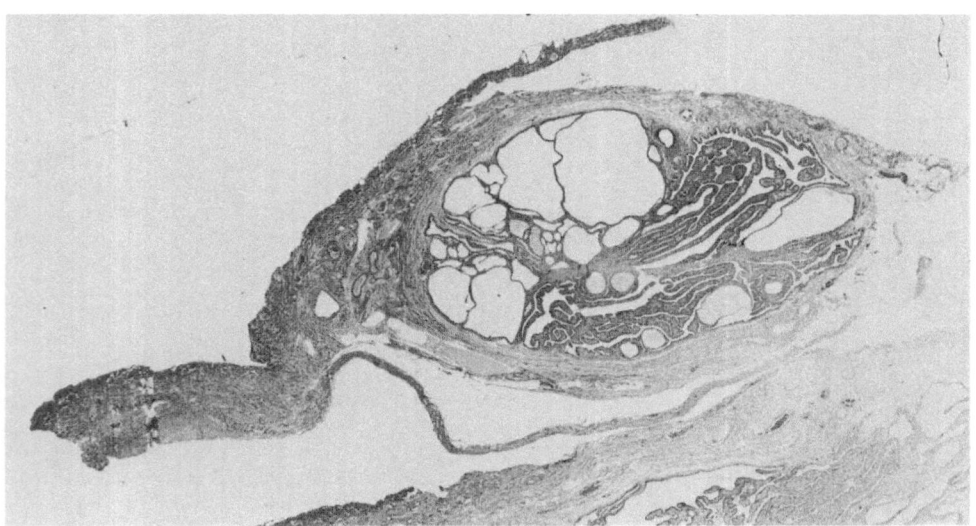

Figure 2. Follicular salpingitis. Fusion of mucosal folds with no active inflammation.

fimbriated end of the Fallopian tube is occluded while the central lumen is patent.

Grossly, the tube with hydrosalpinx appears enlarged to various proportions. Its wall remains thin, and the lumen is filled with serous fluid. The fimbriated end has a ''clubbed'' appearance with a bulblike bulge replacing the normally everted fimbria (Fig. 3). On microscopic sections, the wall of the hydrosalpinx appears thin with remarkable absence of inflammatory infiltrate. The mucosal plicae become flattened and short with focal areas of follicular salpingitis (Fig. 4). On pelvic examination, hydrosalpinx presents as a cystic, nontender mass similar to a cystic ovarian tumor. It is either asymptomatic or causes mild pelvic pressure or pain. If there is no exacerbation of infection, hydrosalpinx frequently regresses spontaneously. The accumulated fluid either becomes reabsorbed or drains into the uterine cavity.

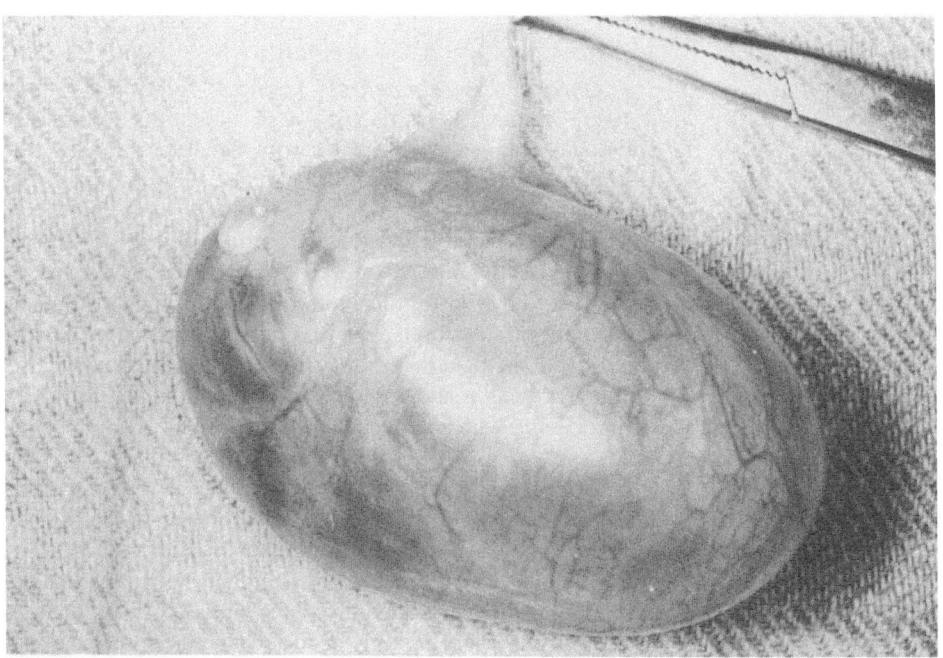

Figure 3. Hydrosalpinx, gross.

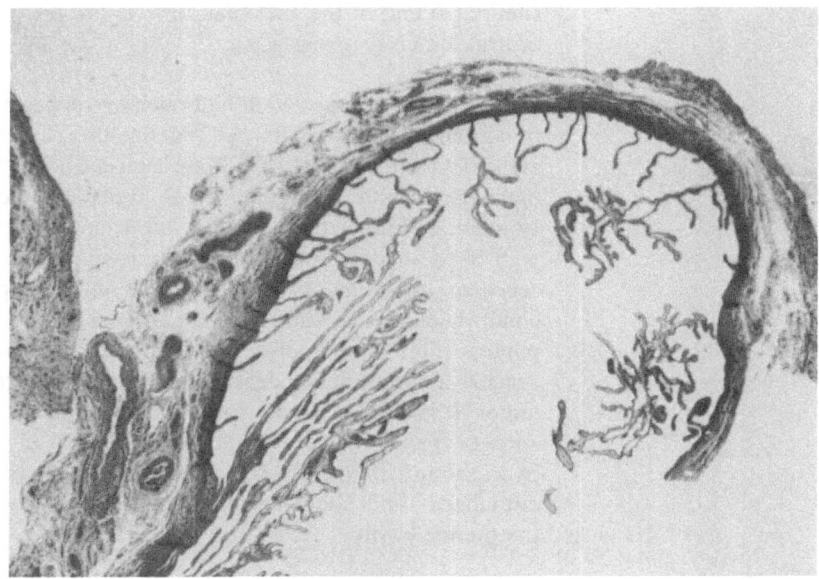

Figure 4. Hydrosalpinx, microscopic.

Chronic Perisalpingitis. Peritubal adhesions often develop during the healing stage of salpingitis, when inflammatory exudate on tubal serosa becomes invaded by fibroblasts.

The adhesions seen after the initial episode of salpingitis are usually fine, membranous, or fiberlike, but they may create a barrier for the ovum pickup mechanism. Dense perisalpingeal adhesions, seen more frequently after recurrent infections, may distort the shape of the tube, producing kinking or torsion and compromising the lumen of the tube or interfering with its muscular contractility.

Not all peritubal adhesions originate from salpingitis. Some follow operative trauma from conservative pelvic surgery such as oophorectomy, excision of the ovarian cysts, salpingectomy for ectopic pregnancy, ovarian wedge resection, excision of endometriotic implants, and tubal reconstructive surgery.[6] Nongynecological abdominal surgery for appendicitis or diverticulitis may also contribute to pelvic adhesions.

Peritoneal Inclusion Cyst. Adhesions may lead to formation of cystlike spaces lined by mesothelium and filled with serous fluid. Peritoneal inclusion cysts may attain considerable size and are often mistaken for ovarian cystic tumors. At surgery, resection is usually futile because the cyst capsule is very thin, and cleavage space between the cyst wall and surrounding organs is hard to find. Consequently, the cyst ruptures during the attempt at resection, and the clear serous content is spilled into the peritoneal cavity. Cyst wall examined microscopically appears as fibrous membrane lined by mesothelium. The mesothelial cells found in pelvic peritoneal adhesions often proliferate and form papillary or alveolar patterns, reproducing epithelia of paramesonephric organs such as endosalpinx or endometrium (Fig. 5). This unusual appearance of mesothelial lining may sometimes create problems for the pathologist in its differential diagnosis from endometriosis or ovarian neoplasms. "Chocolate cysts" are formed when blood from a ruptured Graafian follicle or corpus luteum is trapped in the

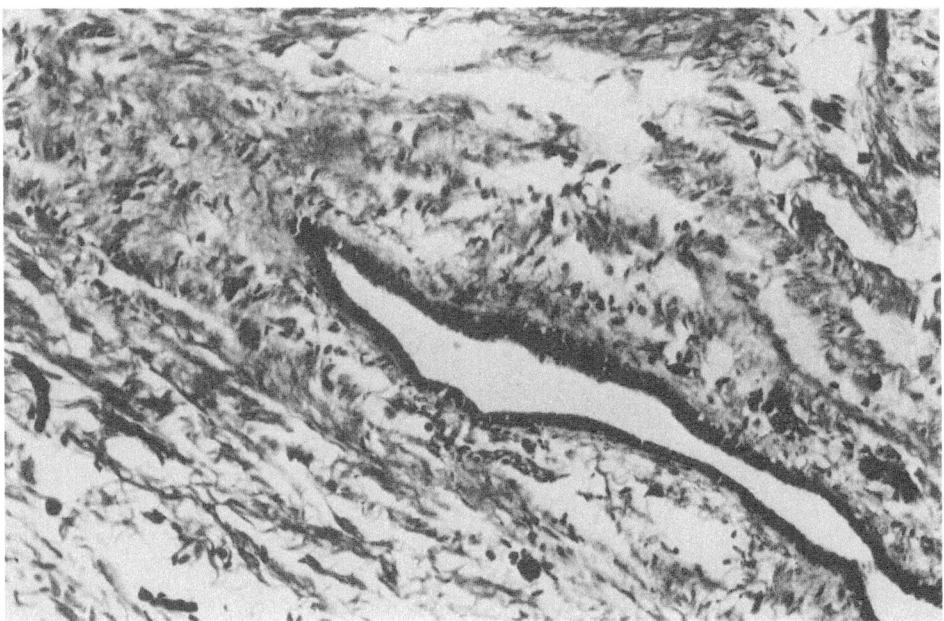

Figure 5. Mesothelial proliferation-simulating endometrial mucosa.

wall of inclusion cysts. The trapped blood may stimulate more adhesion formation, a self-perpetuating process similar to endometriosis. The symptoms of chocolate cysts of inflammatory origin also simulate endometriosis: periodic low abdominal pains, dysmenorrhea, and infertility. Even on microscopic examination, endometriosis may be suspected because of dense fibrous connective tissue and hemosiderin.

Exacerbation of acute infection frequently occurs in a tube with follicular salpingitis or hydrosalpinx. Bacterial flora in recurrent infections are often a nonspecific mixture of aerobic and anaerobic organisms with only occasional presence of gonococci. The mechanism of acute exacerbation of pelvic infection is not entirely clear, but it is possible that stasis of secretions in an obstructed tube promotes multiplication of microorganisms ascending from the cervix and vagina or penetrating from the GI tract. Menstrual discharge, blood, and necrotic endometrium also contribute

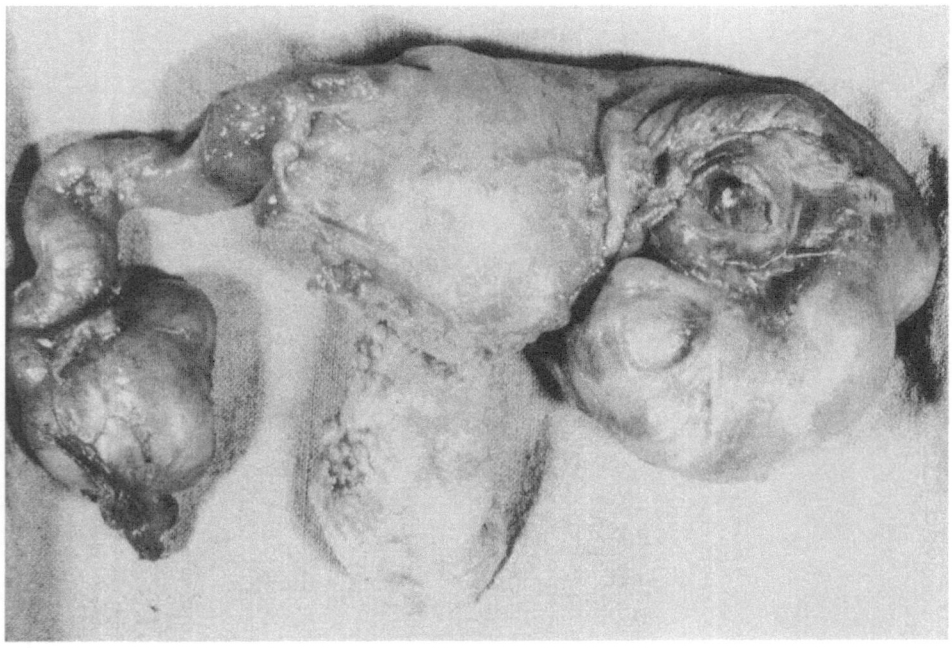

Figure 6. Pyosalpinx, gross.

favorable media for the bacterial growth, which may be the reason why the onset of acute exacerbation of pelvic infection often coincides with the menstrual period.

The following are pathological changes found singly or in combination during various phases of recurrent inflammatory disease.

Pyosalpinx. Pyosalpinx, or a "pus tube," is an accumulation of purulent material in the tube with an obstructed ostium. Pyosalpinx causes marked distention of the tube which nevertheless retains its usual coiled shape (Fig. 6). At this chronic stage of disease, the inflammatory process is no longer limited to the luminal portion of the tube but involves all of its anatomical layers. The wall is thickened, and the serosal surface presents multiple adhesions binding the tube in an immobile position behind the posterior aspect of the broad ligament and the uterus. On microscopic examination, purulent exudate is seen in the tubal lumen. The mucosa and muscularis are also infiltrated with inflammatory cells both of acute and chronic type: polymorphonucleated cells, lymphocytes, plasma cells, and macrophages. The mucosa is partly destroyed by the inflammatory process, but characteristic features of follicular salpingitis may be preserved (Fig. 7). The tubal wall is thickened, and the serosa is distorted by numerous fibrous adhesions lined by mesothelial cells.

Tubo-ovarian Abscess. This serious complication of chronic pelvic inflammation develops when the inflammatory process spreads to the ovaries and other pelvic organs in addition to the Fallopian tubes. Multiple collections of pus are found between the adhesive bands binding the tubes to the ovaries, bowel, omentum, and parietal peritoneum. The normal architecture of pelvic organs is usually distorted beyond recognition, with all organs encased in dense adhesions. Microscopic sections show the characteristic appearance of the abscess wall: granulation tissue with central necrosis and peripheral fibrosis. Within the abscess wall, the component tissue of involved organs may be discerned: ovaries, tubes, omentum, and appendices epiploicae. The inflammatory cells are mostly of chronic type, plasma cells, lymphocytes, foreign body giant cells,

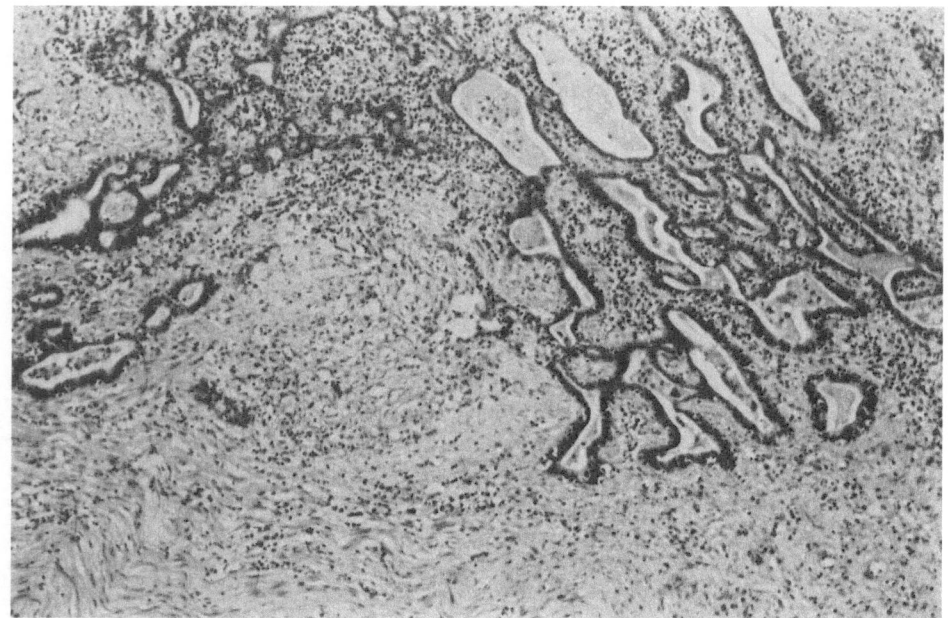

Figure 7. Pyosalpinx, microscopic.

and fat macrophages. Cholesterol crystals may also be found in the area of fat necrosis.

Tubo-ovarian abscess clinically manifests as a serious illness with acute abdomen, intestinal ileus, fever, and elevated white count and erythrocyte sedimentation rate.

Pelvic Abscess. This infrequent serious complication of pelvic inflammatory disease is characterized by a large collection of pus in the pelvis reaching upward toward the abdominal cavity with severe clinical manifestations both local and systemic. Pelvic abscess may drain spontaneously or surgically through the cul de sac or rectum. An unusual complication of pelvic abscess is a rupture into the peritoneal cavity with severe generalized peritonitis and septic shock.

Postpartum and Postabortal Infection

According to the classical concept, the pathogenesis is distinctly different in cases of postpartum or postabortal infections and in those resulting from sexually transmitted disease. Whereas the gonorrheal and chlamydial infections reach the Fallopian tubes along the mucosal surfaces of the cervix and the endometrial cavity, pregnancy-associated infection spreads via lymphatics into the parametrial spaces and usually spares the tubal lumen. The different mode of spread in these two types of infection is explained by the specific predisposition of gonococcus or *Chlamydia* to the columnar epithelium whereas the microorganisms involved in puerperal infection (gram-positive cocci, bacilli, and the anaerobes) favor the lymphatic system. In puerperal and postabortal infections, the usual course of events is endometritis, myometritis, parametritis, and sometimes pelvic abscess or pelvic vein thrombophlebitis. The Fallopian tube is affected in these infections secondarily and only in cases of extensive disease. Clinical experience nevertheless has shown that fertility may be impaired after septic abortion or postpartum infection. The postulated mechanism of infertility in these cases is the probable damage to the interstitial portion of the tube from extension of endometritis and subsequent cornual constriction or occlusion.

Evidence also indicates that fertility may also be adversely affected as a consequence of induced abortion without clinical evidence of infection. Observation of patients 2 years after legal abortion revealed that 7% of these women became infertile and 18% had abnormal hysterogram findings.[7]

Special Types of Pelvic Inflammatory Disease

Infections Associated with Use of Intrauterine Contraceptive Devices

Pelvic inflammatory disease is more frequent in women wearing an intrauterine contraceptive device (IUD) than in those using other forms of contraception. There is no agreement as to whether the IUD may be a direct cause of infection or whether it increases the frequency of sexually transmitted disease through promiscuity and nonuse of barrier contraception.[8] It has been suggested that certain types of IUDs are potentially more "dangerous" than others because their nonmonofilament tails make it easier for the bacteria to penetrate the string and gain access to the uterus.[9] The tubo-ovarian abscess linked to the IUD tends to be more often unilateral than bilateral, unlike the salpingitis of the more common type. Although unilateral tubo-ovarian abscess may occasionally be found in women who do not use the IUD, 50% of such abscesses reported in the literature were associated with the IUD use.[10] Obviously, unilateral adnexal disease interferes less with future reproduction than the bilateral type, because the opposite adnexa are spared both the inflammatory involvement and surgical intervention.

Salpingitis Isthmica Nodosa

This condition is characterized by diverticulilike extensions of endosalpingeal mucosa into the muscular wall of the Fallopian tube. Salpingitis isthmica nodosa is usually found in the absence of any active inflammation and often with no evidence of chronic inflammatory disease. Although some authors classify the salpingitis isthmica nodosa as an inflammatory condition, its exact etiology is not known.[11] On gross inspection, the tube involved in salpingitis isthmica nodosa presents multiple nodular swellings of the isthmic portion. On microscopic examination, isolated spaces are found within the nodular swellings, lined by endosalpingeal type of mucosa. The submucosa and muscularis do not present any pathological changes. The clear role of salpingitis isthmica nodosa in infertility has not been established even though some cases of this condition were found in infertile women.

Granulomatous Salpingitis

Cases of granulomatous salpingitis, although of diverse etiology, share common characteristics such as relatively infrequent occurrence, chronic course, and granulomatous type of tissue reaction. It may be caused by bacteria (tuberculosis and leprosy), fungus (actinomycosis), metazoa (schistosomisis and enterobium), and foreign body (starch or talcum powder).

Tuberculosis. Pelvic tuberculosis is always secondary to tuberculosis in other organs, usually the lungs or GI or GU tract. Pelvic organs become involved during the hematogenous spread of infection, the so-called miliary stage occurring in adolescence shortly after the primary complex. Infection of the genital organs remains latent and asymptomatic for a variable period of time.[12] The Fallopian tube is affected first among the pelvic organs, and therefore, tubercular salpingitis is found in 100% of cases in pelvic tuberculosis. The endometrium is next in frequency among the affected organs and presents tubercular changes in 50% of cases. Cervix and vagina are only rarely involved in pelvic tuberculosis. Twenty percent of patients have a history of pulmonary tuberculosis, and in 30%, extrapulmonary tuberculosis may be found, notably in the GU tract.

In most instances, the gross appearance of TB salpingitis differs little from the pyogenic chronic salpingitis. Rarely seen are the specific features of TB salpingitis such as eversion of the fimbriated end together with distention of the lumen, the so-called "tobacco pouch" appearance or miliary tubercles on the serosal surface. These tubercules must be differentiated from the Walthard rests that are frequently seen in normal tubes. Caseation is observed infrequently, but its presence is diagnostic for tuberculosis. On microscopic examination, typical granulomas may be found containing Langhans-type giant cells surrounded by epithelioid cells within dense lymphocytic and plasma cell infiltration (Fig. 8). Schaumann bodies, birefringent round crystals, are occasionally present in the granuloma. In addition to the granuloma, there is marked proliferation of endosalpingeal folds with numerous points of fusion forming a pseudoacinar pattern. Advanced cases of mucosal proliferation may present difficulties in differential diagnosis from adenocarcinoma. Carcinoma and tuberculosis may coexist

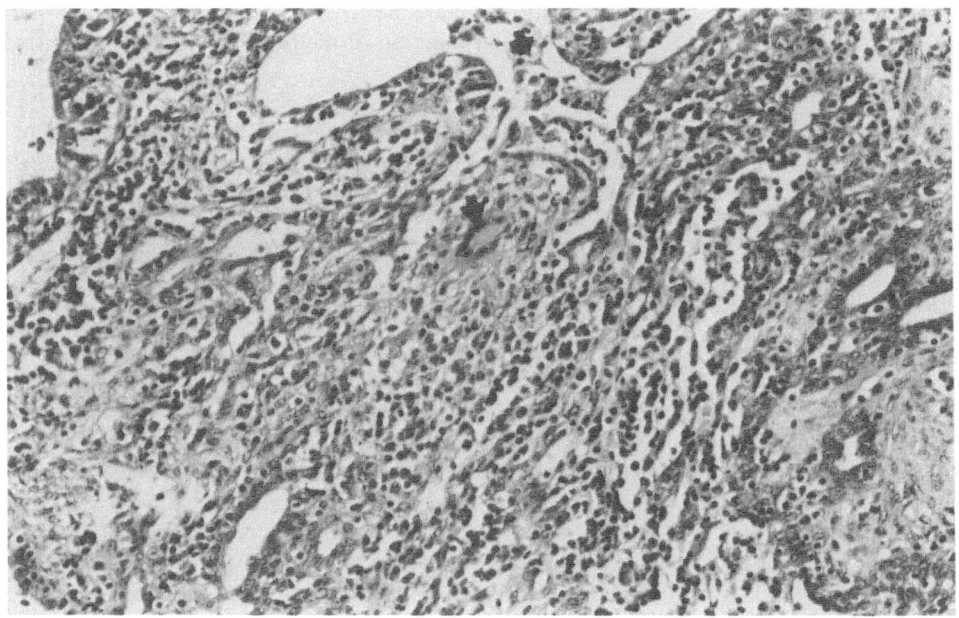

Figure 8. Tuberculosis. Granuloma with giant cell (arrow).

in the Fallopian tube, and therefore, the diagnosis of cancer must not be missed in cases of tuberculosis with intense proliferation. Presence of typical tuberculoid granulomas, although highly suggestive of tuberculosis, is not specific because tubercles may be also found in other granulomatous infections. Definite diagnosis is established only when tubercle bacillus is demonstrated by microbiological methods such as direct Ziehl–Neelsen stain or by cultures and guinea pig inoculation.

Clinical manifestations of tuberculous salpingitis may be totally absent or nonspecific, including low abdominal pain and infertility, but the enlarged Fallopian tubes may be palpated on pelvic examination.

The diagnosis of tuberculus salpingitis is usually made directly at laparotomy or laparoscopy, although it may also be established indirectly when tuberculous granulomas are found on endometrial biopsy specimens. Tuberculous salpingitis affects both tubes extensively and causes infertility. If pregnancy occurs, it is much more likely to be an ectopic one than intrauterine. Antituberculous treatment, effective in arresting the infection, will not restore the normal morphology and function of the organ and will not reverse infertility.

In the United States, tuberculosis is a rare cause of infertility, but it is common in other countries and accounts for 20% of infertility in women.

Leprosy. Leprosy is extremely rare in this country. The gross and microscopic features of lepromatous salpingitis are indistinguishable from the tuberculosis.

Actinomycosis. Actinomyces israeli are the pathogenic fungi of human infections, usually associated with foreign bodies. Recently, several cases of tubo-ovarian abscess have been reported in the wearers of IUDs with the recovery of *Actinomyces* from the abscess cavity.[13] *Actinomyces* have also been identified in 10% of material attached to the expelled or removed IUD. The risk of adnexal disease is probably small in women with *Actinomyces* in the cervix and the vagina, judging from frequent colonization by these fungi of the lower genital tract and the rarity of

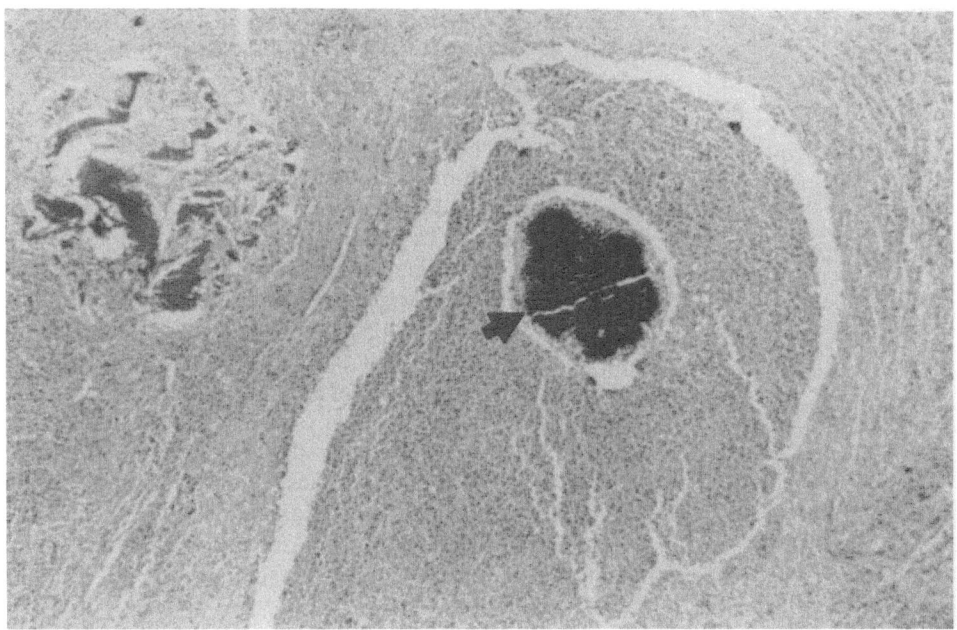

Figure 9. Actinomycosis. ''Sulfur granule'' (arrow).

pelvic abscess. Grossly, the tubo-ovarian abscess caused by actinomycosis has the same appearance as an abscess of other etiology; it is usually multiloculated and contains purulent material. The affected Fallopian tube is thickened with distorted architecture. On microscopic examination, typical ''sulfur granules'' may be identified (Fig. 9). The sulfur granules consist of central colonies of branching, gram-positive hyphae surrounded by purulent exudate and characteristic lipid histiocytes.

Oxyuris vermicularis (pinworm). The Fallopian tube is affected by pinworms in its serosal layer and only rarely in the intraluminal portion. Discrete nodules are found on gross examination of the serosa. On microscopic examination, ova are seen in these nodules. They are surrounded by purulent exudate in which eosinophils predominate. Occasionally, there may be giant cell reaction with tuberculoid granuloma. The pathogenesis of tubal infestation is explained by migration of pinworms up the cervical canal and into the endometrial cavity in cases of fecal contamination of the vagina.[14] No link between pinworm infestation and infertility has been established.

Schistosomiasis. *Schistosoma* is an infrequent form of granulomatous salpingitis. Microscopically, the granuloma resembles tuberculosis in that it contains giant cells together with epithelioid and lymphocytic infiltration. Typical ova in the granuloma provide the diagnostic clue (Fig. 10). Schistosoma infests through the portal vein system. The *S. mansoni* species found in the Western hemisphere attack the lower colon and the organs supplied by colic branches of the superior and inferior mesenteric veins. The *S. hematobium* species found in the Middle East and Africa lodge mostly in the GU tract supplied by vesical branches. Pelvic organs are more frequently involved in schistosomiasis of *hematobium* species than in *S. mansoni* infection. Because of its rarity, little is known about clinical manifestations and the impact on infertility of this parasite.[15]

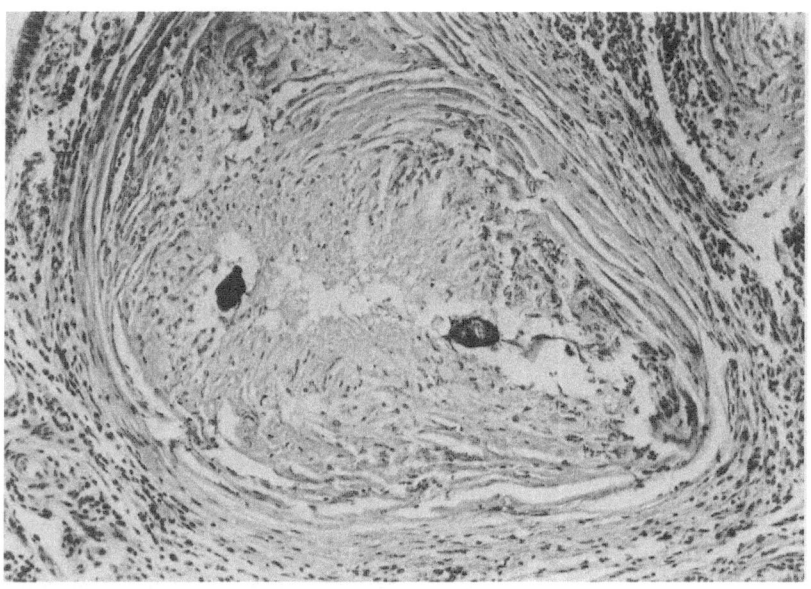

Figure 10. Schistosomiasis. Granuloma with the ova.

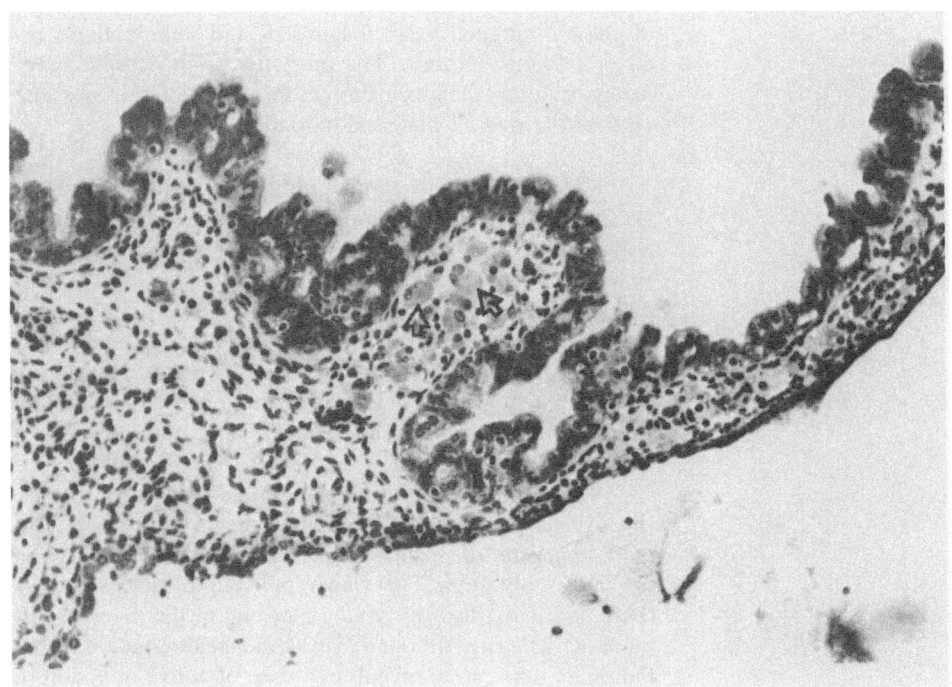

Figure 11. Lipoidal granuloma. Fat macrophages (arrow).

Foreign Body Granuloma. Starch and talcum granuloma are occasionally encountered on the serosal surfaces of the uterine tubes after previous abdominal operations during which the powder was carried into the abdominal wound by surgical gloves. Characteristic talc crystals may be identified on microscopic examination. There is no convincing evidence that these granulomas are an important cause of infertility. Oil granuloma has been reported in the endosalpinx when oil radioopaque media were used for hysterosalpingograms. On microscopic examination, there is a foreign body–giant cells reaction and fat macrophages (Fig. 11).

ECTOPIC PREGNANCY

Tubal Pregnancy

Extrauterine implantation occurs in one of every 100 pregnancies. The true incidence of ectopic pregnancy is probably even higher than one in 100 because not all cases of ectopic pregnancy are diagnosed, and some patients recover without surgery. The mortality from ectopic pregnancy is high. Deaths from ectopic pregnancy constitute 10% of the overall maternal mortality.

The frequency of ectopic pregnancy depends on geographic location and demographic characteristics of the population. The highest rate of ectopic pregnancy, one in 28 of term pregnancies, was reported from Jamaica.[17] The ampulla is the most common location of tubal pregnancy, probably because it has the widest diameter and is the site of ovum fertilization. The densely muscular isthmic portion is a less frequent site of ectopic pregnancy, and both the interstitial portion and the fimbria are the least common.

The fertilized ovum implants in the tube when its passage is delayed, most frequently by a mechanical block. The most important obstacle to tubal transport of the embryo is follicular salpingitis, in which pocketlike spaces act as traps, allowing the embryo to enter one of the recesses but blocking its exit. Although pathological examination of the Fallopian tube rarely reveals evidence of active infection in association with ectopic pregnancy, it does show chronic inactive salpingitis in more than 75% of cases in the affected and the contralateral tube.[18] It is not surprising, therefore, that the rate of repeat ectopic pregnancy is high (15–20%). The link between tubal infection and ectopic pregnancy has also been supported by epidemiologic studies and the follow-up of patients after salpingitis.[4]

Possible noninfectious causes of ectopic pregnancy are: congenital tubal diverticuli,[17] tubal dysfunction, postoperative adhesions, and transmigration of the ova from the opposite ovary, especially in cases of absence of one of the tubes.[19] The transmigration theory is not universally accepted because it is not known how often ova transmigrate in normal pregnancies.

Tubal pregnancy remains intact for only a short period of time, usually no longer than 8–12 weeks. There are only few reports of pregnancy in the Fallopian tube carried to term. The usual outcome of ectopic pregnancy is either a tubal abortion, rupture, or the so-called "chronic ectopic pregnancy."

Tubal Abortion

In tubal abortion, the nonviable conceptus is expelled through the tubal ostium into the peritoneal cavity. Tubal abortion is more common than rupture, because the implanation is most frequent in the ampulla which is distensible and less prone to rupture than is the rigid isthmus.

Bleeding into the tube continues from the placental site after detachment of the conceptus because the weak musculature of the oviduct is not capable of constricting vessels for effective hemostatis. Continuing bleeding produces hematosalpinx and hemoperitoneum.

Rupture

Rupture, which usually occurs in the narrow isthmic portion of the tube, disrupts the wall and lacerates anastomotic utero-ovarian vessels, causing massive bleeding. If the rupture site is in the portion of the tube between two layers of the broad ligament, hemorrhage may be contained in the intraligamental space.

Chronic Ectopic Pregnancy

Chronic ectopic pregnancy is an outcome of failed diagnosis and nonintervention, usually in cases with limited amount of bleeding and nonspecific symptoms. In such cases, blood spilled into peritoneal cavity becomes partly reabsorbed, and the clots become organized. Local inflammatory reaction, occasionally complicated by secondary infection, causes symptoms and signs similar to chronic inflammatory disease and may be often mistaken for this condition.

Tubal Pathology in Ectopic Pregnancy

On gross examination, the Fallopian tube with ectopic pregnancy is enlarged, and the serosa is hyperemic with blood clots adhering to its surface. A rent through all layers of the tubal wall may be identified in cases of rupture, with products of gestation extruded through the rent. In cases of tubal abortion, the products of gestation accompanied by clots may be found in the tubal ostium or in the cul-de-sac. In some of these cases, the tube may return to its normal size and appear ''empty,'' with only blood exuding from the fimbriated end. On microscopic examination, the normal architecture of the mucosa and muscularis is disrupted by the rupture, hemorrhage, or invasive action of the advancing trophoblasts. The lumen of the tube is filled with fresh or hemolyzed blood with placental villi free in the lumen, adherent to the mucosal folds, or penetrating into the tubal wall. In those cases where the conceptus had been expelled from the tube prior to surgery, multiple sections at various levels of the tube may be necessary in order to demonstrate the placenta. On rare occasions, no villi are found in the lumen of the fallopian tube, and the diagnosis of ectopic pregnancy is established only when conceptus is recovered from among the clots in the peritoneal cavity. The trophoblasts in ectopic pregnancy have more proliferative activity

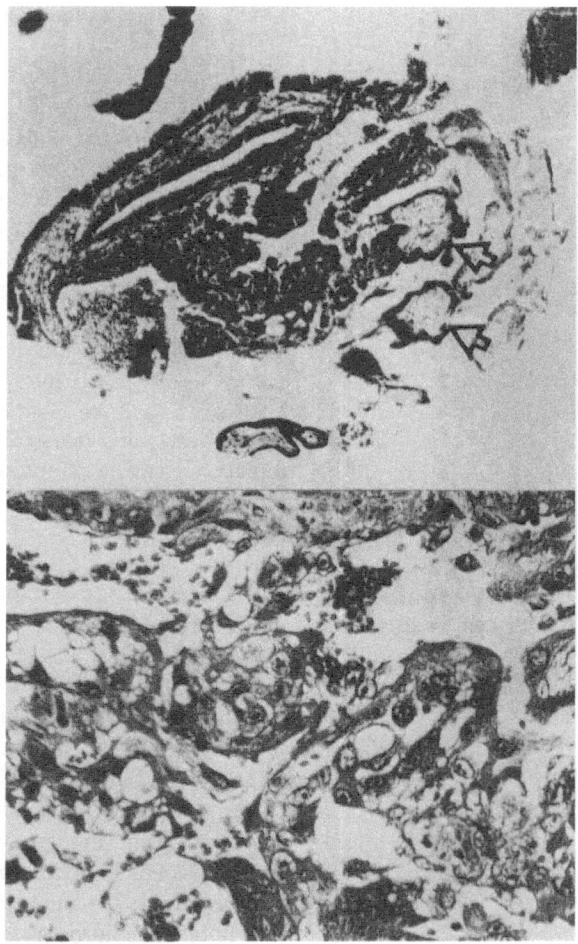

Figure 12. Tubal pregnancy. Villi attached to the mucosa (top). Immature trophoblast with lacunar spaces (bottom).

than in an intrauterine location. Solid clusters of syncytium and cytotrophoblastic cells are common, often with features of immaturity such as lucunar spaces (Fig. 12). Decidual transformation in the tubal mucosa is either totally lacking or very poorly expressed. Evidence of follicular salpingitis, the sequela of previous infection, is found in 75% of cases.[18]

Endometrial Changes in Ectopic Pregnancy

Endometrium stimulated by steroid hormones of placental origin develops into a "hypersecretory state" with decidual transformation and Arias–Stella phenomena. "Hypersecretory endometrium," an exaggeration of secretory phase of the ovulatory cycle with marked gland tortuousity and active secretion of mucus, is evidenced by cytoplasmic vacuolization and free mucus in the gland lumen. Mucus secretion normally ceases after day 20 of the normal cycle. The compacta layer of endometrium undergoes decidual transformation characterized by enlarged

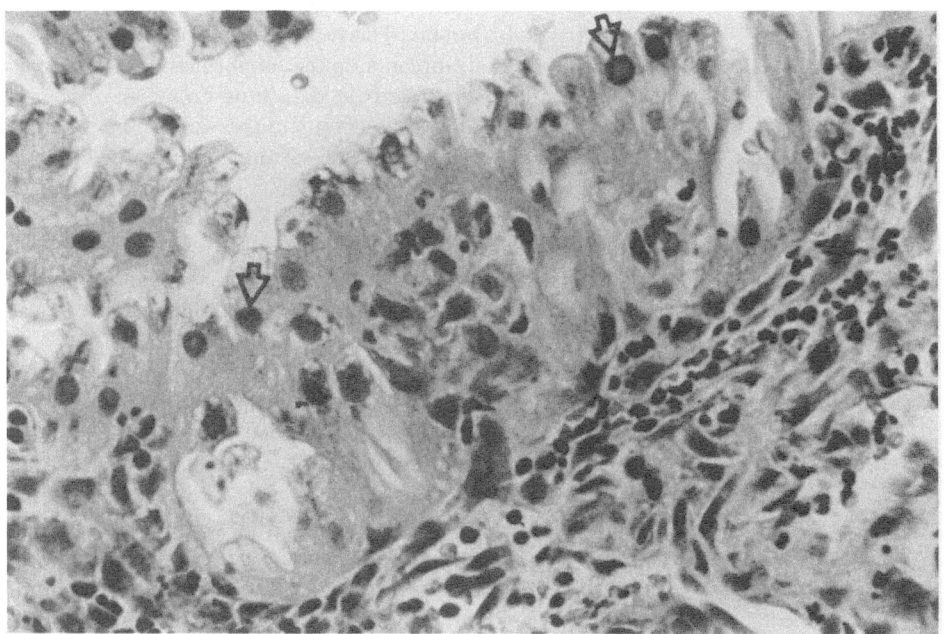

Figure 13. Arias–Stella phenomena. Hyperchromatic cell nuclei (arrow).

stroma cells with abundant granular cytoplasm and vesicular nuclei with prominent nucleoli. Arias–Stella phenomena, frequently observed in ectopic pregnancy and also present with intrauterine pregnancy, may be recognized by nuclear hyperchromasia with hobnailing in the glandular epithelial cells (Fig. 13). The classical endometrial effects of ectopic pregnancy can be found in only 30% of cases; in the remaining cases, they are presumably lost in the process of endometrial shedding. If present in the curettings, the gestational changes are helpful for diagnosis of ectopic pregnancy, especially if no products of gestation are identified in the specimen. Nonetheless, a finding of basal or proliferative endometrium does not rule out the ectopic pregnancy.

ENDOMETRIOSIS

According to the Sampson theory, the tube serves as a conduit for endometrial fragments carried during retrograde menstruation to the pelvic cavity where they subsequently implant and cause endometriosis. Although the Fallopian tube comes in contact first with endometrial fragments outside the uterine cavity, endometriosis is rarely found in the Fallopian tube lumen. The tube is involved only secondarily. Endometrial implants on the tubal serosa can be recognized by their characteristic dark blue color. In advanced cases, implants penetrate deep into the wall of the tube and form dense adhesions with the surrounding organs. On microscopic examination, endometrial glands and endometrial stroma are seen within the tubal musculature (Fig. 14). Hemosiderin-laden macrophages may also be seen. Endometrial elements may diminish or disappear in chronic cases; microscopic findings are then dominated by dense connective and hemosiderin-laden macrophages.

Endometriosis plays an important role in infertility.[20] It has been stated that endometriosis was found in 30–50% of all infertility laparotomies. The exact mechanism of infertility in patients with endometriosis is not clear. The tubal lumen is usually patent, but the architecture may be distorted by peritubal and periovarian adhesions. One postulated mechanism of infertility is the possible impairment of the ovum pickup mechanism because of inadequate motility of the tube and ovary.

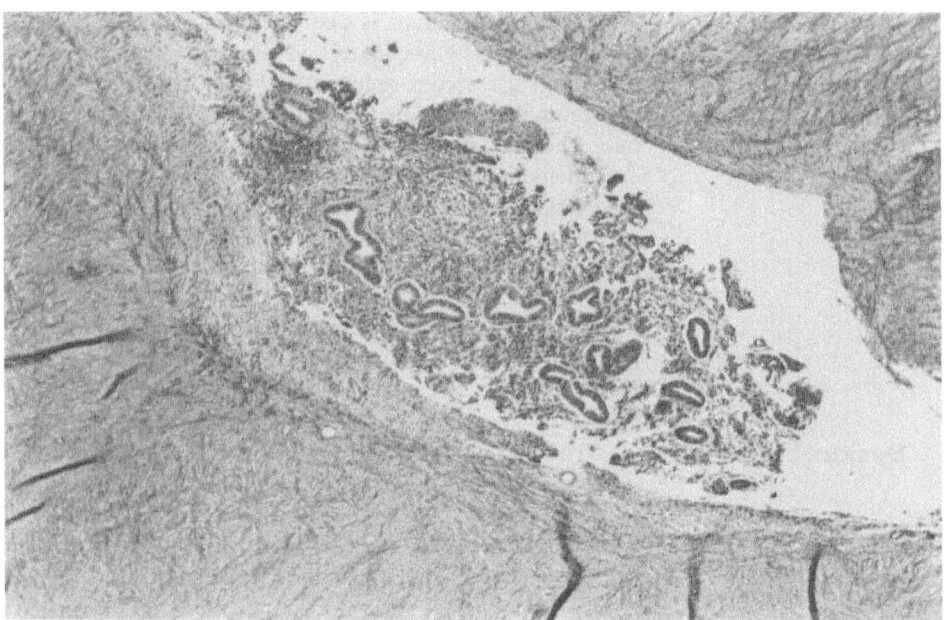

Figure 14. Endometriosis. Endometrial glands and stroma in the muscularis.

The following conditions must be considered in differential with endometriosis:

1. Peritoneal inclusion cysts with hemosiderin deposits from corpus luteum. The inclusion cysts may be differentiated from endometriosis by the absence of endometrial glands and stroma in the cyst wall and the lack of endometriosis in other locations.
2. Metaplasia of pelvic peritoneum with formation of glandlike spaces resembling endometrium lacks the endometrial stroma and the hemosiderin and may thus be differentiated from endometriosis.
3. Adenomyosis tubae has been described mostly in older literature as endometrial ingrowths into the interstitial portion of the tube.[21] Unlike true endometriosis, the continuity of endometrial implants and endometrial cavity is usually maintained in adenomyosis tubae. The clinical implications of adenomyosis tubae are poorly understood.

PATHOLOGY OF STERILIZATION AND TUBAL RECONSTRUCTIVE SURGERY

Tubal sterilization is one of the most frequently performed surgical procedures in this country, and consequently, a resected segment of Fallopian tube is one of the commonest specimens in the surgical pathology laboratory. The main purpose of pathological examination of such specimens, is to ascertain that the submitted tissue actually represents the full thickness of the tube rather than an incomplete segment of tube, the round ligament, an adhesive band, or a vessel.

In the course of examination of the specimens, the following normal variations or pathological changes may be noted:

Decidual Reaction

The decidual transformation in the stromal cells of tubal mucosa is frequently observed in puerperal sterilization specimens. The involved cells closely resemble endometrial decidua and become markedly enlarged, oval, or polygonal with abundant pale basophilic granular cytoplasm

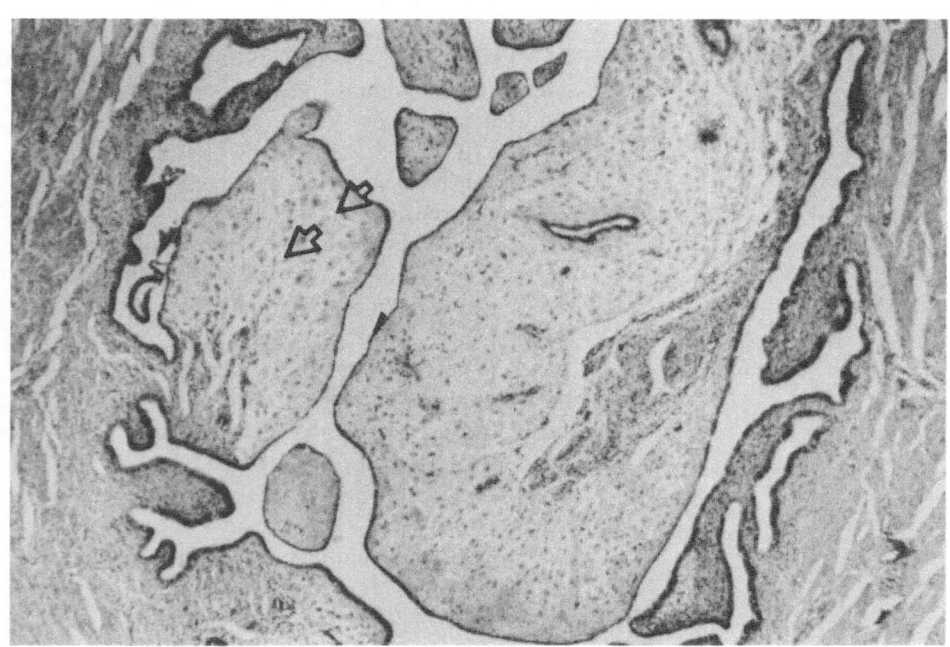

Figure 15. Decidual changes in tubal mucosa.

and enlarged vesicular nuclei and prominent nucleoli (Fig. 15). Decidual reaction, although commonly seen in puerperal tube, is conspicuously absent in early gestation, notably in ectopic pregnancy.

Walthard Rests

These embryonal rests are a constant feature of tubal mucosa. Grossly, they present as multiple 1- to 2-mm nodules scattered on the tubal surface, resembling miliary tuberculosis. On microscopic examination, the Walthard rests appear as solid clusters of squamous cells, occasion-

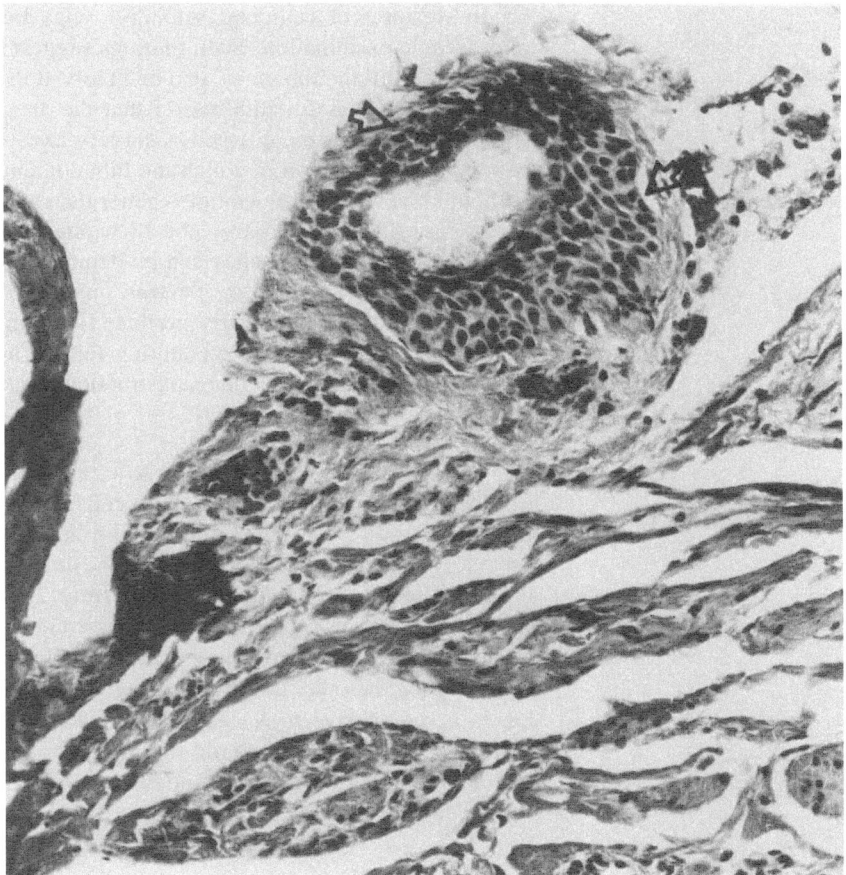

Figure 16. Walthard rest in tubal serosa. Cystic space within the cluster of squamous cells.

ally with a central cavity lined by cuboidal or columnar cells (Fig. 16).

Physiological Salpingitis

Mild inflammatory cells, infiltration of mucosa, and free exudate in the tubal lumen are frequently seen in puerperal sterilization specimens. This type of salpingitis is considered to be an expression of postpartum involution rather than infection.[22]

Chronic Inactive Salpingitis

The changes consistent with chronic inflammation may be found in specimens from sterilization procedures but more often in the excised portions of the tube during reconstructive procedures. If tubal occlusion is of infectious origin, features of follicular salpingitis may be found on microscopic examination. Such findings suggest that the remaining part of the tube may also be involved in inflammatory changes. It is for this reason that the success rate is generally low after reconstructive surgery except for cases of reversal sterilization in which the tubal damage is local. Although the results are two times better than average in the reversal sterilization surgery, not all women achieve conception after restored patency can be demonstrated on hysterogram. Recent scanning electron microscopy studies showed that tubal ligation may produce flattening of folds, deciliation, and polyposis, accounting for the lack of success in some of the cases of reconstruction surgery.[23]

TUMORS
Adenomatoid Tumors

An adenomatoid tumor is a rare benign growth originating from the mesothelial cells of the pelvic peritoneum and found predominantly on the surface of the uterus or the Fallopian tube.[24] On gross examination, the tumor presents as an irregular nodule from 2 to 10 cm in diameter. On microscopic examination, irregular glandlike spaces are seen lined with low uniform cuboidal cells resembling the mesothelium and separated from each other by bands of connective tissue and smooth muscle of various widths (Fig. 17). Adenomatoid tumor has no capsule, and its borders are diffuse, but in spite of lack of encapsulation, it does not exhibit any malignant potential.

The majority of cases of adenomatoid tumor reported in the literature occurred in postmenopausal women.

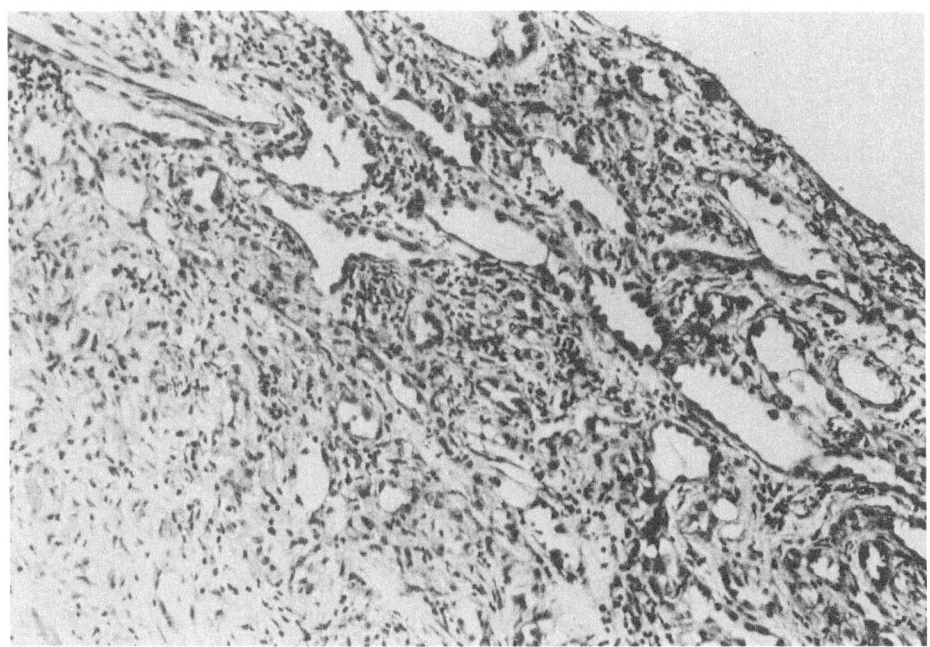

Figure 17. Adenomatoid tumor. Glandular spaces lined with flat epithelium.

Carcinoma   Malignant neoplasms of the Fallopian tube are the least common among all other malignancies of the female genital tract. Tubal carcinoma may occur at any age but approximately one-third of cases are found in women of reproductive age. Carcinoma of the Fallopian tube is usually unilateral but affects both tubes in approximately 20% of cases. Clinical symptoms of cancer of the Fallopian tube are inconstant and nonspecific. The most common symptom is abnormal uterine bleeding, probably caused by an escape of the contents of the hematosalpinx through the utero–tubal junction. Abdominal pain, colicky or dull ache, is the second most frequent symptom. Leukorrhea, often occuring in spurts (hydrops tubae profluens), is also believed to be of tubal origin. Malignant cells may be recovered on a Papanicolaou smear in 30% of cases of tubal cancer. Grossly, the tumor originates in the endosalpinx and causes distention of the affected organ. On sectioning of the Fallopian tube, the papillary tumor may be found in the lumen,

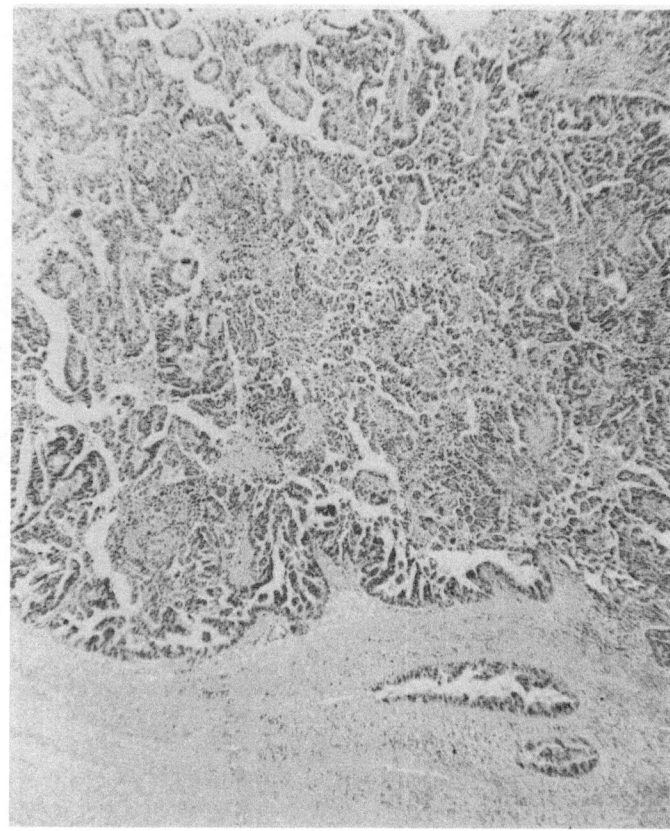

Figure 18. Carcinoma. Papillary, alveolar pattern.

frequently accompanied by hematosalpinx. Advanced tumor may involve adjacent organs—ovaries and uterus, and in such cases it may be difficult to determine whether the tumor is primarily tubal or ovarian. Histologically, the tumor is adenocarcinoma of the papillary alveolar type (Fig. 18). The overall 5-year survival rate is approximately 38%.[25]

REFERENCES

1. Eschenbach DA, Holmes KK: Acute pelvic inflammatory disease: Current concepts of pathogenesis, etiology and management. *Clin Obstet Gynecol* 18:35, 1975.
2. Schlachter J, Hanna L, Hill EC, et al: Are chlamydial infections the most prevalent venereal diseases? *JAMA* 231:1252, 1975.

3. Mardh PA, Ripa T, Svenson L et al: *Chlamidia trachomatis* infection in patients with acute salpingitis. *N Engl J Med* 296:1377, 1977.

4. Westrom L: Effect of acute pelvic inflammatory disease on fertility. *Am J Obstet Gynecol* 121:707, 1975.

5. Ferenczy A, Richart R: *Female Reproductive System Dynamics of Scan and Transmission Electronmicroscopy.* New York, Wiley Biomedical, 1974, p. 234.

6. Kistner RW: Peritubal and periovarian adhesions subsequent to wedge resection of the ovaries. *Fertil Steril* 20:35, 1969.

7. Joupilla P, Kauppila A, Punto L: Observations on patients two years after legal abortion *Int J Fertil* 19:233, 1974.

8. Ory HW: A review of the association between intrauterine devices and acute pelvic inflammatory disease. *J Reprod Medicine* 20:200, 1978.

9. Tatum JJ, Schmidt FH, Phillips DH, et al: The Dalcon shield controversy. Structural and bacterial studies of IUD tails. *JAMA* 213(7):711, 1975.

10. Golde SH, Israel R, Ledger WJ: Unilateral tubo-ovarian abscess: A distinct entity. *Am J Obstet Gynecol* 127:807, 1977.

11. Woodruff JD, Pauerstein CJ: *The Fallopian Tube.* Baltimore, Williams & Wilkins Co, 1969, p 145.

12. Halbrecht I: Diagnosis, pathogenetic role and treatment of the sequels of female genital tuberculosis, in Rippman ET, Wenner R (eds): *Latent Female Genital Tuberculosis.* Basel, S, Karger, 1966, p 232.

13. Schiffer MA, Elgvezabal A, Sultana M, et al: Actinomycosis infections associated with intrauterine contraceptive devices. *Obstet Gynecol* 45:67, 1975.

14. Schenken OR, Tamisea J: Peritoneal granulomas due to *Enterobius vermicularis.* Arch Surg 73:309, 1956.

15. Sedlis A: Manson's Schistosomiasis of the Fallopian tube. *Am J Obstet Gynecol* 81:234, 1961.

15. Schneider J, Berger GJ, Cattell C, et al: Maternal mortality due to ectopic pregnancy: A review of 102 deaths. *Obstet Gynecol* 49:557, 1977.

17. Persaud V: Etiology of tubal ectopic pregnancy: Radiologic and pathologic studies. *Obstet Gynecol* 36:257, 1970.

18. Sedlis A: *Ectopic Pregnancy in Practice of Surgery. Gynecology* Hagerstown, Maryland, Harper and Row, 1979, chapter 33.

19. Bronson RA: Tubal pregnancy and infertility. *Fertil Steril* 28:221, 1977.

20. Kistner RW: Management of endometriosis in the infertile patient. *Fertil Steril* 26:1151, 1975.

21. Hughesdon PE: Gynecological pathology, in Barber, H (ed): *Systemic Pathology.* New York, American Elsevier, 1967, 881.

22. Rubin A, Czernobilsky B: Tubal ligation: A bacteriologic, histologic and clinical study. *Obstet Gynecol* 36:199, 1970.

23. Vasquez G, Winston RML, Boeckx W, et al: Tubal lesions subsequent to sterilization and their relation to fertility after attempts at reversal. *Am J Obstet Gynecol* 138:86, 1980.

24. Young LH, Taylor HB: Adenomatoid tumors of the uterus and Fallopian tube. *Am J Clin Pathol* 48:537, 1967.

25. Sedlis A: Carcinoma of the Fallopian tube. *Surg Clin North Am* 58:121, 1978.

4 Microsurgical Technical Aids and Instrumentation

John J. Stangel

Department of Obstetrics and Gynecology
Section of Reproductive Endocrinology and Infertility
New York Medical College
Westchester County Medical Center
Valhalla, New York 10595

Approximately 12% of couples of reproductive age are infertile, and Fallopian tube disease is the primary cause of this infertility in 30% of these couples. The result is a vast and increasing number of women requiring surgical intervention for the treatment of infertility. Tubal surgeons using conventional surgery can restore oviduct macrostructure with a high degree of reliability, but the damage to the oviduct microstructure, the tubal endosalpinx and muscle, remains or is actually worsened by such surgery.

Tubal infertility surgery requires meticulous restoration of anatomy, opposing endosalpinx to endosalpinx and myosalpinx to myosalpinx, and covering it all with a smooth, flawless serosal layer. Hemostasis must be meticulous; no clots or oozing or raw surfaces should remain at the completion of the repair. Suture affects the tissue in which it lays, and it is apparent that surgeons must use finer, less reactive suture. The result of such work is a higher pregnancy rate when compared to series using conventional techniques.

The use of very fine sutures to deal with small structures in order to obtain proper restoration of anatomy dictates the use of magnification. Operating loupes offer up to sixfold magnification, and an operating microscope can provide magnification up to 40-fold. The term "microsurgery," as used in this chapter, means surgery performed with the aid of magnification, either a loupe or an operating microscope. Moreover, it implies a greater order of surgical precision using fine, nonreactive suture and gentle tissue handling rather than the "same old" surgery under a lens. Microsurgery is as much a surgical philosophy of minimizing tissue damage as it is a specific series of operating techniques. The use of magnification, however, introduces new problems that must be addressed. This chapter will present technical aids and instruments that allow the surgeon to perform optimally and overcome these problems.

SURGEON

Magnification allows the surgeon to increase his visual acuity, and as visual acuity increases, coordination keeps pace. Although hand coordination can increase with practice, hand tremor, which is constantly present and can be ignored under ordinary circumstances, becomes a major problem for the microsurgeon. Every human being has normal physiological movement of his extremities that is manifest as a tremor. The frequency and amplitude of this tremor vary from individual to individual and within the same individual under different circumstances. Tremor can never be totally eliminated, but circumstances can be controlled to minimize these physiological movements. Because tremor may hamper precise movements such as dissection and suturing, it is essential for the microsurgeon to attempt to diminish it.

The frequency of tremor is association with the heart rate. Therefore, efforts by the microsurgeon to maintain a low heart rate and avoid tachycardia should improve surgical performance. A regular, strenuous exercise program such as running can lower the heart rate and diminish tremor. On the other hand, drugs like atropine and its derivatives increase the heart rate and worsen these hand movements. Thus, the surgeon should carefully evaluate all his medications. Alcohol, caffeine, nicotine, muscular exertion, anxiety, and stress all worsen tremor, and the surgeon should strive to minimize his exposure to these factors. Even a single glass of wine within 24 hr of surgery can affect hand movements. Caffeine-containing drinks also should be avoided within the same period of time. The surgeon should do no heavy lifting prior to surgery. Ideally, the car he drives to the hospital should have power steering so that he need not exert strong pressure with the muscles in his arms. To counterbalance the foregoing list of restrictions for the microsurgeon, Dr. Earl Owen, an Australian microsurgeon, has pointed out that coital activity prior to an operation tends to diminish tremor.

In preparation for microsurgery, the surgeon should have a good night's sleep and arrive at the hospital well before the case to avoid rushing. If the operating room is not on the ground floor, the surgeon should take the elevator rather than using the stairs. The surgeon should not move or position the patient on the operating table himself to avoid strong muscle exertion of the muscles of the hands, forearm, and arm. The operating suite should be a quiet, controlled environment, free from loud or sudden noises. The doors should be kept closed to minimize distractions, extraneous noise, air currents, and outside contamination.

THE MICROSURGICAL TEAM

Microsurgery is optimally performed by a stable group participating on a regular basis in the microsurgical procedures and thus forming the "microsurgical team." This team usually consists of a surgeon and an assistant, a scrub nurse, a circulator, and an anesthesiologist. As their exposure to the surgery increases, the group eventually functions as a unit, frequently acting in unison and even anticipating each other's surgical requirements. When the group functions well as a team, many steps in the surgery will proceed without a single word spoken. The result is total unbroken concentration and, probably, the most ideal surgical environment.

The scrub nurse should learn to load a microsurgical needle in a microneedle holder in the proper way and to pass it to the surgeon by placing the needle holder in his hand. Care must be taken neither to drop the needle nor to pass it over the open incision. Some surgeons prefer to load the needle holders themselves under the microscope, but the scrub nurse must still pass the suture and receive used needles at the completion of suturing. Loading a 100-μm needle requires some practice, and keeping track of the needles to assure correct count is of immense importance.

The surgical assistant learns to contribute toward a successful effort by positioning the tissue to be sutured so that the needle is always passed in an axis that facilitates the suturing. Moreover, he must perform all of the retraction when the abdomen is opened; this permits the surgeon to avoid muscle exertion and diminishes tremor.

Microsurgical instruments require special care. They must be carefully cleaned to prevent corrosion and the accumulation of debris in their pivot points and sliding surfaces. Foreign material can cause a needle holder or a pair of microscissors to stick and thus require greater force to close or to fail to open at the required time. The fine, sharp points of forceps and scissors are easily bent if allowed to slide against a firm surface. Thus, microsurgical instruments should not be carried in a metal pan or basin where inertial movement will often cause the instruments to slide along the bottom so that the tips strike the side. The only way to insure the proper care of microsurgical instruments is to have them handled solely by an experienced, responsible staff. The use of the instruments by other than the microsurgical team should be prohibited. The scrub nurse and circulator should be the only ones allowed to handle and clean the instruments when they are not in use by the surgeon or his assistant. The microsurgical instruments should be stored in a special, lined instrument box which is wrapped and autoclaved separately. The box should be opened only when the instruments are required during the course of surgery. Therefore, if unexpectedly the surgical procedure does not warrant the use of the microinstruments, this precaution prevents their unnecessary handling.

POSITIONING THE PATIENT ON THE OPERATING TABLE

During surgery, the operator should be seated close to the patient's side with his arms on her abdomen and his knees projecting under the operating table. If the patient were placed in the usual position on the table, the surgeon's knees would hit the center supporting column of the table. To avoid this, an extension should be added to the foot of the table, and the patient should be displaced in a downward direction with her pelvis placed closer to the foot of the table. This permits the surgeon to sit easily and get close to the operating table without striking the obstructing column. Before the operator sits, he should position the draped microscope next to the patient and lower it over the incision. After the surgeon is seated, the operating table is tilted toward the operator at a 20–25° angle.

TYPE OF INCISION

The abdominal incision for Fallopian tube, ovarian, or other related pelvic reconstruction must allow adequate exposure to the pelvic side walls with minimal restriction of movement throughout the operative field. In other forms of surgery, it may be permissible for the operator to strain to work around corners and odd angles, but such stress increases the difficulty of microsurgery and lessens the quality of the repair.

It is suggested that the Cherney incision offers the best combination of exposure to the pelvic side walls and cosmetic acceptability. This is a low, transverse skin and fascial incision followed by disattachment of the rectus muscles from their tendonous insertions on the pubis. The muscle is reflected back, and the peritoneum entered in a transverse manner at a level above the bladder. The exposure extends well laterally, offering excellent access to the pelvic organs. The surgeon has adequate room to dissect tubes and ovaries adherent to the side walls or deep in the pelvis. The less cramped the surgical field and the less physical and psychological stress imposed on the surgeon, the less the hand tremor and the better the quality of the surgical repair. A midline incision provides as much exposure as the Cherney, but the Cherney incision frequently offers better exposure of the pelvic side walls and is more cosmetically acceptable than a vertical incision. A Pfannenstiel incision is also cosmetically acceptable but may offer less lateral exposure than the Cherney. At the completion of the procedure, the peritoneum is closed, and the tendons are sutured to the stumps of their insertions on the pubis with 0-Dexon.® The remainder of the abdominal closure is achieved in the conventional manner.

AIDS TO PROPER EXPOSURE

Once the abdomen is opened, the abdominal contents must constantly be kept moist. We use 6% or 10%

dextran 70 or dextran 75 as an irrigation solution. Our research data indicate that it has a definite protective effect on peritoneal surfaces. Sponging should be kept to an absolute minimum, but whenever a sponge or a laparotomy pad is used, it must never be dry. A dry rough surface causes extensive abrasion of the serosal surfaces which results in adhesion formation. The bowel should be packed back with moistened laparotomy pads, and additional pads are to be placed to form a gasket around the edge of the abdominal incision. A self-retaining abdominal retractor can then be inserted; the O'Connor-O'Sullivan retractor is quite adequate. It is suggested that the retractor be released for 5 min every hour to prevent substained compression of the femoral nerves and the associated postoperative leg weakness.

Other steps may be taken to facilitate optimal exposure. A Foley catheter can be inserted into the bladder to prevent its distention during surgery. If the patient has a deep pelvis, it may be helpful to pack the posterior fornix and the vagina with moistened laparotomy pads prior to the laparotomy. This will raise the uterus out of the pelvis toward the anterior abdominal wall and facilitate surgery. The pouch of Douglas should be packed with a moistened laparotomy pad to form a ''platform'' or elevated working surface. This raises the ovaries and tubes out of the cul-de-sac and improves exposure. The tube and ovary not being worked on should be covered with a moistened laparotomy pad or a pool of dextran.

Chromotubal perfusion is accomplished via a Foley catheter placed in the uterine cavity. Prior to the laparotomy, the patient should be placed in lithotomy position, and a #14 or #16 Foley catheter is inserted through a slightly dilated cervix into the uterine cavity. The Foley bag is inflated, and the catheter pulled downwards so that the bag is seated tightly against the upper portion of the endocervical canal. The portion of the Foley usually connected to a drainage bag is joined to an intravenous extension tube which is connected to a 50-ml syringe filled with a concentrated methylene blue dye solution. The dye is injected for tubal perfusion during surgery.

After the abdomen has been opened and adequate exposure achieved, the surgeon selects the side from which he will work. The author usually prefers to work on the side opposite the tube that will require the more extensive dissection. If both sides require equal work, the selection of the side is arbitrary.

The table is lowered to the maximum and tilted to a 20–25° angle toward the surgeon. The surgeon should then seat himself comfortably with his feet on the floor, his back and neck straight, and looking forward squarely into the

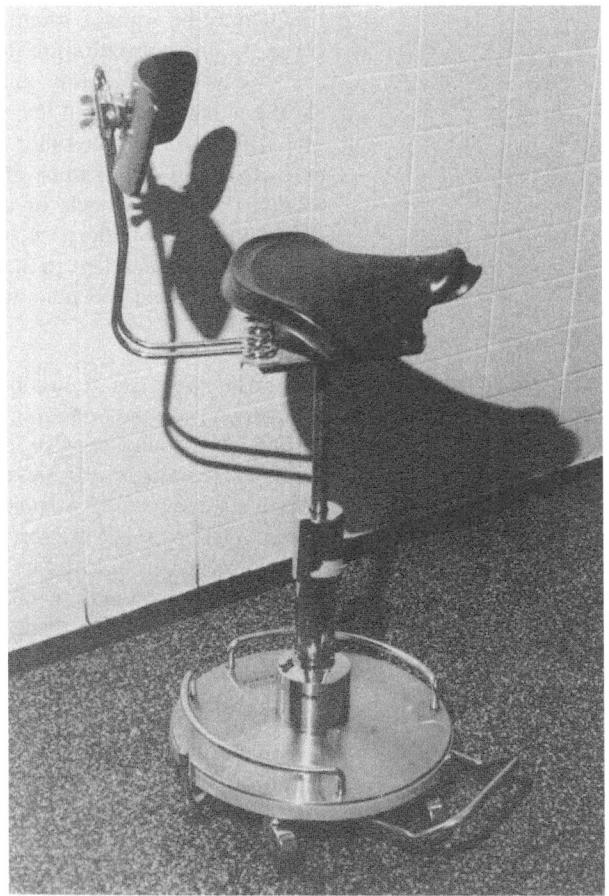

Figure 1. Chair with bicycle-shaped seat. Note the presence of back rest, height adjustment mechanism, and wheel-locking device.

microscope head. His arms should rest on the patient with his forearm and hands supported on the edge of the abdominal retractor. Because the forearm and hands are supported, contraction of the muscles in his upper extremities is lessened, and tremor at the fingertips is diminished. The height of the table and the seat should be adjusted to allow the body and arm position described.

THE CHAIR

The chair used must be comfortable for the surgeon, for he may be required to sit for several hours. The seat itself may be square, round, or shaped like a bicycle seat (Fig. 1); the configuration does not appear to be important as long as the surgeon is comfortable. Some chairs provide arm and hand rests, but the author does not find them helpful. Backrests, on the other hand, do add to the comfort of the chair. The chair must also be adjustable in height and stable. If it has wheels or casters, it must have a built-in locking device. Otherwise, the surgeon must use the muscles in his feet and legs to maintain the position and stability of the chair, and this adds to operator fatigue.

SELECTION OF MAGNIFICATION

The two most commonly used forms of magnification for surgery are the operating loupe and the operating microscope. The loupe consists of a matched set of telescopes with a fixed magnification and working distance attached to a pair of eyeglass-type frames which are worn by the surgeon. The operating microscope is a microscope containing a series of lenses that allows variability in magnification and working distance and attached to an outside support which maintains the position of the microscope relative to the patient. Each device offers advantages and disadvantages.

Operating Loupe

The operating loupe is portable and readily available whenever required. If a surgeon carries his own loupe, he avoids concern over operating in a hospital without any form of magnification or the instrument being unavailable because of concurrent surgery. The loupe is worn by the operator and therefore requires neither draping nor special positioning. There is nothing large and extraneous to be brought into the operative field that may interfere with the movements of the surgeon's hands and instruments. As the surgeon directs his attention from one part of the operative

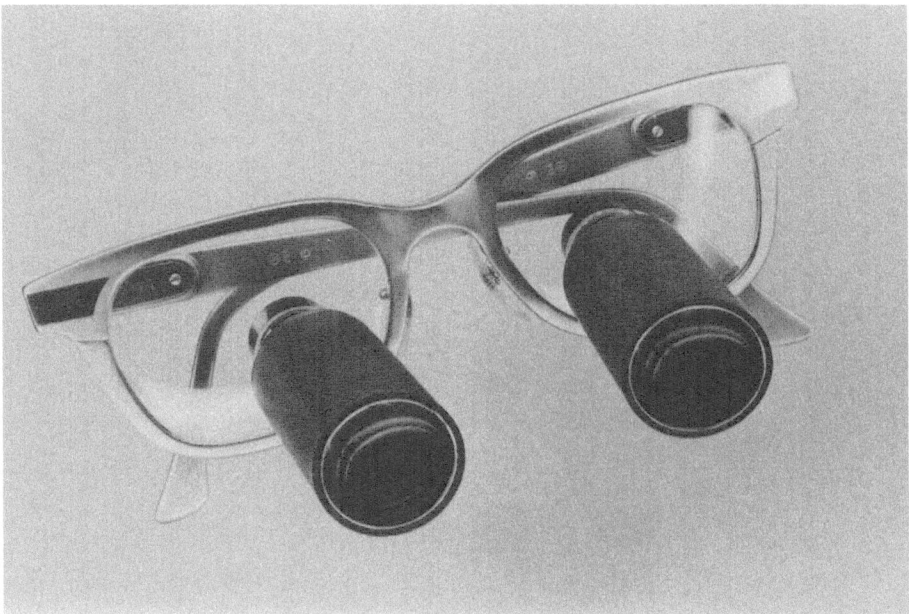

Figure 2. The highest magnification available with loupes, ×6 (Designs for Vision). Note that the loupes are fixed to the frames.

field to another, he simply moves his head rather than making adjustments on an extension arm and column to shift a microscope. Finally, loupes are much less expensive than microscopes.

Unfortunately, loupes also have disadvantages. The loupe must be held in one place to maintain a fixed optical field. This is done by the surgeon maintaining the position of his head by using head, neck, and shoulder muscles. This can be very fatiguing and can lead to headaches and dizziness. Furthermore, as fatigue grows, the surgeon may develop a tremor of the neck, causing the field to shift and shake and making concentration difficult.

Loupes have a lower top magnification than a microscope. The highest magnification known to the author is ×6 in loupes made by Designs for Vision, New York (Fig. 2). Microscopes, on the other hand, can achieve up to ×40 magnification. Furthermore, a loupe of higher magnifica-

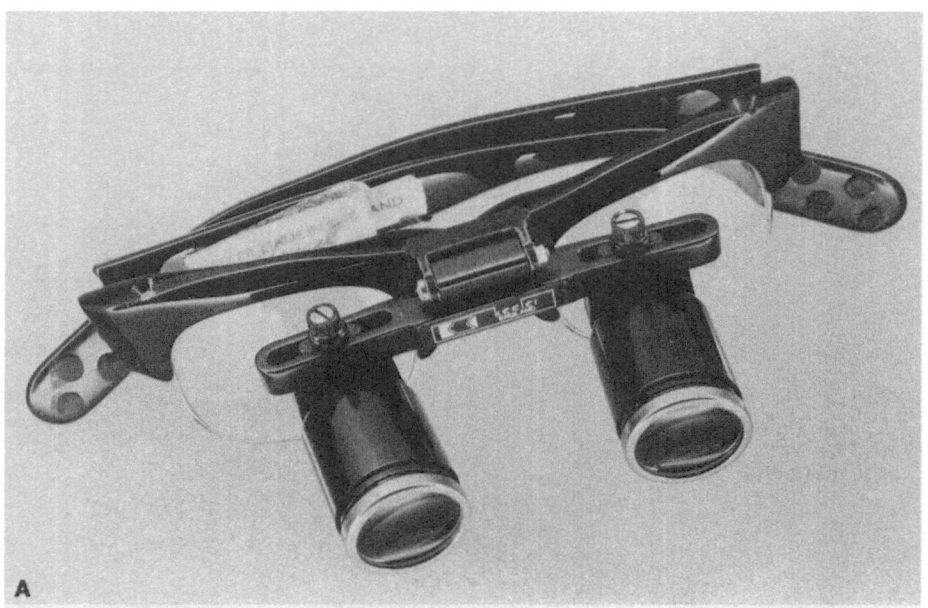

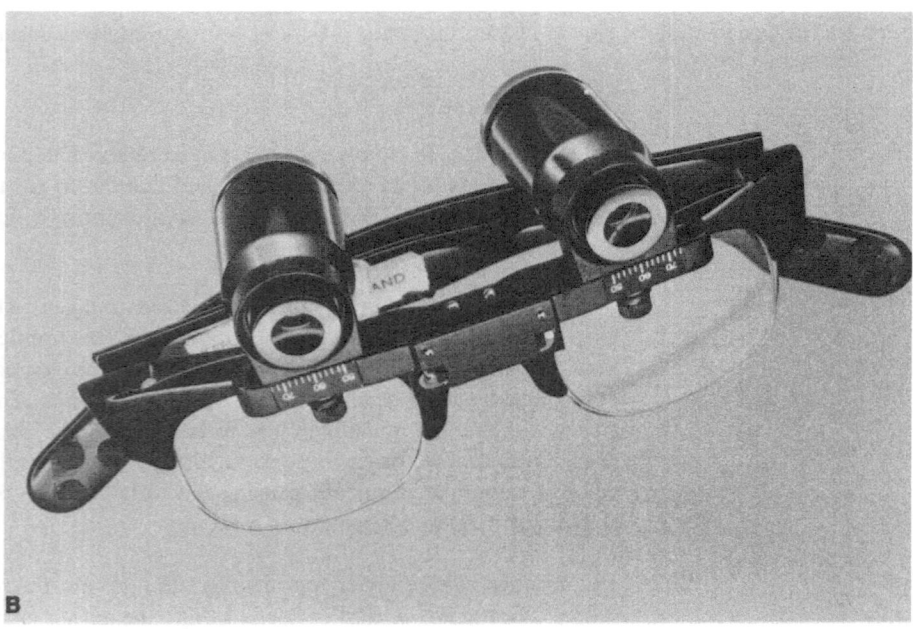

Figure 3. Adjustable loupes by Keeler. (A) The telescope is shown in place. (B) The telescope is flipped upward out of the way; this permits ordinary vision without removal of the loupes.

tion requires a greater degree of stability to maintain the optical field and produces greater fatigue. Loupes provide a small optical field with less depth than do microscopes. The author recommends operating loupes made by Keeler of England and Designs for Vision, New York. The Keeler loupes are ready-made and come in a variety of magnifications (Fig. 3). The Designs for Vision loupes are customized and can be made to fill almost any special specification.

Operating Microscope   The operating microscope provides a much larger optical field with greater depth of field and magnification than does the loupe. The surgeon can change magnification during surgery, and many microscopes have a "zoom" control that permits the operator to obtain the precise magnification required. Moreover, the microscope is supported by a column and extension arm and has a built-in coaxial light source; this reduces the surgeon's fatigue and frequently enhances his operative performance. Microscopes can be equipped with beam splitters that divide the light rays. Channeling a portion of this light to another microscope head allows an assistant to see precisely what the surgeon sees. Alternatively, this light can be directed to a camera, film, or video tape, and the surgery can be recorded. It is not possible to photograph or observe exactly what the surgeon sees with a loupe.

On the other hand, microscopes do have disadvantages. They are far more expensive than loupes. It should be noted that newer, inexpensive microscopes of acceptable quality are being developed, and price may soon be eliminated as a major stumbling block. Microscopes are much less portable than loupes and do not provide the surgeon with the freedom to do microsurgery anywhere at any time. This is a disadvantage with greater application for surgery in underdeveloped countries than in the United States.

Some surgeons feel that use of a loupe is a good introduction to microsurgery, and after gaining some experience with a loupe, they will advance to the use of a microscope. In reality, there is minimal carryover from loupe to microscope. Precise surgery under a microscope necessitates as much work with the microscope as with surgical technique. One cannot gain experience positioning, draping, and focusing a microscope by using a loupe. Even the surgical technique differs somewhat between the microscope and the loupe because of the differences in field size, depth of field, magnification, and color perception. The two forms of magnification are similar and parallel. Each has its own advantages and disadvantages, but it is counterproductive to consider a loupe preparation for a microscope. The author strongly prefers the use of the operating microscope for Fallopian tube surgery.

The most tedious aspect of microsurgery may be draping the microscope with a sterile covering prior to moving it

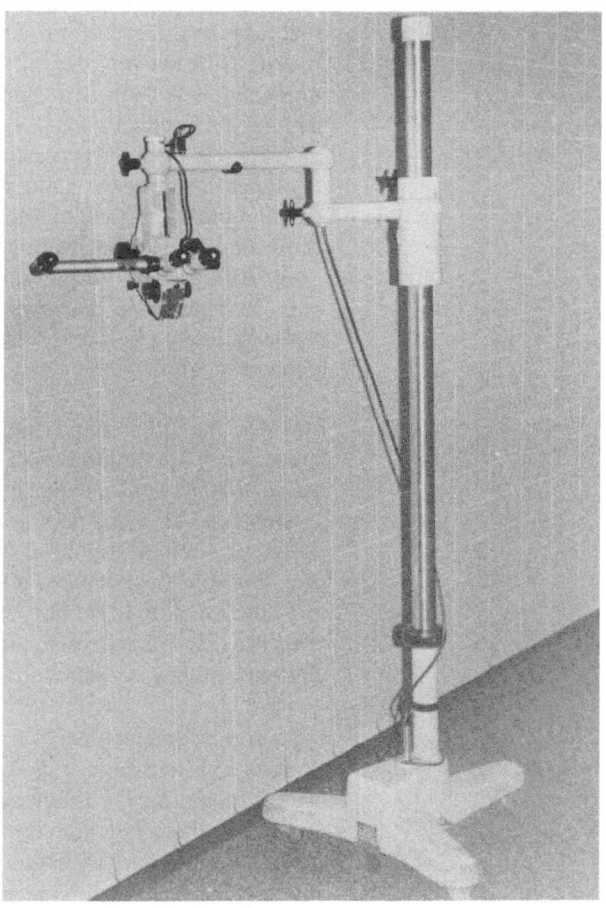

Figure 4. The manually operated microscope, Zeiss OP Mi-1.

into the operative field. Although this is not standard technique in some countries, such as the United Kingdom, it is standard practice in the United States. Once again, with some practice even draping can go smoothly.

The microscope, mounted on a base and column, is moved next to the surgeon. The operating microscope used for gynecologic microsurgery should have a long carriage arm or an extention to the existing carriage arm to allow the surgeon to bring the microscope into the operating field while the base and column remain well out of the field. The

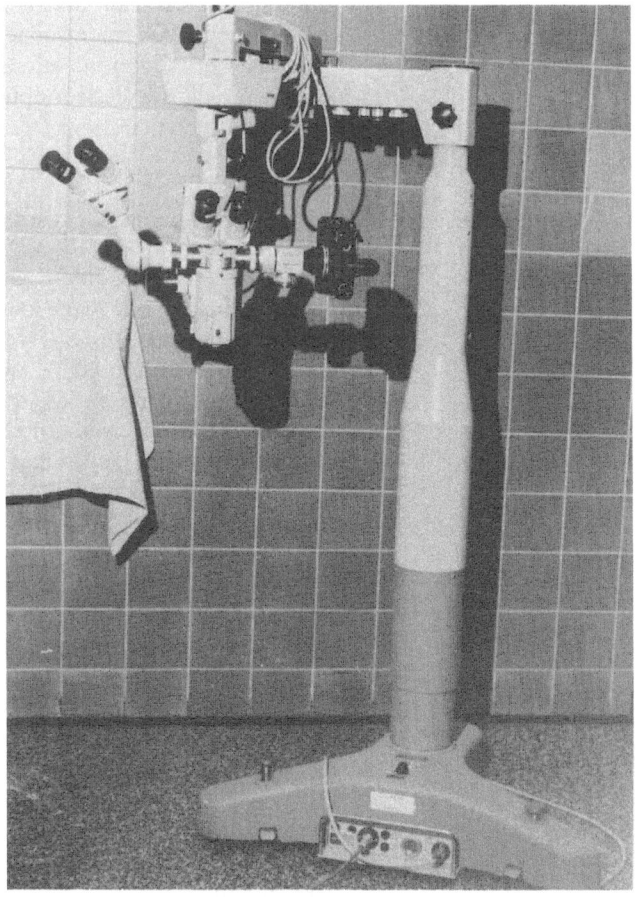

Figure 5. The motorized operating microscope, Zeiss Op Mi-6. Note the large base on the column.

microscope should have an objective with a 250- to 300-mm working distance. This provides sufficient distance between the microscope and operating field to allow manipulation of instruments without hitting the microscope. Ideally, the microscope should have a heavy-duty floor stand. As the extention arm brings the microscope further from its stand, the whole structure becomes less stable and potentially more apt to tip. A heavy-duty stand compensates for the extended arm and anchors the entire structure. It is also helpful to have a motorized column with a foot pedal to allow the surgeon to adjust magnification or focus without removing his hands from the operative field. This also allows the surgeon to maintain concentration with less distraction. The author's surgical team uses a Zeiss Op Mi-1 (Fig. 4) basic, manually operated microscope and the Zeiss Op Mi-6 (Fig. 5) with all of the modifications described above. The Zeiss system provides excellent optics with the ability for future growth and modification.

INSTRUMENTS

Some surgeons suggest that Fallopian tubes and adhesions are best held by Pyrex® glass rods, whereas others believe that tissue should be handled by a well-moistened, gentle, gloved hand. After some brief experience with glass rods during animal surgery, we found no difference in tissue reaction compared to gentle, moist-gloved, digital manipulation. Furthermore, a glass rod shattered in an animal during surgery. In our hands, the use of glass rods appeared to offer no advantage and might entail risk to the human patient, and we have decided not to include them in our surgical protocol.

Two needle holders are suggested for use. The first is a Stangel-modified Barraquer microsurgical needle holder (Sklar Surgical Instrument Company, New York) (Fig. 6). It is 13 cm in length and used for standard microsurgical suturing. The needle holder is light in weight and can be held in a closed position with minimal pressure, conserving the surgeon's energy and minimizing fatigue and tremor. The needle holder tip tapers to a fine, slightly blunted point to allow easier handling of 9-0 and 10-0 suture and fine microsurgical needles. The fine tip and slight closing pressure minimize the chance of bending and breaking a microsurgical needle. Finally, the instrument surface has a dull

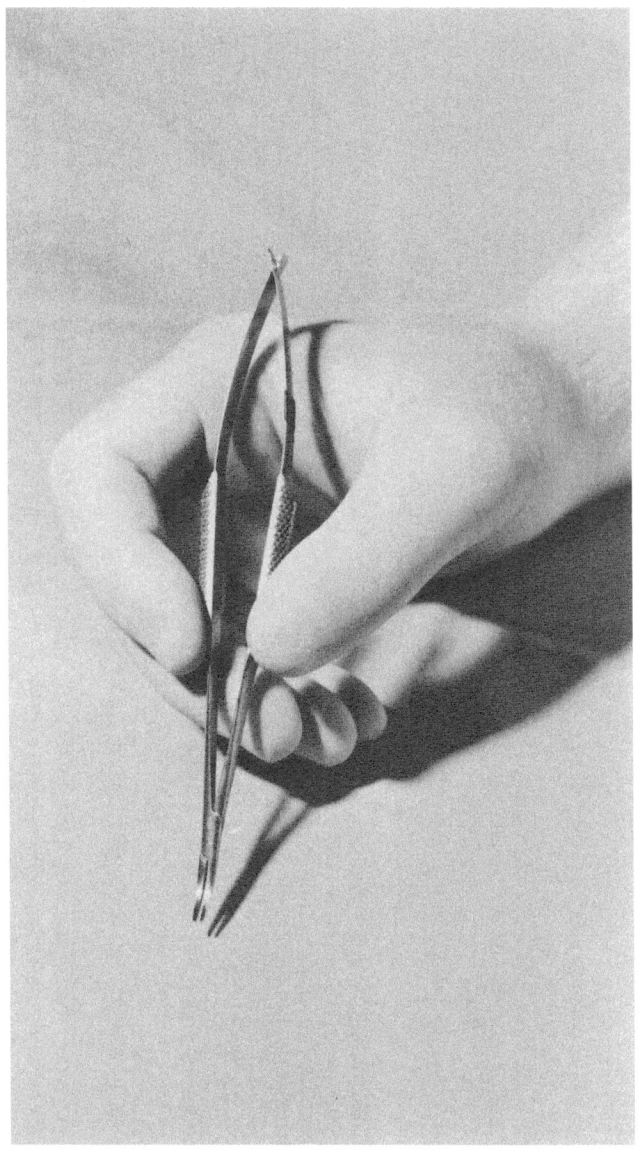

Figure 6. The Stangel-modified Barraquer microsurgical needle holder (Sklar Instrument Company). Note the proper hand and finger position for the utilization of this instrument.

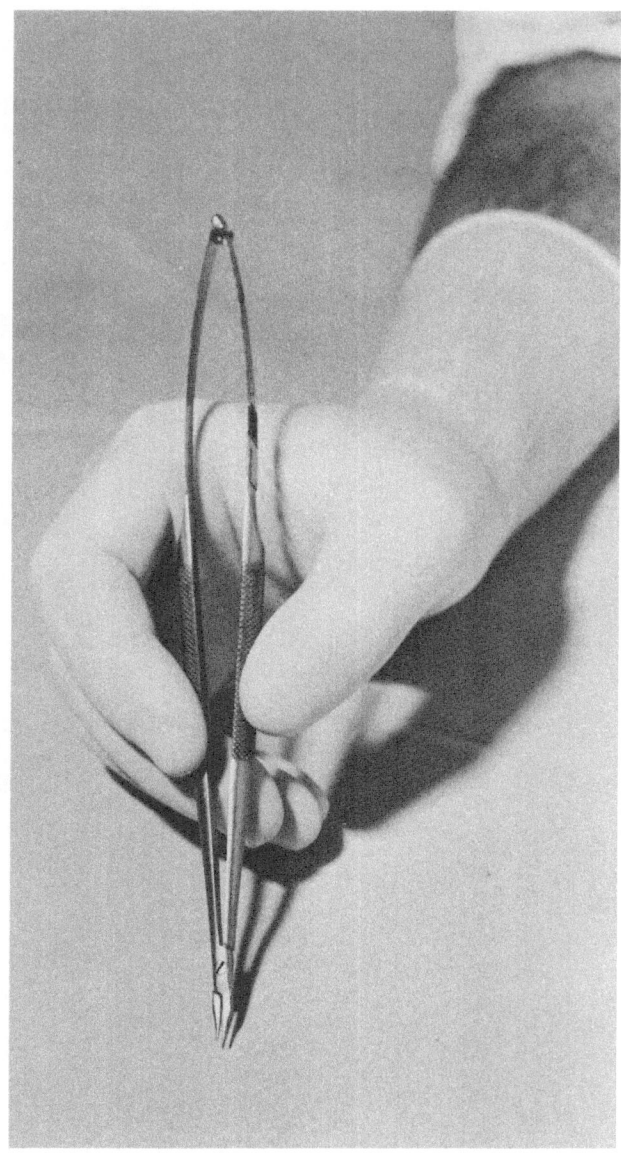

Figure 7. The long microscopic needle holder used for suturing tissue deeper in the pelvis.

rather than a shiny, polished finish. This prevents reflective glare under the light of the operating microscope, thereby diminishing eye fatigue. Suturing tissue deeper in the pelvis requires a similar but longer needle holder, Model 22-9506 (Moria of France and marketed in the United States by Cameron-Miller) (Fig. 7).

Both needle holders have neither locks nor catches. A lock secures the needle in place by holding the needle holder closed but may shake the instrument when released. The result can be small tear rather than a puncture at the point

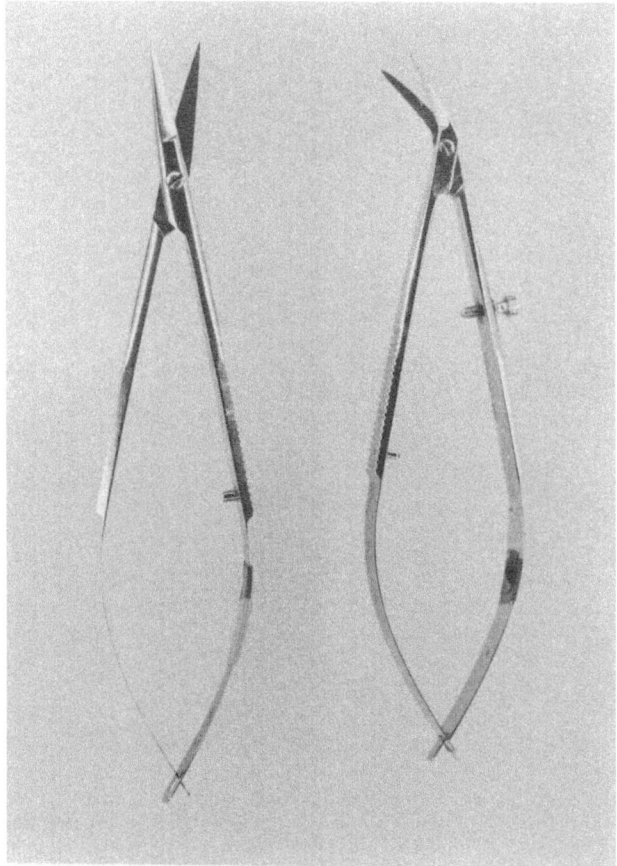

Figure 8. Straight and angled iris scissors.

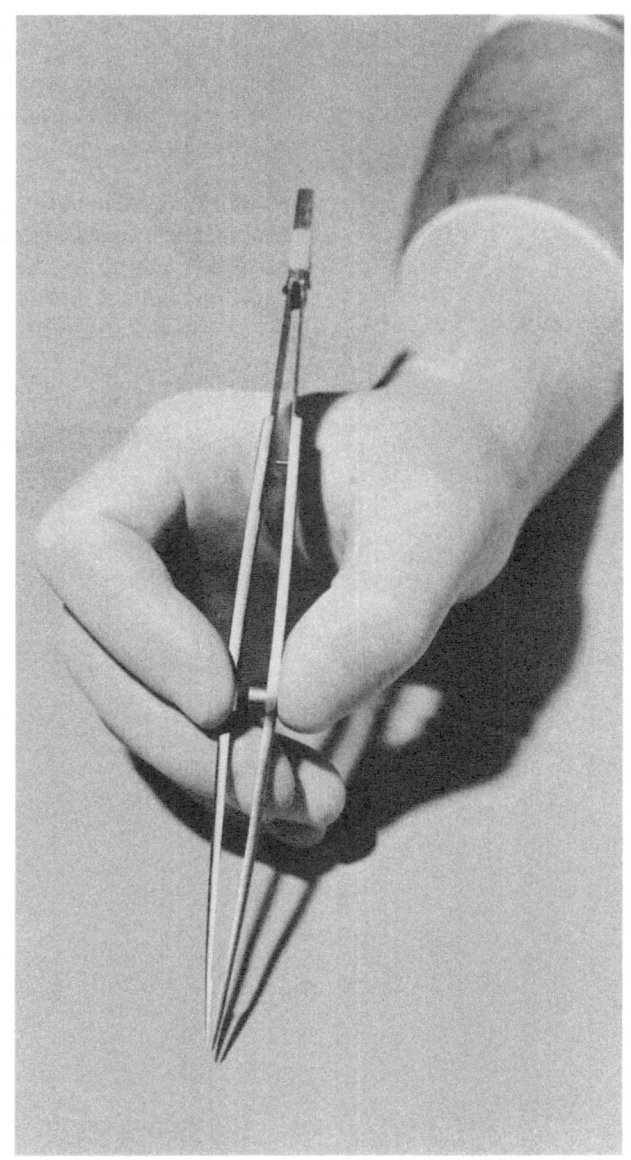

Figure 9. Long tying forceps.

the needle enters the tissue. A lock can actually give the surgeon less, rather than more, control.

Fine Westcott scissors are suggested to cut tissue and suture (Fig. 8). The small Westcotts can be reserved only for tissue, and the larger ones used to cut sutures. Cutting sutures tends to dull the cutting edge of scissors; therefore, the Westcott used for tissue should not be used to cut suture.

A long Moria tying forceps, Model 22-9503 (Moria of France, marketed in the United States by Cameron-Miller) (Fig. 9) may be used for both tissue handling and tying. A small straight and a small curved jeweler's forceps are also important. The jeweler's forceps are used for tissue handling and can be particularly helpful for grasping and dividing fine fimbrial adhesions under the microscope. When the forceps tip becomes damaged the instrument can be discarded and replaced rather than repaired.

Microsurgical tubal anastomosis is facilitated by the stabilization of the tubal segments on both sides of the func-

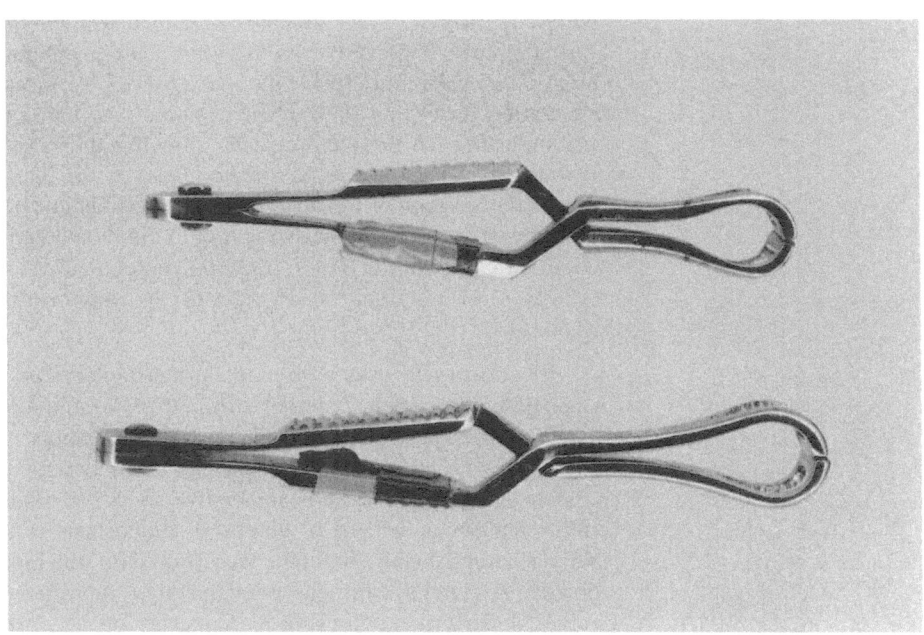

Figure 10. Fallopian tube stabilization miniclamps.

tion site. The Fallopian tube stabilization miniclamp (J. Sklar Manufacturing Company) is designed to stabilize the tube without unnecessary trauma to tissue surfaces (Fig. 10). During end-to-end anastomosis, a miniclamp is placed on either side of the anastomosis site, and the suture approximation of the exposed side is accomplished. The miniclamps are then flipped over, exposing the posterior surface of the tube, and the remainder of the anastomosis is completed. The weight of the clamps stabilizes the tissue throughout the procedure. Similarly, during a salpingoneostomy, a miniclamp is placed just proximal to the terminal end of the hydrosalpinx. The end then can be directed up toward the microscope and stabilized by the miniclamp in that position during the dissection and suturing.

Retrograde Fallopian tube perfusion cannulae (J. Sklar Manufacturing Company) are also useful. These cannulae come in four sizes and are designed to demonstrate oviduct patency or to facilitate the location of tubal obstruction (Fig. 11). The cannula, connected to a syringe containing a concentrated dye solution, is inserted through the fimbria, and the dye is gently injected into the tubal lumen in a retrograde manner. The cannula is advanced while the surgeon continues to inject dye. In this way, a gentle column of fluid precedes the more rigid tube and separates the tissue in preparation for the passage of the cannula. The intact oviduct may then be transilluminated, allowing the point of obstruction to be located. In addition, use of the cannula permits the surgeon to evaluate the fimbrial folds under the operating microscope by allowing him to direct and control a fluid stream onto the fimbrial tissue, perpendicular to its surface, with minimal obstruction to the microsurgical field.

Electrosurgery uses both unipolar and bipolar current. A needle-point unipolar microelectrode is preferable for the dissection of scar tissue and opening of hydrosalpinx. The needle-point electrode can be connected to almost any unipolar coagulation unit. It is imperative to use a minimal cutting current with little or no spark. Hemostasis is optimally accomplished by bipolar coagulation with fine bipolar forceps. A jeweler's forceps with fine tips, modified and marketed fairly inexpensively by Concept, Inc., is usable with most bipolar units. The author uses units made by Codman and Valleylab.

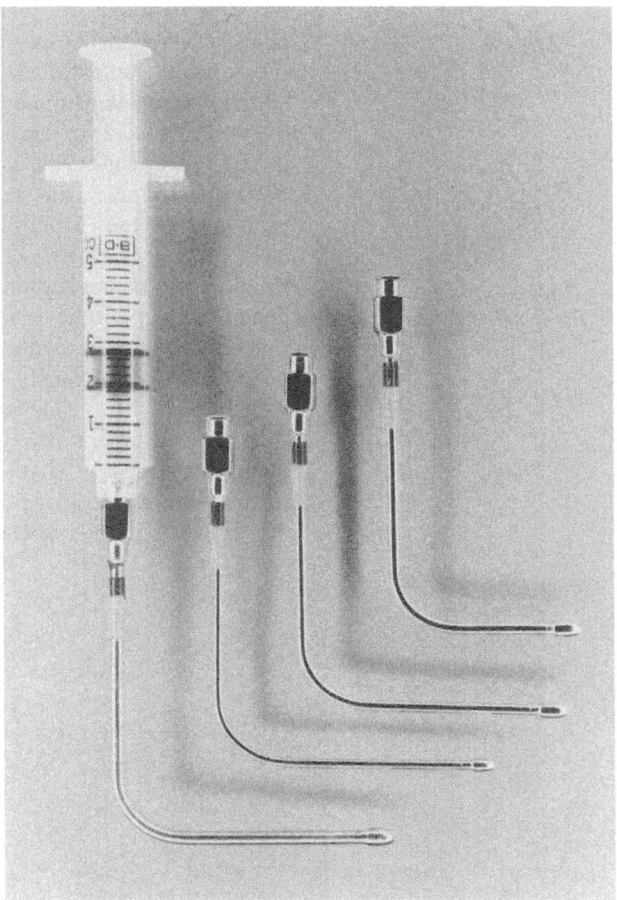

Figure 11. The four sizes of retrograde perfusion cannulae shown with perfusion syringe.

There is much discussion concerning the best materials for and the general structure of microsurgical instruments. Should they be made of stainless steel or titanium? Should the instruments be long or short? Titanium is a very hard, nonmagnetic, noncorrodable metal that is lighter in weight than stainless steel. Instruments made of stainless steel are said to be heavier in the surgeon's hand and become magnetic after many autoclavings. When an instrument becomes magnetic, a microneedle may adhere to a needle holder making it difficult to load and position the small needle, for it seems to move or "dance" about as the needle holder approaches. For this reason, the virtues of titanium instruments have been extolled. In fact, we have found steel to be superior instrument material. Titanium is the harder metal and more difficult to machine than steel. Therefore, if there are two identical needle holders, one made of titanium and the second of steel, the steel instrument will open and close with greater ease. Moreover, the slightly heavier weight of steel gives it a better feeling in the surgeon's hand. The problem of magnetization of the steel instruments can be dealt with by periodic demagnetizing with a degausser. This procedure rids the needle holder of its magnetic pull on a needle for several weeks.

An instrument box (Fig. 12) is as important as the instruments (Fig. 13) it contains. Keeping microsurgical instruments in one place helps insure their protection. The box should only be handled by members of the microsurgi-

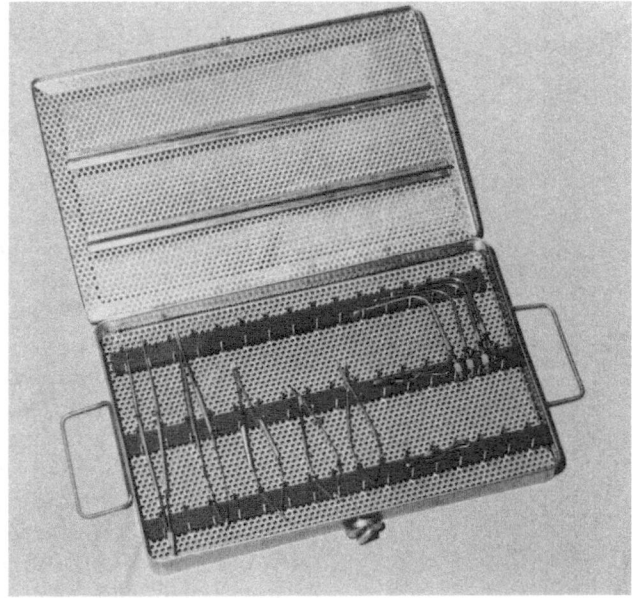

Figure 12. Instrument box for storage and autoclaving of microsurgical instruments.

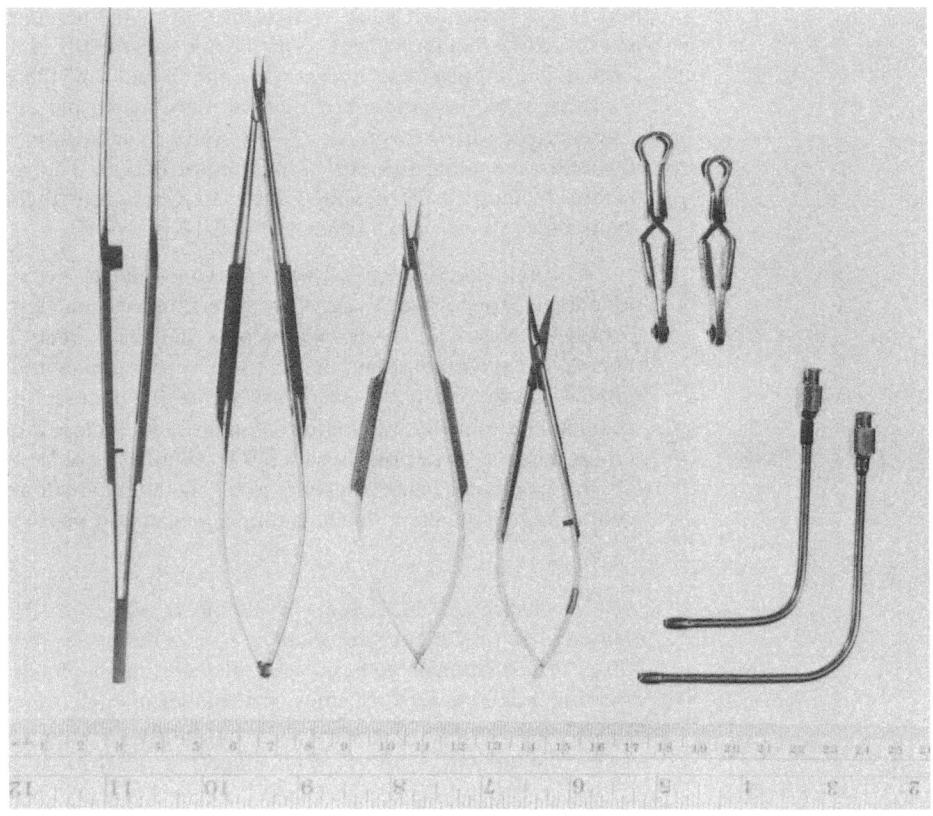

Figure 13. The basic instruments used for microsurgical tubal reconstruction. They are (left to right) tying forceps, long and short needle holders, iris scissors, tubal stabilization miniclamps, and perfusion cannulae.

cal team to avoid abuse of the fine-tipped delicate instruments. The box should protect the instruments during transport and autoclaving and still allow the circulation of air to minimize the amount of condensation to occur after autoclaving. Condensation encourages corrosion, even of stainless steel instruments. The author's surgical team uses an 8 in. × 12 in. sterilizing tray, Model Number 24-0812 (Linaire Instruments), and finds it satisfactory.

SUTURE Suture selection is one of the more important factors in microsurgery. The diameter, composition, and configuration of the suture material as well as the size, wire diameter, and the cross-sectional shape of the needle must all be considered. Suture produces a reaction in the tissue in which it is placed, and the amount of reaction depends in part on characteristics of the suture. An 8-0 suture is the largest diameter acceptable for most tubal reconstruction. The reduction in the degree of scar tissue does not appear to be significant as one goes to finer 9-0 and 10-0 sutures.

Chromic gut is very tissue reactive, whereas nylon, prolene, Dexon®, and Vicryl® produce minimal reaction. Current research in our laboratory indicates that a monofilament suture produces less tissue reaction than does braided suture. We use 8-0 Dexon® suture for microsurgical tubal anastomosis, salpingoneostomies, and the repair of serosal defects. Experiments with a 9-0 monofilament Dexon® are in process, and it appears to be an excellent suture with good tensile strength and minimal scar tissue production.

Microsurgical needles are available in varying wire diameters and different wire shapes. A wire diameter from 100 to 145 μm appears to be adequate for most human Fallopian tube microsurgery. Needles of a smaller diameter tend to bend, and needles of a larger diameter produce too much tissue trauma and scarring. We suggest a TE-100 or a TE-145 needle by Davis and Geck.

HOLDING OF INSTRUMENTS

Microsurgical instruments should be held in a manner that gives the surgeon the maximum control and ability to stabilize the instrument while preserving the greatest proprioceptive sense of the tip of the instrument. Ideally, the instrument should be held in such a way that it becomes a mechanical and sensory extension of the surgeon's hand.

The optimal instrument position is achieved by holding the instrument between the thumb and second and third fingers and leaning it against the webbed space of the hand as one would hold a pencil. The thumb and index finger have the greatest representation on the sensory cortex of the brain; thus, the "normal" writing position maintains a proprioceptive sense. The instrument is balanced between the three fingers and the hand and is therefore mechanically able while still capable of intricate three-dimensional movements.

POSITIONING OF TISSUE

After the instrument is positioned in the hand, the hand must be positioned relative to the incision to be closed. Suturing cannot be performed efficiently in all planes or axes. Most surgeons suture most efficiently by passing the needle toward themselves. Moreover, a right-handed person should pass the needle in an axis at 45° to his own body, starting with the needle entering the tissue at the upper right and leaving the tissue in the lower left. This may be illustrated by imagining the face of a clock lying in front of the surgeon; 12 o'clock is away from, and 6 o'clock is closest to the operator. A right-handed surgeon passes his needle most efficiently if it enters between 1 and 2 o'clock and exists between 7 and 8 o'clock. The axis of the incision to be closed should be from between 10 and 11 o'clock to between 4 and 5 o'clock. A left-handed surgeon simply reverses positions.

The surgeon should always attempt to suture in the axis previously described. The tissue should be gently moved, packed, and stabilized to attain this position. If the position is not right, the surgeon, the patient, or the tissue should be moved to achieve the proper relationship. As the surgeon gains more experience, the need to maintain ideal positioning decreases. Nevertheless, every surgeon has days when movements are perceived as clumsy and suturing does not go well. At these times, even the most experienced surgeon should check the basics by checking the position of the surgical instrument in the hand and the relative position of hand and body to the incision being sutured.

CONCLUDING THOUGHTS

One of the key factors in successful microsurgery is a comfortable interface of man and mechanical devices. The author has described techniques and instruments that work well for his surgical team. This is presented as a beginning—a starting point. Helpful suggestions may be selected and techniques modified as required. The basic principles discussed in the chapter, however, should be kept in mind when changes are being made. Arm and hand support and the minimum amount of muscle contraction in the arm and forearm must be maintained. Normal tissue must be protected, and the surgeon must cause as little trauma as possible.

5 Patient Selection and Preoperative Counseling

Niels H. Lauersen

Department of Obstetrics and Gynecology
Mount Sinai School of Medicine
New York, New York 10029

Prior to consideration of microsurgery for the treatment of infertility, the prospective patient should be thoroughly evaluated to determine that the cause of the infertility is indeed surgically correctable. The physician should also familiarize the patient with the expense and the extent of infertility evaluation required prior to surgery and thoroughly explain the chance of success attributable to the microsurgical procedure under consideration.

INTRODUCTION

The number of infertile couples has dramatically risen over the past decade. The postponement of parenthood until more mature years may contribute to the problem, but, with increasing frequency, this infertility can be corrected by modern surgical techniques.

A woman faces an increased possibility of acquired tubal damage with increased age because she simply has more opportunity to contract infection and develop peritubal adhesions. The use of an intrauterine contraceptive device may render a patient susceptible to one-sided salpingitis or other forms of uterine infection resulting in infertility. The sexual revolution has resulted in the spread of venereal disease with subsequent pelvic inflammatory disease, and much infertility may be a result of previous gonococcus infection. More than one million abortions are performed annually in the United States, and postabortion endometritis can lead to tubal-ovarian infection or abscess with resulting tubal damage. Infections from other sources such as pelvic tuberculosis can also be a causative factor in infertility.

Endometriosis, which affects approximately three million women in the United States, is frequently characterized as the "career woman's disease." The increase in the incidence of pelvic endometriosis is believed to be partly caused by the delay in childbearing. Endometriosis is frequently the cause of infertility in women when no other cause can be identified.

Women with a history of appendectomy, particularly when the surgery was precipitated by a ruptured appendix, often develop extensive pelvic adhesions that may cause infertility.

Male infertility susceptible to microsurgical correction could result from anatomic disorders of the external genitalia caused by congenital malformations, trauma, or previous surgical damage.

Finally, the number of voluntary surgical sterilizations of both men and women has risen dramatically over the past decade. The clinician is now frequently faced with the problem of reversing this induced infertility.

CANDIDATES FOR MICROSURGERY

Potential candidates for microsurgery include women with tubal problems such as peritubal or periovarian adhesions secondary to pelvic infection, previous abdominal surgery, or pelvic endometriosis. Microsurgery may be indicated in women with a history of previous ectopic pregnancy resulting in the removal of a portion of the Fallopian tube, congenital tubal abnormalities, or previous tubal sterilization. Severe pelvic adhesions may not obstruct Fallopian tube patency but still cause infertility, particularly if they are dense and interfere with tubal-ovarian mobility. Such adhesions may be corrected by microsurgery (Fig. 1).

Microsurgery may correct infertility in males resulting from damage or trauma to the vas deferens or congenital

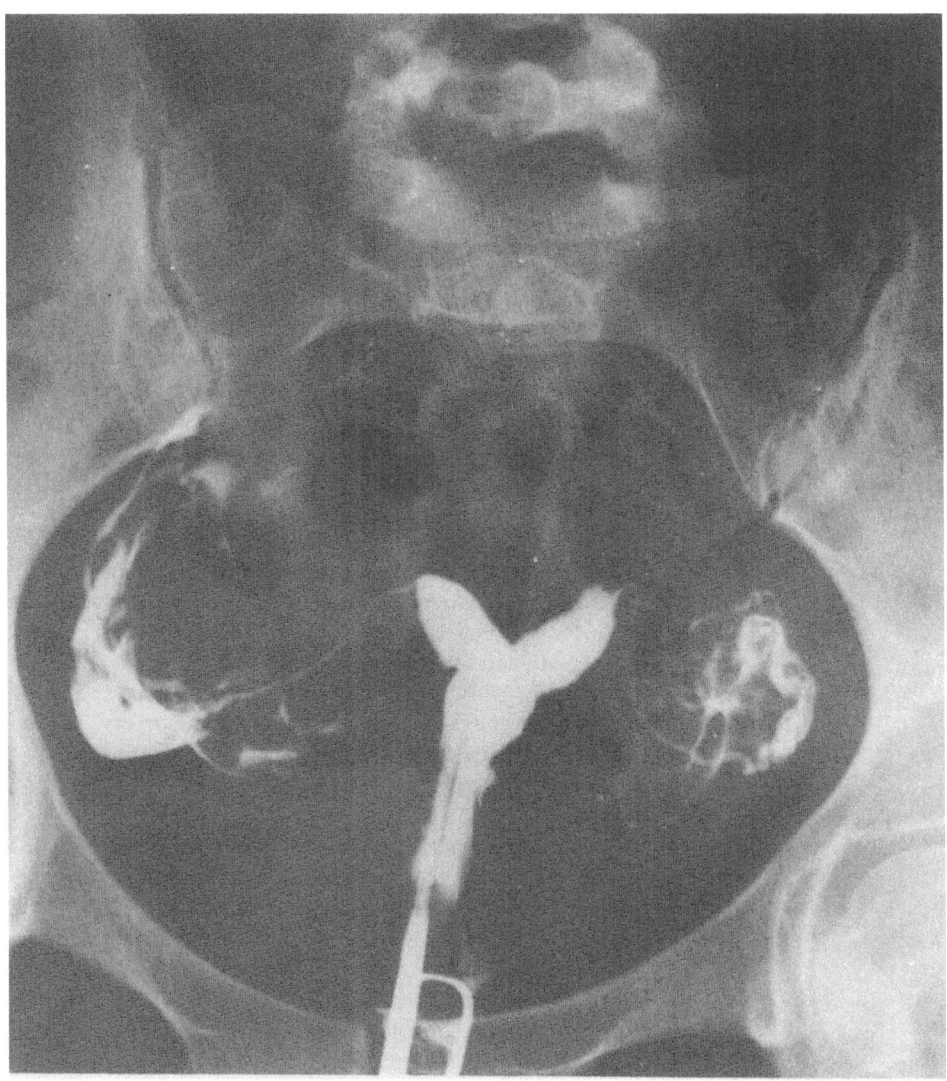

Figure 1. A hysterosalpingogram that reveals a uterine septum and normal Fallopian tubes but suggests bilateral peritubal adhesions. The probability of success of salpingolysis in this patient can be best assessed by a laparoscopy, but if the fimbriae and the ovaries are normal, the chance of successful pregnancy could be 80%.

abnormalities. Surgery may be required in patients in whom infertility is caused by varicocele or undescended testes.

Demand for reversal of previous surgical sterilization is on the increase, and microsurgery is particularly efficacious in this area. The time lapse between original sterilization and the demand for reversal reportedly ranges from 1 week to 16 years.[1] The two chief reasons for the reversal request are a change in marital status resulting in a new marriage partner or the loss of a child.[1]

Men and women with infertility caused by one of the abovementioned pathophysiologies may be potential candidates for microsurgery and should be referred for consultation with an infertility specialist fully trained in microsurgical techniques. The probability of reversing infertility resulting from these problems can be greatly enhanced by utilizing these advanced and sensitive techniques.

PATIENT COUNSELING

The preliminary consultation for consideration of a microsurgical corrective procedure should allow sufficient time for detailed explanation, and this initial interview is best conducted in the presence of both the patient and his or her spouse. During this interview, the physician should determine the couple's motivations for microsurgery, particularly in a request for sterilization reversal. The couple's degree of commitment should be assessed.

The patient should bring all previous medical records to this first visit. This is particularly important in a female patient who has undergone a tubal sterilization. The physician must determine the exact sterilization technique to assess accurately the chance of successful reversal. Tubal sterilization carried out in the midportion of the Fallopian tube offers a reasonable chance of reversal. Similarly, patients sterilized by the Pomeroy method, the single-burn technique, or the Fallop ring may also have a good prognosis for reversal. However, a subtotal salpingectomy or a fimbriectomy with excision of the long distal segment of the tubes offers minimal reversal potential.[1]

A male candidate for microsurgical reversal of sterilization should also supply all relevant medical records, particularly the semen analyses obtained prior to previous vasectomy.

The complete picture of the previous surgery is not usually available from the operative report, and it is important that the patient supply all available previous reports and X rays during the initial interview. The goal of the first interview is to provide a clear picture of the nature and the extent of infertility that forms the basis of the judgment as to the appropriate corrective microsurgery. The female patient must also be informed that she will need genetic counseling and amniocentesis if she should conceive after the age of 35.

During the initial interview, the infertile couple should be informed as to the extent of the additional infertility work-up necessary to rule out concurrent infertility problems. The couple should understand the surgery involved, the possibility of success, and the amount of money and time required for repeated visits and preoperative work-up. The physician must then determine if the couple remains sufficiently motivated to proceed with the surgery (Fig. 2).

The prospect of an extensive fertility work-up coupled with a discouraging chance of complete success may dissuade many patients from the further pursuit of microsurgery. Gomel[1] estimated that approximately 25% of the couples seeking reversal of female surgical sterilization decided to forego microsurgery after the initial interview had provided a more realistic understanding of the necessary preoperative examination and the procedure itself. Couples with living children or older couples may reassess the expense and reevaluate its worth for them. Patients automatically will be excluded when it is determined that their previous sterilization procedure does not permit a successful reversal. Gomel[1] found that approximately another 20% of patients were excluded from microsurgical tubal sterilization reversal because of the presence of other absolute factors of infertility or social or psychological problems discovered during the period from the initial interview to the planned surgery.

Forty to 50% of infertility patients initially interviewed as potential candidates for microsurgery may be finally dis-

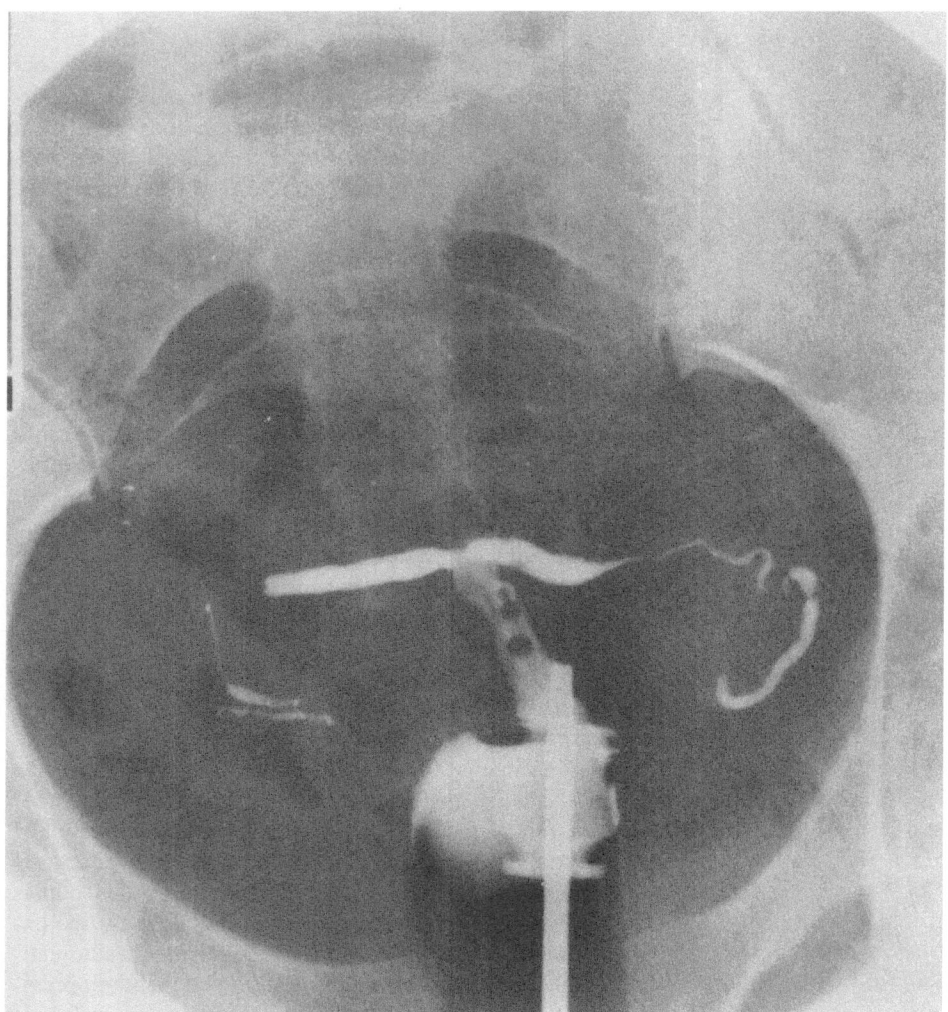

Figure 2. A hysterosalpingogram that shows a bicornuate uterus with occluded Fallopian tubes bilaterally. A laparoscopy would be indicated to evaluate the extent of the damage to the fimbriae and the ovaries. A salpingoneostomy would be the corrective microsurgery indicated with an estimated success rate of about 20%. The chances of success in this patient might even be lower because of the severely birconuate uterus. This should be discussed honestly with the patient.

qualified because of either lack of motivation or other causes of infertility.[1] Every surgeon should be aware of this realistic figure and should not pressure those patients who are not strongly motivated toward surgery which can involve both emotional and financial burdens.

CHANCE OF SUCCESS

Success in the surgical treatment of infertility should be strictly judged by its ultimate outcome, namely, the term delivery of an infant. A number of factors significantly affect this success rate, and one of the major factors is the surgical technique employed. The difficulties involved in a direct comparison of the success rates of microsurgery and macrosurgery for infertility must be acknowledged. Discrepancies exist in the reported number of cases and the time period when surgery was performed, and, importantly, there are differences in patient selection. An important difference is the type of infertility surgery attempted (Table I). The reported success rate for macrosurgery, however, forms an information base against which the success of microsurgery can be judged. Microsurgery in women for all of the types of infertility surgery categorized by the American Fertility Society gives the patient almost twice the chance for successful term pregnancy as macrosurgery (Table II).

The reports of microsurgical techniques employed for salpingolysis, fimbrioplasty, cornual implantation, and

Table I
Comparison of Effectiveness of Macro- and Microsurgical Techniques

	Macro				Micro			
Procedure	No. of cases	Patients pregnant	Patients with tubal pregnancies	Patients to term	No. of cases	Patients pregnant	Patients with tubal pregnancies	Patients to term
Implantation	1037	329	10 of 273	163 of 625	13	1	1	0
Anastomosis	308	125	15 of 138	66 of 233	262	167	5	157
Salpingostomy	653	167	22 of 522	39 of 215	112	44	14	29
Fimbrioplasty	225	42	11 of 198	19	9	6	1	5
Salpingolysis	412	205	17	173	6	3	1	2
Combinations	38	8	2	5	15	6	2	4
Totals	2673	876 (33%)	77 of 1581 (5%)	465 of 1748 (27%)	417	227 (54%)	24 (6%)	197 (47%)

Table II
Classification of Surgical Techniques[a]

I. Implantation
  A. Isthmus
  B. Ampulla
II. Anastomosis
  A. Intramural (interstitial)
    1. Isthmus
    2. Ampulla
  B. Isthmus
    1. Isthmus
    2. Ampulla
  C. Ampulla
    1. Ampulla
III. Salpingoneostomy (salpingostomy)
  A. Terminal
  B. Midampulla (medial)
  C. Isthmus (including linear salpingoneostomy)

IV. Fimbrioplasty
  A. Deagglutination and/or dilation
  B. Incision of peritoneal ring
  C. Incision of tubal wall
V. Lysis of adhesions (classified according to adnexa with mildest adhesions)
  A. Mild (less than 1 cm of tube or ovary involved in band or strings)
  B. Moderate (partially surrounded tube or ovary)
  C. Severe (encapsulating peritubal or periovarian adhesions)
IV. Combinations
  A. Different operations on right or left tubes
  B. Multiple operations on same tube (i.e., implantation and anastomosis)

[a] *Ad Hoc* Committee of the Ninth World Congress of Fertility and Sterility, April 12–16, 1977, Miami Beach, Fla.[19]

combination operations are very scant, totaling only 43 cases from two different surgical teams.[2,3] In contrast, there were more than 1700 cases of macrosurgery reported for these techniques from numerous investigators over a period of 30 years.

Salpingolysis (Table III) performed by macrosurgical techniques has afforded a fairly good success rate of 42% term pregnancies.[2,4−10] This success rate, coupled with the fact that in certain cases of pelvic adhesions the use of optical magnification technique might not offer any real advantage, has limited the application of the new technique. On the other hand, in cases of peritubal or fimbrial adhesions, microsurgery might yield a greater chance of success than gross surgery.

Damage to the fimbriated end of the Fallopian tube is very difficult to correct surgically. The mean reported success rate for gross fimbrioplasty is only 8%[2,9−16]; the highest reported success rate is that of Moore-White in 1960[13] of ten term pregnancies in 30 patients (Table IV). *Fimbrioplasty* may be considered a fertile new field for the expansion of microsurgery. Siegler and Kontopoulos[2] reported a success rate of four term pregnancies in 11 patients with mac-

Table III
Comparison of the Effectiveness of Macro- and Microsurgical Techniques in Salpingolysis

	Macro				Micro			
Reference	No. of cases	Pregnancy	Tubal	Term	No. of cases	Pregnancy	Tubal	Term
Martius[4]	138	68	7	57				
Arronet et al.[5]	46	21	1	20				
Young et al.[6]	47	18	2	15				
Spangler et al.[7]	101	52	0	47				
Horne et al.[8]	33	20	2	14				
Umezaki[9]	24	14	2	11				
Siegler and Kontopoulos[2]	15	6	3	3	6	3	1	2
Spadoni[10]	8	6	0	6				
Total	412	205 (50%)	17 (4%)	173 (42%)	6	3 (50%)	1 (17%)	2 (33%)

rosurgery, but this success was improved to five term pregnancies in nine patients when the fimbrioplasty was performed by microsurgical techniques (Fig. 3).

Cornual implantation has been widely reported as infertility surgery, achieving a success rate of approximately

Table IV
Comparison of the Effectiveness of Macro- and Microsurgical Techniques in Fimbrioplasty

	Macro				Micro			
Reference	No. of cases	Pregnancy	Tubal	Term	No. of cases	Pregnancy	Tubal	Term
Ingersoll[11]	18	0	0	0				
Palmer[12]	44	2	2	0				
Moore-White[13]	38	15	1	10				
Hanton et al.[14]	32	6	1	1				
Crane and Woodruff[15]	34	8	2	2				
Siegler[16]	27	2		2				
Umezaki[9]	18	4	3	1				
Siegler and Kontopoulos[2]	11	4	2	2	9	6	1	5
Spadoni[10]	3	1	0	1				
Total	225	42 (19%)	11 of 198 (6%)	19 (8%)	9	6 (67%)	1 (11%)	5 (56%)

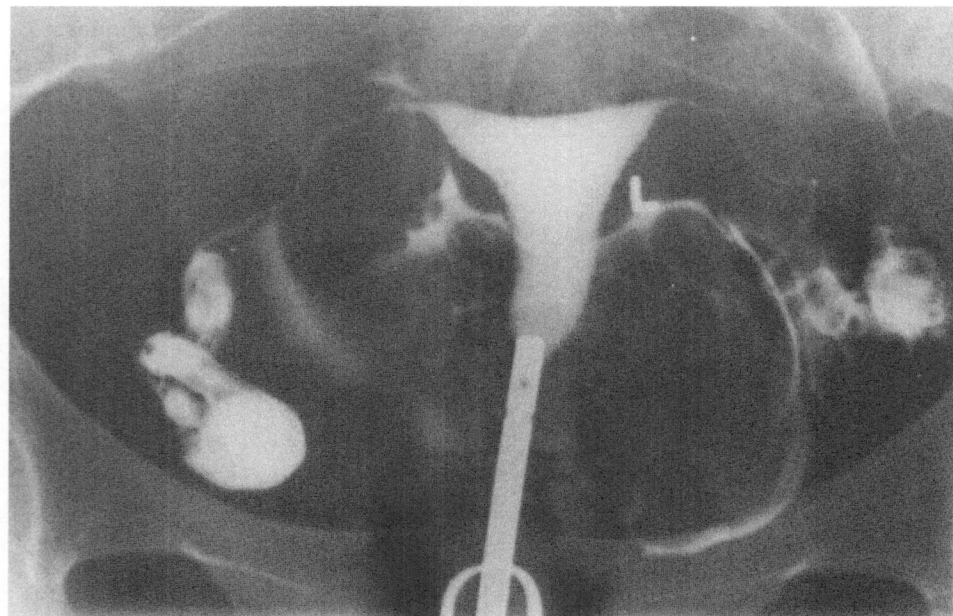

Figure 3. This hysterosalpingogram shows a normal uterine cavity, a patent left Fallopian tube with peritubal adhesions, and a right tubal occlusion with hydrosalpinx. This patient might not be a candidate for microsurgery since the right Fallopian tube is patent. However, if the patient remains infertile after the hysterosalpingogram, a laparoscopy would be indicated to determine the degree and extent of damage. Salpingolysis in association with salpingoneostomy might be indicated.

one term pregnancy for every four patients with macro-technique (Table V).[2,9,10,17–24] There are only 13 cases of cornual implantation using microsurgery reported by Siegler and Kontopoulos,[2] and Silber and Cohen[3] and no reported term pregnancies. The reason for so few reported cases may lie in the fact that cornual implantation is, by nature, a gross surgical technique.[17] In contrast, microsurgery offers the greatest advantages when there are workable proximal and distal segments of the tube extant.

Reports of combination procedures that involve different operations on different tubes or multiple operations on the same tube are scant for both macro-[2,10,19] and microsurgical[2] techniques (Table VI). Siegler and Kontopoulos[2] reported, however, that a success rate of 10% was

Table V
Comparison of the Effectiveness of Macro- and Microsurgical Techniques in Implantation

	Macro				Micro			
Reference	No. of cases	Pregnancy	Tubal	Term	No. of cases	Pregnancy	Tubal	Term
Vartan[17]	13	5	0	5				
Umezaki[9]	8	3	0	0				
Kistner and Patton[18]	646	204	N.R.	70 of 234				
Siegler and Perez[19]	124	23	2	16				
Palmer[20]	118	52	N.R.	45				
Peterson et al.[21]	16	8	0	8				
Wheeless[22]	10	1	0	1				
Diamond[23]	37	15	5	5				
Rock et al.[24]	52	15	2	11				
Siegler and Kontopoulos[2]	9	1	1	0	11	1	1	0
Silber and Cohen[3]					2	0	0	0
Spadoni[10]	4	2	0	2				
Total	1037	329 (32%)	10 of 273 (4%)	163 of 625 (26%)	13	1 (8%)	1 (8%)	0 (0%)

increased to 27% when they employed microsurgical rather than macrosurgical techniques in combination operations.

Salpingostomy (salpingoneostomy) is the surgical technique employed to deal with tubal occlusions, often the sequelae of pelvic inflammatory disease. Macrosurgical techniques have been reported since the 1940s and have achieved

Table VI
Comparison of Effectiveness of Macro- and Microsurgical Techniques in Cases Requiring Combinations of Treatment

	Macro				Micro			
Reference	No. of cases	Pregnancy	Tubal	Term	No. of cases	Pregnancy	Tubal	Term
Siegler and Perez[19]	23	3	0	2				
Siegler and Kontopoulos[2]	10	3	2	1	15	6	2	4
Spadoni[10]	5	2	0	2				
Total	38	8 (21%)	2 (5%)	5 (13%)	15	6 (40%)	2 (13%)	4 (27%)

varying success rates; the mean is 18%, 39 reported term pregnancies in 215 patients (Table VII).[2,6,8-10,25-35] Microsurgery has improved this success rate to 26%, but this still may be considered a fairly low chance for successful pregnancy. The prospect of success depends on the degree of tubal damage that the surgery seeks to correct, and often, such damage is severe and extensive.[36] Novy[35] has the largest reported series with salpingostomy performed through microsurgery and achieved 12 term pregnancies in 50 patients; the reported results for the three remaining microsurgical teams attempting this technique were similar and fairly consistent[2,32,34] (Fig. 4).

Tubal anastomosis, where there is at least part of the distal and proximal tubes extant, has received the most at-

Table VII
Comparison of Effectiveness of Macro- and Microsurgical Techniques in Salpingostomy

Reference	Macro				Micro			
	No. of cases	Pregnancy	Tubal	Term	No. of cases	Pregnancy	Tubal	Term
Mulligan[25] (1949–1954)	21	3		2				
Mulligan[25] (1955–1959)	45	16		9				
Buxton and Mastroianni[26]								
No splint	31	4	2	2				
Hoods	9	3	1	2				
Garcia[27]	25	10	2	7				
Crane and Woodruff[28]	17	3	1	1				
O'Brien et al.[29]	57	14	1	N.R.				
Young et al.[6]								
No splint	24	9	2	6				
Hoods	18	3	0	3				
Grant[30]	103	16	3	N.R.				
Grant[30]	53	22	0	N.R.				
Lamb et al.[31]	37	4		N.R.				
Horne et al.[8]	52	20	2	N.R.				
Umezaki[9]	18	1		N.R.				
Swolin[32]					33	15	6	9
Cognat and Rochet[33]	118	28	5	N.R.				
Gomel[34]					50	18	5	12
Novy[35]					6	2	0	2
Siegler and Kontopoulos[2]	15	5	3	2	23	9	3	6
Spadoni[10]	10	6		5				
Total	653	167 (26%)	22 of 522 (4%)	39 of 215 (18%)	112	44 (39%)	14 (12%)	29 (26%)

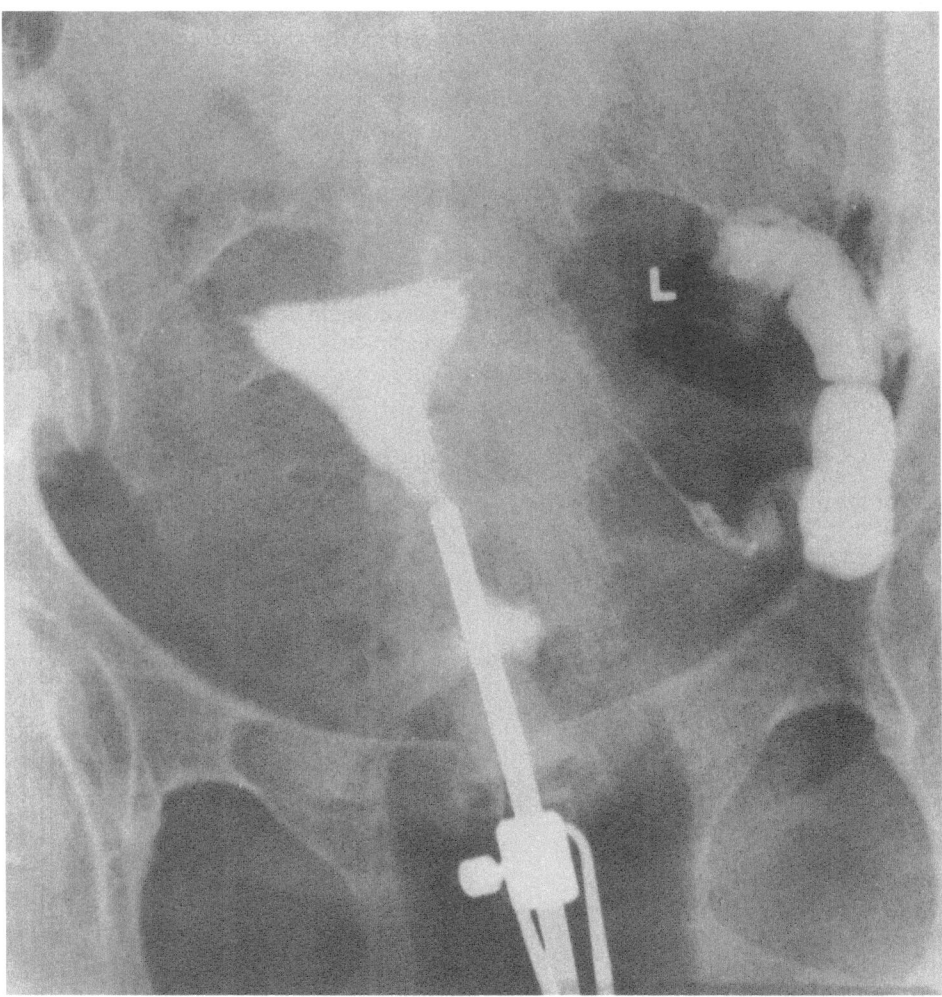

Figure 4. A hysterosalpingogram in which the uterine cavity appears normal; the right Fallopian tube is not visualized; the left Fallopian tube is visualized with evidence of severe hydrosalpinx and tubal occlusion. The probability of surgical success cannot be estimated in this patient without laparoscopy. If the right fimbriae and ovary are normal, microsurgery would not be indicated. If the right tube is also damaged, the chance of surgical success will depend on the degree of damage to the endosalpinx. The chance of successful microsurgery is minimal in this patient.

tention from the microsurgeons. This technique is utilized to repair congenital and acquired tubal defects and to reverse voluntary tubal sterilization. The reported number of cases of tubal anastomosis involving microsurgical technique, 262,[1-3,23,37-39] approaches the number reported for macrosurgical technique, 308,[2,9,14-16,19,26,27,31,40-45] and permits a degree of statistical analysis (Table VIII). Although the rates of pregnancy are not statistically different, the incidences of tubal pregnancy, 11% for macrosurgery versus 2% for microsurgery, and the success rates in term pregnancies, 28% for macro versus 60% for micro, are significant differences. The availability of microsurgical techniques offers the appropriate candidate more than twice the chance of achieving term pregnancy while cutting her risk of an ectopic pregnancy by 80%.

Table VIII
Comparison of the Effectiveness of Macro- and Microsurgical Technique in Anastomosis

Reference	Macro				Micro			
	No. of cases	Pregnancy	Tubal	Term	No. of cases	Pregnancy	Tubal	Term
Helman[40]	3	1		1				
Buxton and Mastroianni[26]	1	1		1				
Hanton et al.[14]	2	1		0				
Timonen and Nieminen[41]	68	26		12				
Garcia[27]	53	13						
Crane and Woodruff[15]	6	2						
Siegler[16]	7	4		3				
Lamb and Moscovitz[31]	8	2		2				
Garcia[42]	16	8						
Williams[43]	5	0	0	0				
Umezaki et al.[9]	6	3		3				
Siegler and Perez[19]	46	18	1	14				
Hodari et al.[44]	14	7	3	3				
Owen and Pickett-Heaps[37]					10	6	0	6
Diamond[23]					28	21	0	18
Winston[38]					45	25	1	24
McCormick et al.[45]	53	34	8	25				
Siegler and Kontopoulos[2]	20	5	3	2	16	9	1	8
Vammen et al.[39]					20	14	1	11
Gomel[1]					118	77	1	76
Silber and Cohen[3]					25	15	1	14
Total	308	125 (41%)	15 of 138 (11%)	66 of 233 (28%)	262	167 (64%)	5 (2%)	157 (60%)

One important factor to be considered when choosing the appropriate female candidate for microsurgical tubal anastomosis is the length of the tubal segments. Gomel[46] demonstrated that there is an inverse relationship between the total length of the reconstructed tube and the time interval from surgery to pregnancy. Nine patients who became pregnant within the first postoperative cycle in Gomel's series had oviducts of 5.5 cm or longer. The length of the oviduct is related not only to *when* a patient may become pregnant but *whether* she may become pregnant. Silber and Cohen[3] reported that 100% of 11 patients with tubal length of 4 cm and beyond achieved intrauterine pregnancy. This dropped to 43% when the tube was 3–4 cm, and, when the tube was less than 3 cm long, there were no intrauterine pregnancies in a series of seven patients (Fig. 5).

To aid in the rational selection of the appropriate female candidate for microsurgery, Hoffman[47] offers the following classification of risks:

Class I: Acceptable risk

1. Patient otherwise displays adequate criteria for fertility without therapy.
2. Adequate mobility of oviducts with minimal tubal or periovarian adhesions.
3. Overall length of oviduct is at least 8 cm, with isthmus at least 2 cm in length.
4. Luminal disparity is not more than 3 : 2 in the anastomosed segments.

Class II: Moderate risk

1. All of the above are true, but there is only one reparable tube.
2. Where any one of the Class I factors is subliminal and must receive therapy (e.g., borderline semen, ovulation induced, dense adhesions lysed).
3. Age over 34.
4. Endometriosis, minimal or small leiomyomata.

Class III: Poor risk

1. Where any two of the Class I criteria are not satisfied.

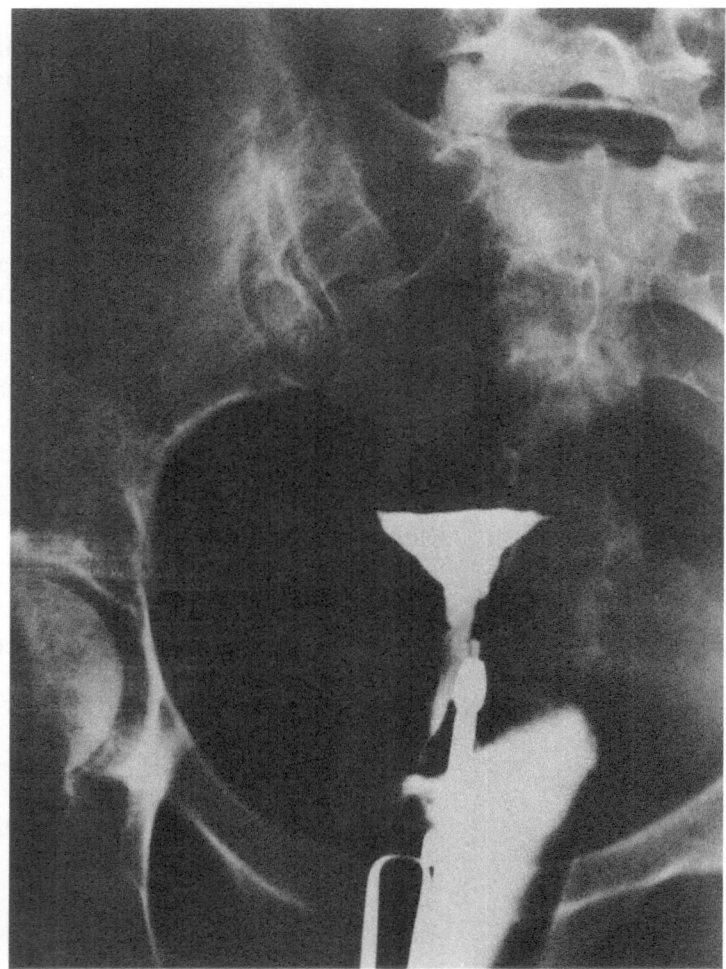

Figure 5. This hysterosalpingogram shows that the patient has previously undergone a bilateral tubal sterilization. Tubal length of more than 4 cm is required for optimal success of tubal reanastomosis. If the tubal length is less than 4 cm, tubocornual anastomosis could be attempted; however, tubal reimplantation might be the treatment of choice although this technique has a low success rate. Laparoscopy would be indicated to determine the condition of the distal segments of the Fallopian tubes and the ovaries.

2. Age over 37.
3. Large leiomyomata or extensive endometriosis.

Class IV: Unacceptable for statistical classification

1. Regardless of circumstances, where each tube is subjected to a different modality of treatment (e.g., fimbriolysis on one side and anastomosis on the other).

The application of microsurgical techniques to male fertility problems is a promising new area of medical exploration. Microsurgical techniques, as suggested by Silber,[48] include cryptorchidism and testicular autotransplantation, testicular homotransplantation, vascularized transplant of vas deferens and even penile reimplantation following trauma. Other techniques include vasoepididyostomy and creation of an artificial spermaconduit. At the present time, however, there are insufficient numbers of reported cases utilizing microsurgery in these procedures to permit a profitable analysis of the chances of success.

Table IX

Comparison of the Effectiveness of Macro- and Microsurgical Techniques in Vasovasostomy

	Macro			Micro		
Reference	No. of cases	Pregnancy	Spermatazoa postvasovasostomy	No. of cases	Pregnancy	Spermatazoa postvasovasostomy
Massey and Nation[49]	4	1	3			
Humphreys[50]	3	2	3			
Dorsey[51]	20	5	18			
Waller and Turner[52]	10	1	6			
Phadke and Phadke[53]	76	42	63			
Hanley[54]	35	10	27			
Derrick et al.[55]	1630	303	620			
Dorsey[56]	129	24	114			
Pardanani et al.[57]	50	11	31			
Gupta et al.[58]	50	N.R.	17			
Schmidt[59]	117	53	94			
Silber et al.[60]				36[a]	N.R.	31
Silber[61]				400	30 of 42	N.R.
Total	2124	452 of 2059 (22%)	996 of 2084 (48%)	400[a]	30 of 42 (71%)	31 of 36 (86%)

[a] The 36 patients are included in the later figure of 400.

The major field for reported microsurgery involves the reversal of vasectomy and vasovasotomy. There have been more than 2000 reported cases of attempted vasectomy reversal utilizing macrosurgery (Table IX). Gross surgical techniques resulted in postoperative spermatazoa in 48% of patients, but a pregnancy incidence, the stricter measure of success, in only 22%. Silber et al.,[60] employing microsurgical techniques, achieved spermatazoa in 86% of 36 patients.

In a separate report, Silber and Cohen[3] state that more than 400 patients have submitted to microsurgical vasectomy reversal. There was a pregnancy rate of 71% among the first 42 cases. This appears to be a significant improvement over the chances of success offered by macrosurgery. One fact that may also be considered when estimating the chances for successful reversal of vasectomy is the time interval from the original operation. The chances for success decrease with time, and there may be only a very poor chance after 10 years.

PREOPERATIVE INFERTILITY INVESTIGATION

The preoperative investigation should follow a definite plan and include a complete infertility work-up of both partners. The complete regime may require 4 to 6 months. The microsurgery candidate and his or her partner should, during this time, be seen in the office five to six times at approximately monthly intervals. The physician should utilize all information gleaned from previous medical records, X rays, and operative reports obtained during the initial interview. The purpose of the preoperative work-up is to detect any major infertility problem that exists apart from the reason for the microsurgery. These unrelated problems must be discovered and should be resolved, if possible, prior to the microsurgery. If complete resolution is not possible, its contribution to the patient's infertile status must be assessed. In certain instances, such as primary ovarian failure, plans for microsurgery must be abandoned. But in less severe cases, such as a subfertile sperm count in the male or pelvic endometriosis in the female, the influence of this additional problem must be taken into account when determining chances of success.

Preoperative Investigation in Men

The male patient, either as a candidate for microsurgery himself or as the partner of the candidate, must undergo a complete physical examination with special emphasis on the genitalia. An integral part of the male work-up is a semen analysis. A sperm count of 20 million per milliliter is the lower limit of fertility; in addition, there must be good progressive motility in at least 40% and normal morphology in at least 60% of the total sperm population.[61] If the sperm count reveals infertility or subfertility, the male patient should have thyroid function tests as well as determination of total gonadotropin excretion (FSH/LH). Abnormal results in these tests may indicate the need for a testicular biopsy.

When a male microsurgery candidate desires vasectomy reversal, it is important to determine his prevasectomy fertility. If a prevasectomy record of a sperm analysis is unavailable, the physician must learn if the candidate had fathered children. A low sperm count or fertility problems prior to the vasectomy will, of course, affect the patient's chance of fertility following reversal. The occurrence of any major disease such as mumps or exposure to hazards such as radiation that could adversely affect fertility during the intervening period since the vasectomy must be determined. The problem of any physically or psychologically induced impotence should also be detected, explored, and resolved prior to consideration of microsurgery for male infertility.

Preoperative Investigation in Women

The female patient, either as potential microsurgery candidate or partner of the candidate, must be interviewed for a detailed medical history. Information to be obtained includes age, marital history, menstrual history, and history of any previous abdominal surgery or infection that might indicate the presence of pelvic adhesions adversely affecting subsequent fertility. The patient's obstetrical history is of prime importance. If she has previously become pregnant and carried that pregnancy to term in the near past, this indicates a good chance of a normally functioning endocrine and reproductive system. If the obstetrical history, however, reveals a number of unsuccessful pregnancies that resulted in spontaneous abortion, missed abortion, intrauterine fetal demise, or premature labor, the possibility of genetic problems and congenital or acquired reproductive defects should be considered.

The physical examination naturally should assess general physical health with special attention to any indication .of endocrine problems and the presence of abnormal development of the genitalia. The physician should look for hirsuitism and obesity, and their presence might demonstrate the need for a more extensive endocrinology work-up including blood levels of estradiol, progesterone, testosterone, LH, and FSH, as well as thyroid function tests. The female patient should keep a monthly record of basal body temperature to provide evidence of ovulation. An endometrial biopsy is also only presumptive evidence of ovulation, but it may be required when other procedures have not provided sufficient information. It should be performed

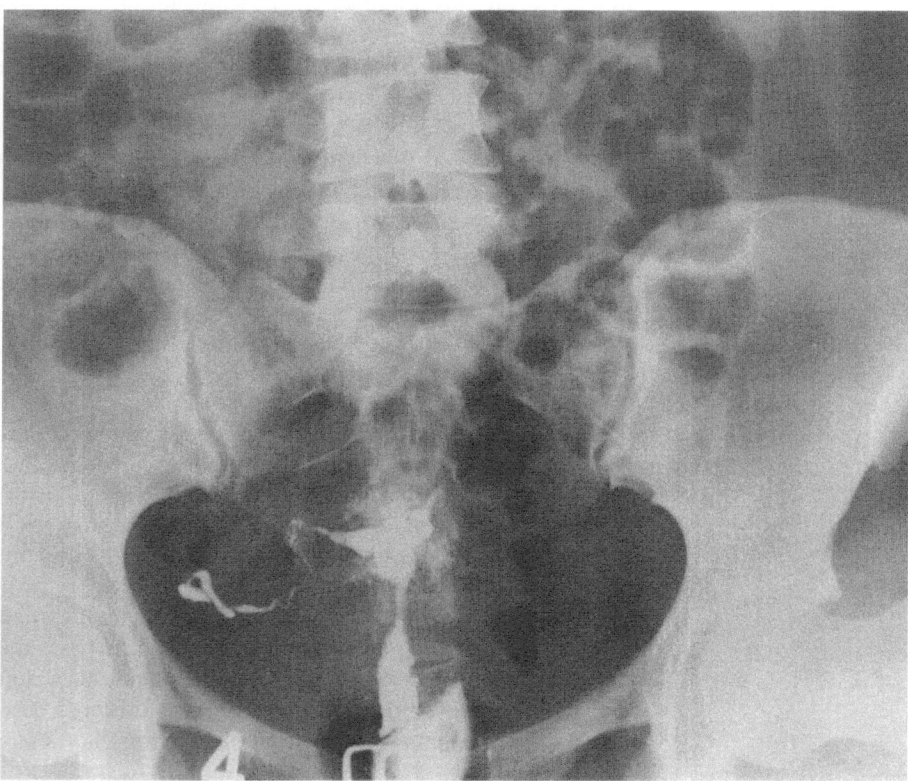

Figure 6. A hysterosalpingogram reveals the appearance of intravasation of the myometrium in combination with occluded right Fallopian tube; there also is no filling of the left tube. This condition will only offer minimal chance of surgical success. A laparoscopy would be indicated to evaluate the extent of damage to the left Fallopian tube and fimbriae. Lysis of uterine synechea could be performed via hysteroscopy, and a right salpingoneostomy might be successful since it appears that the damage of the endosalpinx is minimal on the right side.

under local anesthesia to minimize discomfort and on day 22, 23, or 28 of the cycle. A postcoital test might occasionally be indicated to rule out immunologic incompatability of the cervical mucus and semen.

A *hysterosalpingogram* must be performed when a female patient requests reversal of surgical sterilization and may be suggested in certain other instances such as history of pelvic inflammatory disease, pelvic adhesions, endometriosis, or previous ectopic pregnancy. The hysterosalpingogram is best carried out immediately after menstruation by the gynecologist himself with the use of a fluoroscope. It is required to evaluate the uterine cavity and the Fallopian

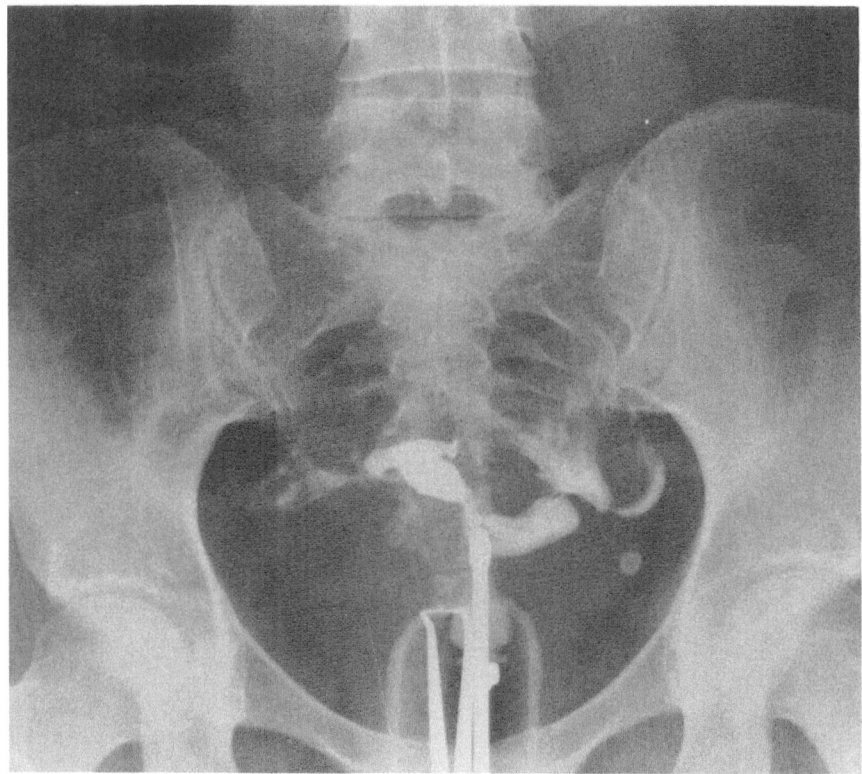

Figure 7. This hysterosalpingogram shows a typical hammerhead shark uterus; the Fallopian tube is not visualized on the right side. Left tube shows evidence of perifimbrial adhesions. The chance of successful surgical correction of this condition is minimal.

tubes (Figs. 6 and 7). It provides the most accurate information on the level of the sterilization procedure in case of previous tubal "ligation," and it gives an indication of the length and patency of the proximal Fallopian tubes (Fig. 5). This information is absolutely essential for an intelligent assessment of the chances of successful microsurgery.

Prior to microsurgery, a female patient should undergo a laparoscopy which provides a clear visualization of the pelvic organs and allows inspection of the distal portion of the Fallopian tubes and the ovaries (Fig. 8). A laparoscopy, furthermore, gives a clear picture of any pelvic pathology such as endometriosis, peritubal adhesions, or acute infections.

CONCLUSION   Any attempt to outline a procedure for the counseling of microsurgery candidates can only provide relevant data and define the broad boundaries of the problem. The patient and his or her partner must be approached by the physician

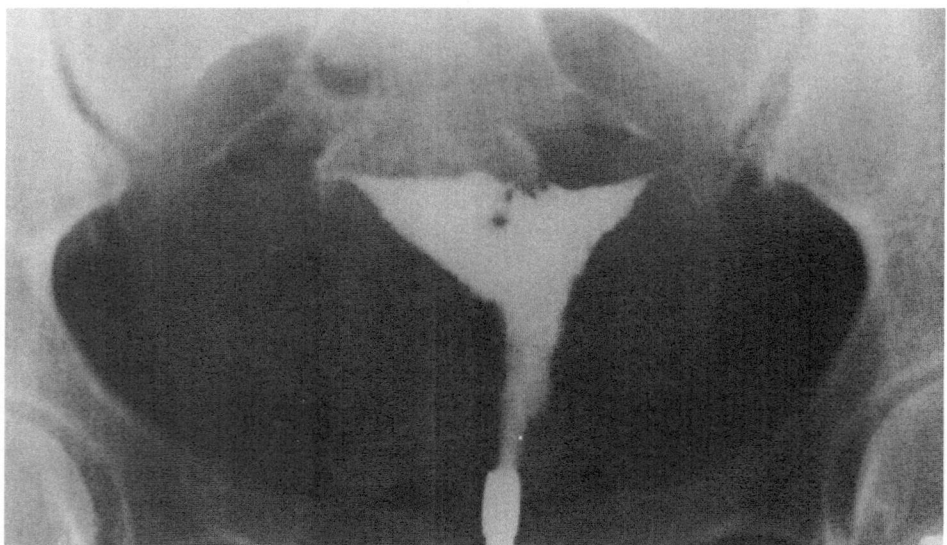

Figure 8. A hysterogram showing intrauterine synechea and visualization of proximal segments of Fallopian tubes. Hysteroscopy for diagnosis and correction of intrauterine defect should be combined with laparoscopy to assess the status of the tubes.

on an individual basis. The fertility problem will alter significantly from patient to patient with the numerous factors to be considered, increasing or diminishing the chance of surgical success in terms of full-term pregnancy. Although the patient has the final choice of pursuing or abandoning the proposed microsurgery, the physician has the responsibility of guiding the patient's decision with accurate information as to the chances of success in general and his own informed judgment as to this individual's particular chance of success. The benefits provided by microsurgery will accrue only when that surgery is desired by the patient and indicated by the patient's condition.

REFERENCES

1. Gomel V: Microsurgical reversal of female sterilization: A reappraisal. *Fertil Steril* 33:587, 1980.
2. Siegler AM, Kontopoulos V: An analysis of macrosurgical and microsurgical techniques in the management of the tuboperitoneal factor in infertility. *Fertil Steril* 32:377, 1979.
3. Silber SJ, Cohen R: Microsurgical reversal of female sterilization: The role of tubal length. *Fertil Steril* 33:598, 1980.
4. Martius H: Surgical techniques in the treatment of sterility in woman. *Int J Surg* 4:70, 1959.
5. Arronet GH, Eduljee SY, O'Brien JR: A nine-year survey of Fallopian tube dysfunction in human infertility: Diagnosis and therapy. *Fertil Steril* 20:903, 1969.
6. Young PE, Egan JE, Barlow JJ, et al: Reconstructive surgery for infertility at the Boston Hospital for Women. *Am J Obstet Gynecol* 108:1092, 1970.
7. Spangler DB, Jones GS, Jones NW: Infertility due to endometriosis. *Am J Obstet Gynecol* 109:850, 1971.
8. Horne HW, Clyman M, Debrovner C, et al: The prevention of postoperative pelvic adhesions following conservative operative treatment for human infertility. *Int J Fertil* 18:109, 1973.
9. Umezaki C, Katayama P, Jones HW Jr: Pregnancy rates after reconstructive surgery on the Fallopian tubes. *Obstet Gynecol* 43:418, 1974.
10. Spadoni LR: Tubal and peritubal surgery without magnification: An analysis. *Am J Obstet Gynecol* 137:189, 1980.
11. Ingersoll FM: Plastic operation on the Fallopian tube. *N Engl J Med* 241:686, 1949.
12. Palmer R: Salpingostomy: A critical study of 396 personal cases operated upon without polyethylene tubing. *Proc R Soc Med* 53:357, 1960.
13. Moore-White M: Evaluation of tubal plastic operations: Classification of tubal disease. *Int J Fertil* 5:237, 1960.
14. Hanton EM, Pratt JH, Banner EA: Tubal plastic surgery at the Mayo Clinic. *Am J Obstet Gynecol* 89:934, 1964.
15. Crane M, Woodruff D: Factors influencing the success of tuboplastic procedures. *Fertil Steril* 19:80, 1968.

16. Siegler AM: Salpingoplasty: Classification and report of 115 operations. *Obstet Gynecol* 34:339, 1969.

17. Vartan K: Tubal sterilization and its reversal. *Br Med J* 1:552, 1973.

18. Kistner RW, Patton GW Jr: *Atlas of Infertility Surgery*. Boston, Little, Brown 1975, p 132, 144.

19. Siegler AM, Perez RJ: Reconstruction of Fallopian tubes in previously sterilized patients. *Fertil Steril* 26:383, 1975.

20. Palmer R: Presented to the Ad Hoc Committee on Tubal Surgery. Thirty-Third Annual Meeting of The American Fertility Society, Miami, Fla., 1977.

21. Peterson EP, Musich JR, Behrman SJ: Uterotubal implantation and obstetric outcome after previous sterilization. *Am J Obstet Gynecol* 128:662, 1977.

22. Wheeless CR Jr: Problems with tubal reconstruction following laparoscopic sterilization using the electrocoagulation and resection technique. *Fertil Steril* 28:723, 1977.

23. Diamond E: A comparison of gross and microsurgical techniques for repair of cornual occlusion in infertility: A retrospective study, 1968–1978. *Fertil Steril* 32:370, 1979.

24. Rock JA, Katayama KP, Martin EJ, et al: Pregnancy outcome following uterotubal implantation: A comparison of the reamer and sharp cornual wedge excision techniques. *Fertil Steril* 31:634, 1979.

25. Mulligan WJ: Results of salpingostomy. *Int J Fertil* 11:424, 1966.

26. Buxton CL, Mastroianni L: Surgical treatment of infertility. *Obstet Gynecol* 20:844, 1962.

27. Garcia CR: Surgical reconstruction of the oviduct in the infertile patient, in Behrman SJ, Kistner RW, (eds): *Progress in Infertility*. Boston, Little, Brown, 1968.

28. Crane M, Woodruff D: Factors influencing the success of tuboplastic procedures. *Obstet Gynecol Surv* 24:458, 1969.

29. O'Brien JR, Arronet GH, Eduljee SY: Operative treatment of Fallopian tube pathology in human fertility. *Am J Obstet Gynecol* 103:520, 1969.

30. Grant A: Infertility surgery of the oviduct. *Fertil Steril* 22:496, 1971.

31. Lamb EJ, Moscovitz W: Tuboplasty for infertility. *Int J Fertil* 17:53, 1972.

32. Swolin K: Electromicrosurgery and salpingostomy: Long term results. *Am J Obstet Gynecol* 121:418, 1975.

33. Cognat M, Rochet Y: Notre experience de la salpingoplastie. *J Fr Gynaecol Obstet Biol Reprod* 6:839, 1977.

34. Gomel V: Salpingostomy by microsurgery. *Fertil Steril* 29:380, 1978.

35. Novy MJ: Tuboplasty after fimbriectomy, in Sciarra JJ, Zatuchni GI, Speidel JJ (eds): *Reversal of Sterilization*. New York, Harper & Row, 1978, p 143.

36. Gomel V, McComb P: Microsurgery in gynecology, in Silber SJ (ed): *Microsurgery*. Baltimore, Williams & Wilkins, 1979, p 162.

37. Owen ER, Pickett-Heaps AA: The microsurgical fallopian tube reconstruction. *Aust NZ J Surg* 47:300, 1977.

38. Winston RML: Tubal anastomosis for reversal of sterilization in 45 women, in Brosens I, Winston RML (eds): *Reversibility of Female Sterilization*. London, Academic Press, 1978, p 55.

39. Vammen AN, Gideon WP, Elkins JP: Reanastomosis of the previously ligated Fallopian tube. *Fertil Steril* 32:652, 1979.

40. Hellman LM: Tubal plastic operations. *J Obstet Gynaecol Br Commonw* 63:852, 1956.
41. Timonen S, Nieminen V: Tubal pregnancy: Choice of operative method of treatment. *Acta Obstet Gynaecol Scand* 46:327, 1967.
42. Garcia CR: Sixth Annual Postgraduate Course on Infertility Surgery. Presented at the 12th Annual Meeting of the American Fertility Society, San Francisco, April, 1973.
43. Williams GFJ: Fallopian tube surgery for reversal of sterilization. *Br Med J* 1:599, 1973.
44. Hodari AA, Vibhasiri S, Isaac AY: Reconstructive tubal surgery for midtubal obstruction. *Fertil Steril* 28:620, 1977.
45. McCormick WG, Torres J, McCanne LR: Tubal reanastomosis: An update. *Fertil Steril* 31:689, 1979.
46. Gomel V: Causes of failed reconstructive tubal microsurgery. *J Reprod Med* 24:239, 1980.
47. Hoffman JJ: Sterilization reversal: Assessment of demand and results, in Brosens I, Winston R (eds): *Reversibility of Female Sterilization.* London, Academic Press, 1978, p 161.
48. Silber SJ: Microsurgery of the male genitalia: Vascular, in Silber SJ (ed): *Microsurgery.* Baltimore, Williams & Wilkins, 1979, p 259.
49. Massey BD, Nation EF: Vas deferens anastomosis: A report of four consecutive successful cases. *J Urol* 61:391, 1949.
50. Humphreys RH: Vas deferens anastomosis: A review of the literature and a report of three consecutive successful cases. *West J Surg* 61:658, 1953.
51. Dorsey JW: Surgical correction of postvasectomy sterility. *J Int Coll Surg* 27:453, 1957.
52. Waller JI, Turner TA: Anastomosis of the vas after vasectomy. *J Urol* 88:409, 1962.
53. Phadke GM, Phadke AG: Experiences in the reanastomosis of the vas deferens. *J Urol* 97:888, 1967.
54. Hanley HG: Results of vasal anastomosis following voluntary vasectomy. *Br J Urol* 40:721, 1972.
55. Derrick FC, Yarbrough W, D'Agostino J: Vasovasostomy: Results of questionnaire of members of the american urological association. *J Urol* 110:556, 1973.
56. Dorsey JW: Surgical correction of postvasectomy sterility. *J Urol* 110:554, 1973.
57. Pardanani DS, Kothari ML, Parulkar GB, et al: Surgical reversal of vasectomy by vas anastomosis. *J Reprod Fertil* 41:321, 1974.
58. Gupta I, Dhawan S, Goel GD, et al: Low fertility rate in vasovasostomized males and its possible immunologic mechanism. *Int J Fertil* 20:183, 1975.
59. Schmidt SS: Vas anastomosis: A return to simplicity. *Br J Urol* 47:309, 1975.
60. Silber SJ, Galle J, Friend D: Microscopic vasovasostomy and spermatogenesis. *J Urol* 117:299, 1977.
61. Silber SJ: Microsurgery of the male genitalia: Non-vascular, in Silber SJ (ed): *Microsurgery.* Baltimore, Williams & Wilkins, 1979, p 332.

6

Endoscopy in the Evaluation of Infertile Patients

Martin S. Goldstein

Department of Obstetrics and Gynecology
Mount Sinai School of Medicine
New York, New York 10029

The introduction of microsurgery for infertility represents a significant improvement over the previously disappointing results of conventional surgical techniques. The greatest potential for success, however, is realized by a thorough patient evaluation prior to surgery. This evaluation establishes a rational basis for both patient selection and the estimation of probability of success in any single patient. Endoscopy is a most important part of this preoperative patient work-up and should not be bypassed prior to microsurgery. It permits the infertility surgeon to evaluate thoroughly the condition of the oviduct, the extent of pelvic adhesion, endometriosis, or any Müllerian duct malformations and to assess their surgical correctability.

The gross description of the uterus and tubes was first and most eloquently given by their discoverer, Gabriele Fallopius, in 1561:

> That slender and narrow seminal duct rises, fibrous and pale, from the horns of the uterus itself, becomes, when it has gone a little bit away, appreciably broader, and curls like a branch until it comes near the end, then losing the horn-like curl, and becomes very broad, has a distinct extremity which appears fibrous and fleshy through its red color, and its end is torn and ragged, like the fringe of a

well-worn garment, and it has a wide orifice which lies always closed through the ends of the fringe falling together, and if these be carefully separated and opened out, they resemble the orifice of a brass trumpet.

This original description of the Fallopian tubes remains important to the microsurgeon of today. The gross visual evaluation of the ectosalpinx may provide an indication of the etiology of infertility when conditions such as peritubal adhesions and malformations are detected through endoscopy. Preoperative endoscopy provides information that can eliminate unnecessary laparotomies and futile reparative procedures and permits the tubal surgeon to discuss prognosis and scope of proposed tubal surgery with the patient. Endoscopy performed after infertility surgery can provide an objective evaluation of results and an opportunity to diagnose and lyse postoperative adhesions (Fig. 1).

The evaluation of the anatomic etiologies of infertility presently relies on the techniques of hysteroscopy, laparoscopy, and hysterosalpingography. These three diagnostic modes are complementary procedures for determining how deviations from the normal anatomy of the reproductive system correlate with infertility. The hysteroscope permits us to directly visualize the endometrial cavity and tubal ostia, whereas the laparoscope enables us to confirm the extent of peritubal adhesions, fimbrial pathology, endometriosis, and uterine anatomy including myomata, tubal patency, and ovarian abnormalities. Visual external inspection is not sufficient, and hysterosalpingographic findings must be included. The hysterosalpingogram pictures the endometrial cavity, defines patency, and is our only way to visualize the endosalpinx.

The ideal preoperative diagnostic evaluation would provide visualization of the Fallopian tube in its entirety and permit correlation of its anatomic features with its physiological role. At present, the majority of the endosalpinx cannot be visualized without physically invading the uterine musculature and tubal structure and altering the tube's physiology. The interstitial intramural portion of the tube, which lies within the musculature of the uterine cornua, is visible only at the tubal ostia by hysteroscope. This part of the tube may follow either a straight or convoluted

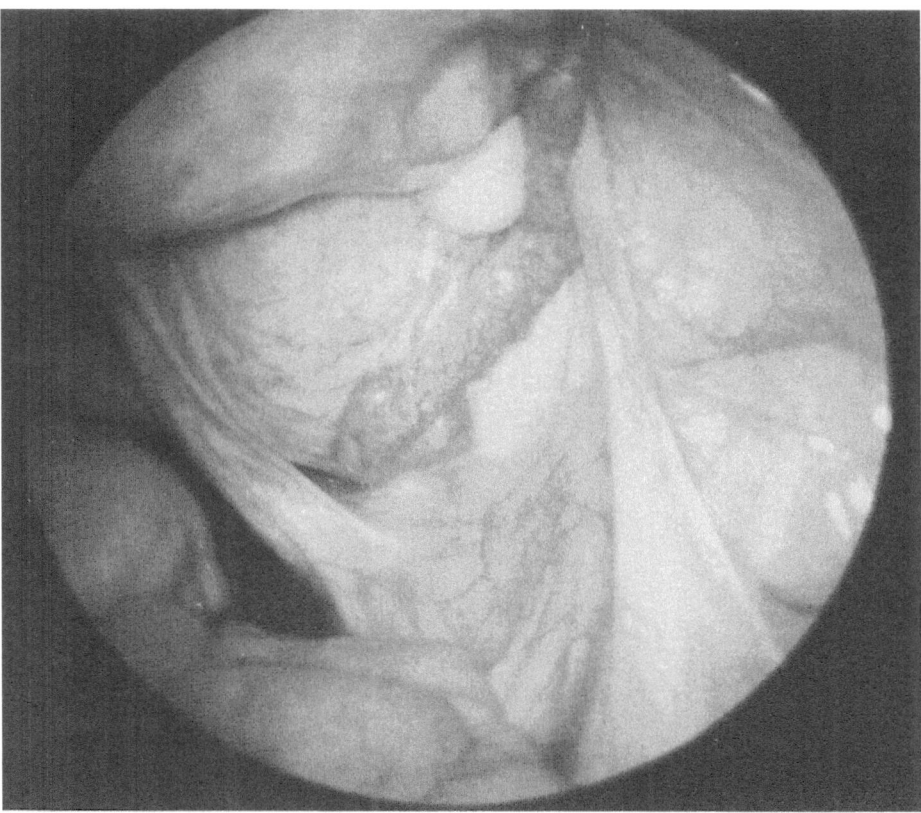

Figure 1. Second-look laparoscopy 1 year after salpingostomy. The uterus is seen superior to the right ovary and tube. Tubal patency is demonstrated, but fimbrial architecture is not preserved. Serosal vascularity is increased in the repaired portion of the tube.

route from the tubal ostia to the serosal surface of the uterus; it is 1–1.5 cm in length and approximately 200 μm in diameter. Muscular alterations, perhaps caused by myomata in the tubal or uterine muscle, may lead to tubal occlusion; the correctability of this occlusion may be impossible to assess preoperatively. The *isthmic* portion of the tube, beginning at the uterotubal junction and extending distally for 2–3 cm, contains an inner longitudinal, a middle circular, and an outer longitudinal muscle layer (Fig. 2). The lumen varies from 0.23 to 2 mm in diameter. The muscular development of the *isthmus* suggests that it may act as a

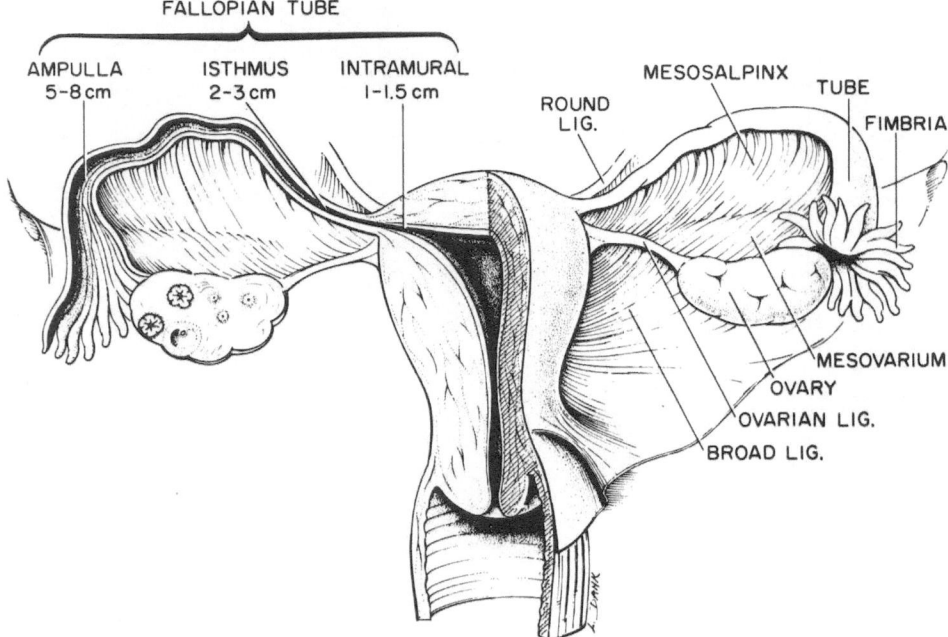

Figure 2. Normal uterotubal anatomy.

sphincter and could be a possible source of spasm leading to tubal occlusion, which may be revealed by hysterosalpingography. The *ampullary* portion of the tube is 5–8 cm long, with the lumen diameter increasing from 2 mm at its *isthmic* junction to 1 cm at its distal end, and terminating in the *fimbria*.[1] The endosalpinx can be visualized at the *fimbria* by laparoscopy. The laparoscope permits gross evaluation of the tubal serosa and the *fimbria*. It is inspection at the microscopic level, however, that could provide more meaningful correlation with tubal physiology.

The ability to predict accurately the success of subsequent tubal microsurgery requires extrapolation of the findings made in the visible portions of the Müllerian system to the tubal functions of sperm transport and capacitation, ovum pickup, ovum transport, fertilization, embryo transport, and zygote maintenance. Successful intrauterine pregnancy provides the most meaningful evaluation of these functions. Tubal patency and external oviduct appearance are, at present, the only available objective measures for evaluating tubal infertility factors which are responsible for 25–50% of all female infertility.[2,3] These determinations concentrate on assessment of tubal patency, the pressure necessary to demonstrate it, tubal length, functional relationship between tube and ovary, peritubal adhesions, and their vascularity and thickness. The techniques of this vital premicrosurgery assessment are laparoscopy, hysteroscopy, and hysterosalpingogram.

LAPAROSCOPY

Preoperative laparoscopy and microsurgical correction can be performed as either a single or a two-staged procedure. The choice depends on suspected pathology and physician/patient preference. Sterilization reversal may be planned in a single stage, although, occasionally, the preoperative laparoscopy will identify cases in which reversal is impossible, and the planned microsurgery must be cancelled. When tuboplasty is unrelated to prior sterilization, a two-staged laparoscopy repair procedure is preferable to provide a basis for determining the advisability of pursuing microsurgical correction and predicting the success of such correction. In salpingostomy for fimbrial occlusion, for example, where success rates are less than 50%,[4] the extent of scarring should be known and discussed with the patient and her husband prior to repair, possibly with the aid of laparoscopic photography or videotape.

Laparoscopy can be performed under either local or general anesthesia. Laparoscopes of from 5 to 10 mm can be utilized. The 6-mm sheath has a cross-sectional area of 28.26 mm^2 compared to 94.98 mm^2 of an 11-mm sheath.[5] The ease of performance that characterizes utilization of the smaller scopes makes them ideal for use with local anesthesia. Premedication of intravenous meperidine, 50 mg, and diazepam, 10 mg, in conjunction with infraumbilical field block with penetration of local anesthesia to the depth of the peritoneum provides adequate anesthesia for the procedure.

The abdomen should be distended with gas. If electrocoagulation is not contemplated, nitrous oxide can be used as the distending gas, for it is less irritating to the patient than carbon dioxide. The key to successful local laparoscopy lies in the careful avoidance of overdistension of the peritoneal cavity. In patients with no previous surgery, adequate pneumoperitoneum can usually be achieved with less than 2 liters of gas. In patients with prior surgery, 2–4 liters of gas should be employed to separate any preexistent adhesions. General anesthesia is preferable in these patients because of the increased degree of pneumoperitoneum required.

After the patient is placed in a lithotomy position and satisfactory local or general anesthesia is established, a vertical or transverse incision is made in the inferior pole of the umbilicus. A Veres needle is introduced while the anterior abdominal wall is manually lifted. The needle is inserted by a rapid thrust perpendicular to the anterior abdominal wall and parallel to the patient's spine. In obese patients or in patients with previous abdominal surgery, a pneumoperitoneum can be created by placing an insufflating needle transvaginally in the cul-de-sac. After creation of a pneumoperitoneum, the laparoscopic trocar is positioned with the same technique as the Veres needle. In patients with previous abdominal surgery, the risk of penetrating adhesions and bowel can be minimized by placing a 14-gauge needlescope through the umbilical incision to assess the status of peritoneal adhesions prior to the placement of the 5- or 10-mm laparoscope. This technique directs placement of the laparoscope to areas free of adhesions.

A probe must always be introduced for accurate tubal measurements, probing of tubal ostia, palpation of the tube, measurement of the fimbria ovarica, and assessment of thickness and vascularity of adhesions as well as any biopsy or lysis of adhesions required during the operative laparoscopy. The 3-mm or 5-mm trocar is inserted at the upper crest of the montine hairline. Transillumination prior to placement will identify vascular areas. An incision is made with a scalpel, and the trocar is introduced. Trocar placement must be under direct laparoscopic vision. Once the trocar tip penetrates the peritoneum, the laparoscope can be used to exert intraabdominal upward pressure adjacent to the trocar to insure control and safety in the placement of the second trocar. When biopsy or laparoscopic lysis of adhesions is not contemplated, use of the 3-mm probe provides

LAPAROSCOPY – OPERATIVE DESCRIPTION

Date ______________________ Patient Age ______________
Clinical Diagnosis ______________________ First
____
Observer ______________________ Repeat

Uterus — Bladder

Right Broad Ligament — Bowel

Right Tube
Right
Right Ovary — Appendix

Left Broad Ligament — Others

Left Tube

Left Ovary — Photo

Cul de Sac — Cine

DIAGRAM

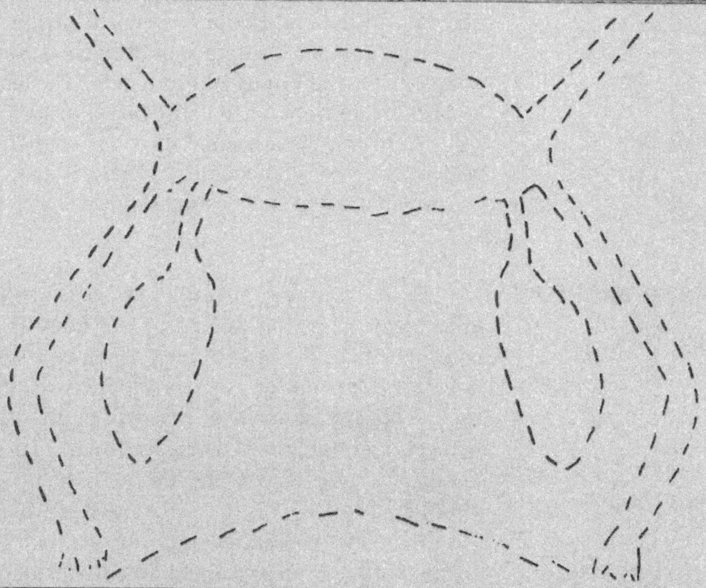

Diagnosis ______________________

Operative Procedure ______________________

Figure 3. Laparoscopic descriptive form as proposed by the American Association of Gynecological Laparoscopists.

easier introduction of the probe. Total security in laparoscoping patients with extensive prior surgery can be gained by visualizing the umbilical trocar site with a 5-mm scope inserted through the lower puncture site. This insures that inadvertent damage in the initial trocar placement has not occurred.

Chromopertubation with indigo carmine should be performed in conjunction with laparoscopic visualization to assess tubal patency and corroborate prior hysterosalpingographic findings. Laparoscopic findings should be described carefully and accurately in diagramatic form (Fig. 3). Photography provides an excellent method of documentation and is beneficial in subsequently describing procedures and chances of success to patients. Photography in conjunction with serial laparoscopy is the best method for monitoring the success of therapy for endometriosis. Successful photography can be performed with an automatic camera, such as the Olympus OM2, modified by replacing the focusing screen with an endoscopic screen to permit increased light for visualization. Camera mounting is accomplished by an adapter ring and 80- to 100-mm lens. The laparoscopic light source is sufficient when using fast film such as Kodak ASA 400. A 10-mm laparoscope provides superior photography. Videotaping of procedures provides the most accurate documentation of pelvic anatomy.

HYSTEROSCOPY   Hysteroscopy is a simpler and less traumatic technique than laparoscopy, as access to the body is provided by a natural orifice, the cervix, rather than by a surgical incision. A pelvic examination is performed to determine the uterine axis. The cervix is then grasped with a tenaculum, and paracervical block is performed with 10–20 ml of 1% lidocaine (Xylocaine®) The uterus is sounded, and the cervix dilated to Hegar 6 (6 mm). The hysteroscope, within its 7-mm sheath, is inserted into the cervix. The insufflating channel of the hysteroscope is filled with a liquid medium to prevent introduction of air bubbles that will interfere with the visualization of the uterus. An insufflating medium is needed to separate the walls of the uterus and permit visualization of the uterine cavity; 32% dextran (Hyscon®) with a molecular weight of 70,000 or 5% dextrose in water can be used. A pressure of less than 150 mm Hg is usually adequate to separate the walls of the uterus. Carbon dioxide can also be used as the dilating medium. In the CO_2 technique, a contracervical cap is applied to the cervix by negative pressure to effect a tight seal. With the CO_2 technique, gas flow must be less than 100 ml/min, and intrauterine pressure must be less than 200 mm Hg to prevent embolization.

The technique of hysteroscopic insertion is uncomplicated, but visualization of the endometrial cavity and the interpretation of findings require significant experience. The hysteroscope can be used to identify polyps, submucus myomata, synechiae, and cavitary irregularities. By visualizing the lateral uterine wall and following its direction superiorly, the cornual cone can be identified. After the cornua is located, the tubal ostia can be visualized. Flow of Hyscon® (dextran 32%) or injected indigo carmine can be identified entering the tubal ostia. Irregularities of the endometrial cavity in proximity to the tubal ostia can be identified. Cavity irregularities such as subseptate or bicornuate uterus can only be confirmed by simultaneous hysteroscopy–laparoscopy to define uterine shape as compared with the shape of the endometrial cavity. The hysteroscope can be used to lyse synechiae and cut the septum of a subseptate uterus. If septolysis is attempted, simultaneous laparoscopy must be performed to monitor the procedure safely.[6,7]

HYSTERO-SALPINGOGRAM

The hysterogram was introduced by Rubin and Carey[8] in 1914 as a test for tubal patency. Hysterosalpingography complements endoscopy in providing significant information prior to all tubal reparative procedures. The gynecologist and radiologist must work closely on both technique and interpretation. Salpingography is useful in determining tubal patency, locating tubal occlusions, and aiding in the diagnosis of congenital uterine malformations, intrauterine adhesions, myomata, polyps, and, at times, adenomyosis. In evaluating the anatomy of the Fallopian tube, the hysterosalpingogram can define hydrosalpinx, tubal diverticula, salpingitis, isthmica nodosa, isthmospasm, and kinks and tortuosity of the tubes. The value of hysterosalpingography in comparison to hysteroscopy and laparoscopy, has recently been questioned.[9-13] Each proce-

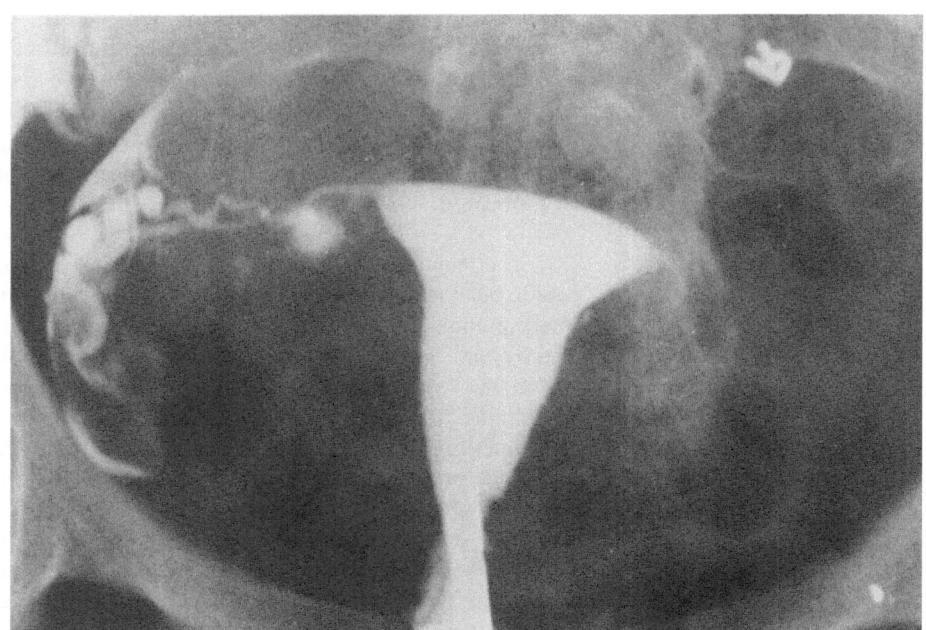

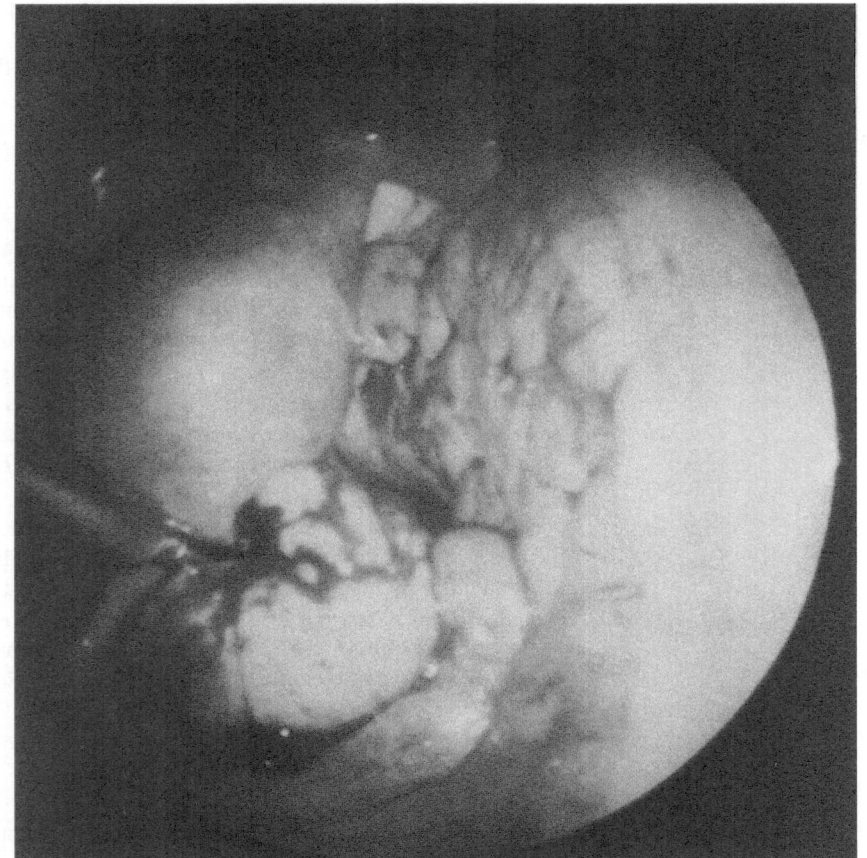

dure, however, has diagnostic advantages in specific areas, and no diagnostic mode should be bypassed if it might yield useful information (Fig. 4).

PREOPERATIVE ENDOSCOPIC EVALUATION BEFORE TUBAL REANASTOMOSIS

The operative report of the prior tubal sterilization must be evaluated. If bilateral fimbriectomy was performed, reanastomosis should not be attempted, and no further diagnostic studies are required. When sterilization was accomplished by another technique, microsurgical reversal may be possible, and evaluation should continue (see Chapter 5).

A hysterosalpingogram should be performed to examine the interstitial portion of the tube. This should ideally be scheduled at least 2 weeks prior to tubal surgery to minimize the risk of operating on a tube that contains any active inflammation.[14] The hysterogram in Fig. 5 demonstrates the right tube filling for a distance of 1.5 cm and the left tube filling for approximately 1.2 cm. This patient had previously undergone unipolar coagulation laparoscopic sterilization. Isthmic–ampullary reanastomosis was successful. If the hysterogram had revealed that the tube was occluded at the ostia, microsurgical reanastomosis would not be possible, and tubal reimplantation with a statistically poorer success rate would be the only alternative.

Laparoscopy must be performed prior to tubal reanastomoses to reveal the condition of the distal Fallopian tube and the fimbria (Fig. 6). The success rate for reanastomosis is poor if less than 3–4 cm of tube is present. A one-stage approach for tubal reanastomoses should be planned. If no contraindications to reanastomoses, such as tube length of less than 3.5 cm, absent or scarred fimbria, concomitant inflammatory disease, or cornual occlusion, exists, the surgeon may proceed with the repair immediately following the laparoscopy.[15–19] In this circumstance, the laparoscopy can

Figure 4. (Top) A hysterosalpingogram demonstrating tortuous left Fallopian tube with free spillage and peritubal adhesions. The uterine cavity is normal, and the right tube is occluded in the proximal isthmic portion. (Bottom) Laparoscopy of the same patient as in A, demonstrating endometriosis as the etiologic factor for tubal tortuosity and right-sided occlusion. Definitive diagnosis in this patient could only be made by laparoscopy.

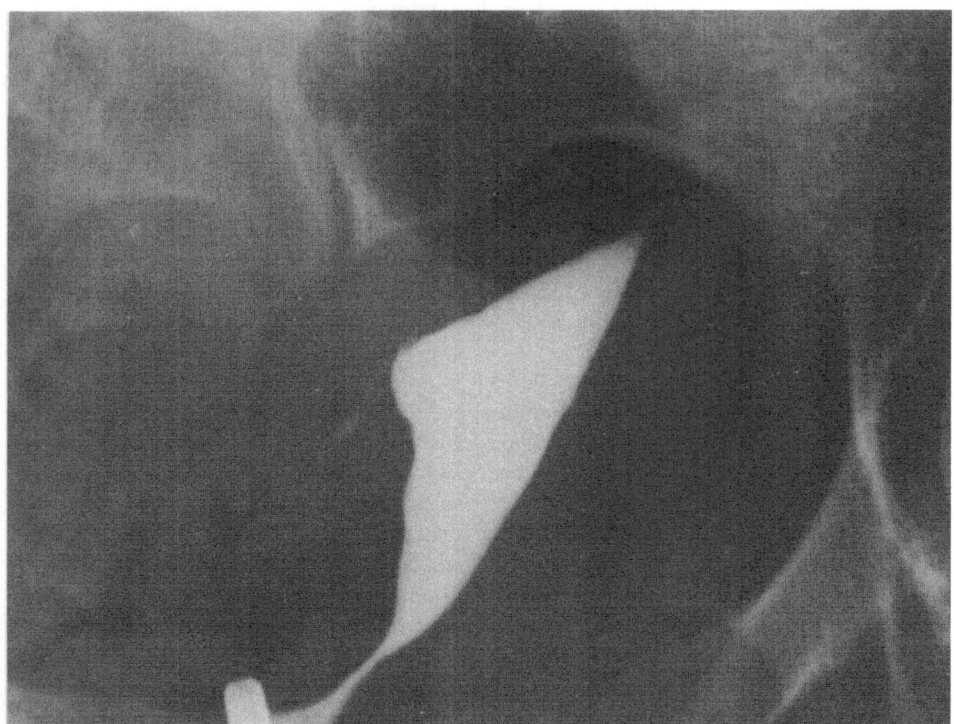

Figure 5. A hysterosalpingogram in a patient prior to tubal reanastomosis. Note the filling of the right tube to 1.5 cm and of the left to 1.2 cm. Subsequent isthmic–ampullary reanastomosis was successful.

be performed with the patient in the lithotomy position and without the use of a uterine elevator. A second puncture site with a 3-mm or 5-mm probe for uterotubal manipulation is necessary. This approach has the advantage of not manipulating the uterus vaginally, thus minimizing the chance of introducing vaginal organisms into the uterus and upper genital tract.

PREOPERATIVE ENDOSCOPIC EVALUATION IN TUBAL OCCLUSIVE DISEASE

Once proximal or midtubal occlusion has been diagnosed by a hysterosalpingogram, preoperative hysteroscopy should be performed to evaluate the tubal ostia and to detect the presence of synechiae and scarring within the cornual cone. Moreover, these adhesions may be lysed at this time.

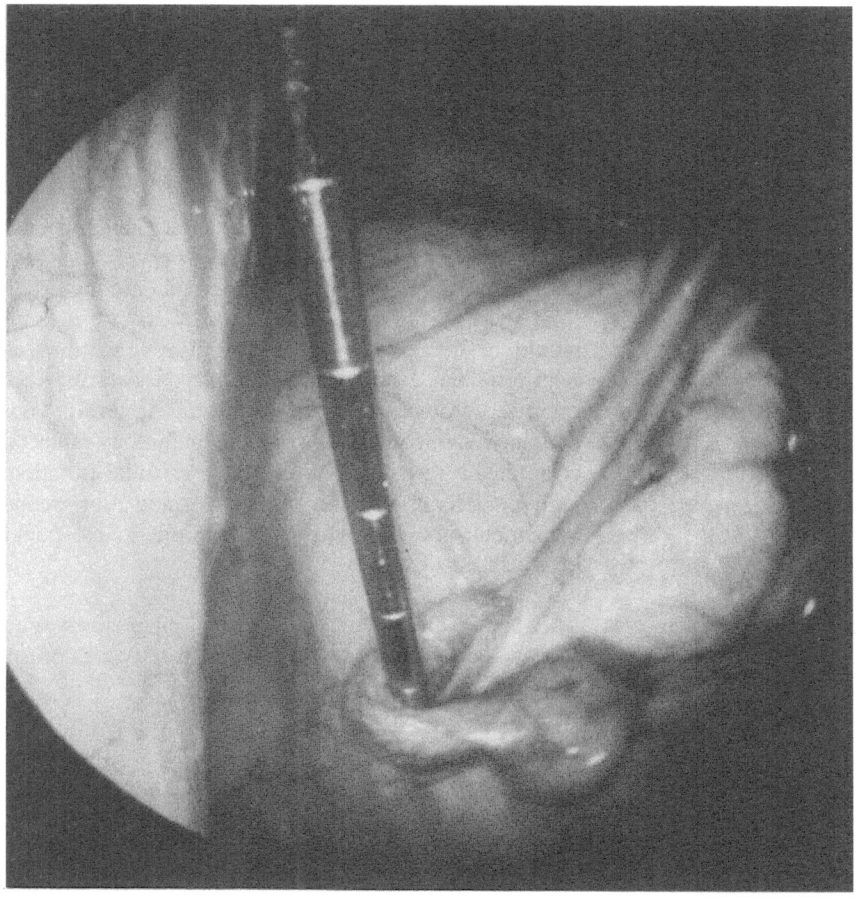

Figure 6. Laparoscopy in patient with previous postpartum Pomeroy tubal ligation. The distal segment of the tube is shown being lifted by a probe. The distal segment of the Fallopian tube is of adequate length for reanastomosis. Note the fibrosis present in the previously ligated segment of the Fallopian tube. Normal ovary is visualized in the lower portion of the illustration.

Proximal or Midtubal Occlusion

A free flow of Hyscon® into the tubal ostia would suggest tubal spasm as the cause of occlusion seen on hysterogram. This evaluation of the cornual cone should include careful inspection for the presence of any small submucus myoma.

Laparoscopy and chromopertubation must be performed to confirm the diagnosis of tubal occlusion made on hysterogram and to exclude tubal spasm as the causative factor. The laparoscopist then seeks the actual etiology of the occlusion; this may be endometriosis, myomata of the cornua or tube, inflammatory disease, salpingitis isthmica nodosa, or tubal neoplasia. Some of these factors, such as endometriosis or cornual myomata, may be treatable without tubal microsurgery.

In cases of proximal occlusion, laparoscopy must evaluate the distal tube and fimbria as well as other pelvic pathology. If the patient had experienced concurrent proximal and distal tubal disease, the success rate of tuboplasty would be decreased. Patency of the distal tubal segment with proximal obstruction could only be determined by retrograde chromopertubation from the fimbria. Tubal appearance and concomitant pelvic pathology must also be correlated to predict the true status of tubal function. Corrective microsurgery should be performed after preoperative presentation of the endoscopic findings to the patient and her husband (Table I).

Distal Tubal Occlusion   The results of microsurgical salpingostomy are worse than in any other type of reconstructive microsurgery.

Table I
Factors to Be Considered in Endoscopic Evaluation
of Tubal Occlusion

1. Extent of hydrosalpinx and extension to tubal ampulla.
2. Thickness and vascularity of adhesions.
3. Fimbrial appearance and possible biopsy to determine a ciliary index.
4. Other pelvic pathology including periovarian inflammatory disease.
5. Tubal serosal culture and possible culture of adhesions by biopsy.
6. Evaluation of concomitant endometriosis.
7. Possible disturbance in tubo-ovarian spatial relationship. Measurement of tubo-ovarian ligament and fimbria ovarica to define the proximity of fimbria and ovary.
8. Tubal length (measured) and tortuosity.
9. Hysteroscopy to exclude inflammation of the tubal ostia and cornual cone.
10. Possible use of prophylactic antibiotics.
11. Preoperative endoscopy performed by the same physician who will perform the definitive surgery.
12. In cases of unequal tubal disease, both tubes carefully evaluated and photographed to determine the applicability of the unilateral or the bilateral approach to correction.

Gomel reported a 30.5% intrauterine pregnancy rate and a 10% ectopic pregnancy rate in 72 patients.[20] Swolin reports a 97% patency rate but only 27% intrauterine pregnancy rate with 9% ectopic rate in a series of 33 patients.[21] When strict criteria for operability are defined and applied to distal occlusion, however, the rate of success should improve dramatically. Laparoscopy assists in the selection of suitable candidates for distal tubal reconstructive procedures. An intelligent evaluation of tubal pathology requires a search for specific abnormalities and their detailed description and illustration to replace the single, vague classification of distal fimbrial occlusion and associated hydrosalpinx. It is the function of preoperative endoscopy to identify and characterize these abnormalities.

Hydrosalpinx frequently begins as an endosalpingitis; therefore, the state of the endothelium is an important factor in postoperative success. Brosens and DeGraef[22] found a decrease in the number of ciliated cells in the fimbria of the Fallopian tube in pathological states. They correlated the ratio of ciliated to nonciliated cells, the ciliary index, with success in subsequent pregnancies. Microbiopsy to determine the ciliary index has been suggested as part of preoperative evaluation.[23] Gomel,[24] however, questioned the value of a single tubal microbiopsy because of the nonuniform appearance of the terminal end of the reconstructed hydrosalpinx.

Intratubal adhesions in the distal ampulla are a poor prognostic sign and frequently are associated with postoperative reocclusion or ectopic pregnancy. In a series by Gomel,[25] 60% of patients achieving pregnancy after salpingostomy did so after the first postoperative year, which suggests that a regeneration of endosalpinx and restoration of tubal function may be temporally related. The extent and vascularity of peritubal adhesions also correlate with reparative success; thick, more vascular adhesions are associated with poor prognosis. When hydrosalpinx extends to the ampulla with ampullary distension, a greater possibility for endosalpingeal damage exists.

Endometriosis as an etiologic factor or coexistent finding in distal tubular occlusion must be evaluated and treated in conjunction with any tuboplasty. Similarly, any progressive or ongoing inflammatory tubal disease must be detected and excluded preoperatively; the altered endothelium in a hydrosalpinx may be more susceptible to reinfection and tubal reocclusion. Intraoperative manipulation and cervical dye instillation immediately prior to tubal repair may introduce new pathogens. Therefore, the diagnostic endoscopy and therapeutic microsurgery should not be performed in the same operative session. Tubal and peritoneal cultures should be obtained to detect aerobic and anaerobic organisms with particular attention directed toward *Chlamydia* and *Mycoplasma*. If inflammatory adhesions can be biopsied during endoscopy, the results of this cultured tissue may be more accurate than swab cultures of the serosa. Prophylactic antibiotics after diagnostic manipulation may decrease the risk of aggravating salpingitis.

ENDOSCOPIC EVALUATION IN UNEXPLAINED INFERTILITY

When hysterosalpingogram fails to reveal the possible cause of infertility, a total preoperative evaluation of the reproductive tract is to be performed. Emphasis should be directed toward evaluating factors such as endometriosis, tuboovarian spatial relations,[26] peritubal adhesions, and tubal distortions such as increased tortuosity, fimbrial scarring, and pelvic scarring, which may suggest prior tubal inflammatory processes as the possible etiology for infertility. If peritubal and periovarian adhesive disease is identified, salpingoovariolysis can be performed by operative laparoscopy.[27] If, however, operative laparoscopy is performed, the basic tenents of microsurgical technique should be observed. Hemostasis must be meticulous; lysis of adhesions must be associated with minimal tissue manipulation. Ancillary operative procedures such as administration of antiobiotics, steroids, and high-molecular-weight dextran lavage of the surgical area may be considered by the surgeon.

If unsuspected endometriosis is encountered, it should be described, photographed, and graded as to severity. The initial status of the endometriosis must be carefully noted as a basis of comparison with the results of second-look laparoscopy to evaluate the success of medical management.

SUMMARY   The pelvic microsurgeon should be an experienced and competent endoscopist. The ability to evaluate pathology and correlate findings with the physiological role of the Fallopian tube will ultimately result in better success rates for microsurgical oviductal surgery. Diagnostically, it is hoped that the future will provide an endoscope that permits magnification at levels that allow evaluation of microscopic damage to the oviduct. At present, careful and thorough preoperative evaluation will eliminate futile reparative procedures and permit the microsurgeon and his patient to be aware of the extent of procedures, the predictive success rate, and the risks of ectopic pregnancy.

REFERENCES

1. Pauerstein CJ: *The Fallopian Tube—A Reappraisal.* Philadelphia, Lea and Febiger, 1974, p 14.
2. Ansari A: Diagnostic procedures for assessment of tubal patency. *Fertil Steril* 31:469, 1979.
3. Dor J, Homburg R, Rabau E: An evaluation of etiologic factors and therapy in 665 infertile couples. *Fertil Steril* 28:718, 1977.
4. Swolin K: Salpingostomy and salpingolysis, in Phillips JM (ed): *Microsurgery in Gynecology.* St. Louis, American Association of Gynecologic Laparoscopists, Department of Publishing, 1977, p 125.
5. Taylor HW: A comparative evaluation of the 5mm laparoscope in gynecologic endoscopy. *J Reprod Med* 15:65, 1975.
6. Lindemann H: Historical aspects of hysteroscopy. *Fertil Steril* 24:230, 1973.
7. Mohr J, Lindemann HJ: Hysteroscopy in the infertile patient. *J Reprod Med* 19:161, 1977.
8. Carey WH: Determination of patency of Fallopian tubes by the use of collargel and X-ray shadows. *Am J Obstet Dis Women Child* 69:462, 1914.
9. Swolin K, Rosencrantz M: Laparoscopy vs. hysterosalpingography in sterility investigation: A comparative study. *Fertil Steril* 23:270, 1972.
10. Correy JF, Scholzman FCM: Laparoscopy and hysterosalpingography in the diagnosis of infertility. *Aust NZ J Obstet Gynecol* 17:205, 1977.
11. Kasten Dieck E, Gani MA, Majewski A: A comparative evaluation of culdoscopy and laparoscopy in gynecology. *Endoscopy* 7:181, 1975.
12. Moghissi K, Sup Sim G: Correlation between hysterosalpingography and pelvic endoscopy for the evaluation of tubal factor. *Fertil Steril* 26:1178, 1975.
13. El-Minani M, Aldel-Hali M, Ibrahim A, et al: Comparative evaluation of laparoscopy and hysterosalpingography in infertile patients. *Obstet Gynecol* 51:29, 1978.
14. Stampf P, Maren CM: Febrile morbidity following hysterosalpingography. *Fertil Steril* 33:487, 1980.
15. Silber S, Cotten R: Microsurgical reversal of female sterilization. The role of tubal length. *Fertil Steril* 33:598, 1980.

16. Leeton J, Selwood T: The tortuous tube: Pregnancy rate following laparoscopy and hydrotubation. *Aust NZ J Obstet Gynecol* 18:259, 1978.
17. Donnez J, Casanas-Roux F, Ferin J: Macroscopic and microscopic studies of Fallopian tube after laparoscopic sterilization. *Contraception* 20:498, 1979.
18. Gomel V: Microsurgical reversal of female sterilization: a reappraisal. *Fertil Steril* 33:587, 1980.
19. Vasquez G, Winston RL, Boecky W, et al: Tubal lesions subsequent to sterilization. *Am J Obstet Gynecol* 138:86, 1980.
20. Gomel V: Salpingostomy by laparoscopy. *J Reprod Med* 18:181, 1977.
21. Swolin K: Electro-microsurgery and salpingostomy: Long term results. *Am J Obstet Gynecol* 121:418, 1975.
22. Brosens IA, DeGraef R: Micro-biopsy of the Fallopian tube. *Int J Fertil* 2:55, 1975.
23. Brosens I, Vasquez G: Fimbrial microbiopsy. *J Reprod Med* 16:171, 1976.
24. Gomel V: Causes of failed reconstructive tubal microsurgery. *J Reprod Med* 24:234, 1980.
25. Gomel V: Salpingostomy for hydrosalpinx. *Fertil Steril* 29:380, 1978.
26. Cohen BM, Katz M: The significance of the convoluted oviduct in the infertile woman. *J Reprod Med* 21:31, 1978.
27. Swolin K: Laparoscopy as an operative tool in female sterility. *J Reprod Med* 19:167, 1977.

7

Reversal of Female Sterilization

J. Victor Reyniak

Department of Obstetrics and Gynecology
Division of Reproductive Endocrinology
Mount Sinai School of Medicine
New York, New York 10029

Voluntary female surgical sterilization has become widely accepted as an effective alternate, but potentially irreversible, method of fertility control (contraception). The spontaneous pregnancy rate, the presenting failure of the procedure, is usually less than 1%. When discussing sterilization with a potential candidate, the physician should stress its irreversible nature and that a temporary method of surgical sterilization is yet to be devised. Furthermore, when performing a sterilization, the physician has the obvious responsibility to assure that a failure does not occur.

It is acknowledged that the overwhelming majority of women will be satisfied with this permanent contraception. Considering, however, the mere increase in sterilization procedures performed annually, it becomes obvious that a significant number of women will consider procedure reversal. In addition, the attention given to the improved successful reversal rate achieved by new microsurgical methods obviously contributes to this trend.[1]

Figures indicate that the most prevalent reason for request of sterilization reversal is a change in marital status.[2,3] Other reasons include death of a child, an improvement in economic situation, or a psychological desire to overcome supposed ill effects of tubal sterilization.[4] It is noteworthy that in a survey of 107 patients, 75.7% admitted to having had an unhappy marriage at the time of sterilization.[3]

For the woman who requests a reversal, a counseling physician should allow ample time for a preliminary discussion that should include the patient's partner. It is helpful to obtain the operative records of the previous sterilization procedure performed, as some methods—salpingectomy, fimbriectomy—are virtually irreversible and therefore exclude the need for further detailed discussion and work-up. Fortunately, the most common procedures include Pomeroy-type tubal ligation, which removes a part of isthmic or ampullary portion of the tube, and a great variety of laparoscopic techniques. Unipolar coagulation, with or without excision of tubal segment, bipolar multiple-coagulation technique, and application of Fallope ring or Hulka clip are all widely used. The bipolar multiple-point coagulation method presents a basically very poor reversal potential in most cases.

Discussion with the candidate couple must include an outline of preoperative work-up, an outline of surgical risk, and a realistic assessment of chances for achieving a term pregnancy. Gomel[1] has stated that about 25% of couples will abandon the reversal plan after this initial discussion. Patients who qualify for the reversal procedure and who decide to proceed must have a preliminary assessment of their fertility potential and of the general health of the woman made. The male partner should have spermanalysis regardless of his previous fertility record. The woman's ovulatory process should be evaluated by means of basal body temperature, plasma progesterone level on postovulatory day 6–10, and/or endometrial biopsy. A hysterosalpingogram is advisable, especially in cases after laparoscopic sterilization, to evaluate the length and internal architecture of the proximal tubal segments and the uterine cavity. Finally, laparoscopy allows assessment of distal tubal segments and detection of possible unsuspected pelvic pathology such as endometriosis, leiomyomata, and hydrosalpinx of the distal tubes.

Several authors[1,5,6] have stressed the need for laparoscopy before contemplated tubal reconstruction. The visualized remaining tubal segments may appear markedly different than expected from the previously analyzed operative report of sterilization. Most importantly, the length of these segments can be accurately measured using a second puncture probe. This measurement is a vital prognostic factor, since an inverse relationship has been noted between the total length of the reconstructed tube and the length of the reconstructed oviduct is directly related to the occurrence of pregnancy.[7] The subsequent pregnancy rate was 100% in 11 patients with tubal length of 5 cm on either side. Fifty percent of the patients with 3–4 cm of tube conceived, and there were no pregnancies when patients' oviducts measured less than 3 cm.

MACRO- AND MICROSURGICAL METHODS OF STERILIZATION REVERSAL

The physician who has taken responsibility for restoring fertility potential in a previously sterilized woman must choose the surgical approach that offers the optimal chance for success. Reported data indicate that a very significant improvement in term pregnancy rate can be achieved with the microsurgical approach as compared with conventional methods (see Chapter 5). Admittedly, evaluation of the result of various surgical methods is difficult. Many confounding factors exist in comparison of a series of patients, such as the variation in type of sterilization, the tubal length, the discrepancy in lumens, and the technique of the individual surgeon, all of which preclude an outline of uniform analysis of reported results.[8]

Instrumentation and Techniques

Instruments, loupes, and microscopes are described in detail in Chapter 4. It is, however, worthwhile pointing out that to ease organization of the working field and to avoid clutter, the minimal necessary instrumentation should be used for tubal anastomosis. The following instruments should be prepared: microneedle holder, straight iris scissors, small suture scissors, two pairs of jeweler's forceps, one microtooth forceps, tubal perfusion cannula. In addition, two 20-cc syringes should always be filled with dextran 70 or isotonic physiological solution for constant irrigation of tissues. A 10-cc syringe with 20-gauge needle for transfundal perfusion should also be ready. Loupes are used for initial preparation of the tubal segments and dissection of adhesions, if present. A microscope is preferred for preparation of occluded segments for anastomosis. The instrument set should also include several glass or plastic rods to facilitate atraumatic tissue manipulation.

Preparation of the Patient

Excellent exposure and access to the tubes is essential. Thus, prior to laparotomy, it is advisable to place a moistened laparotomy or a gauge roll in the vagina, packing it tightly in order to elevate the uterus and stabilize the pelvic organs. This avoids the problem encountered with a widely altering focal plane. Gomel[1] also recommends placing a pediatric Foley catheter in the uterine cavity with extension tubing extending to the sterile field to permit tubal perfusion without the need for transfundal puncture. The abdomen can be entered through a Pfannenstiel incision, and adequate exposure is achieved with a self-retaining retractor. Sufficient elevation and immobilization of the uterus and adnexa can be accomplished by placing moistened laparotomy pads loosely around the uterus. Some surgeons recommend rubber- or plastic-lined packs to avoid possible shedding of lint particles.[9] All exposed surfaces must be kept moist at all times. Isotonic physiological solutions are recommended, and we use[10,11] 6% dextran 70 because its antithrombotic and local "siliconizing" effect[12,13] may be more effective in protecting the tissues and minimizing adhesion formation.[14] The tubal segments are inspected, and any existing adhesions are divided with a microelectric needle, working close to the serosa or ovarian cortex. Glass rods are used to lift the adhesions or put them under tension, allowing for precise cauterization with minimal risk of inadvertent spread of the current to the adjacent structures.

Depending on the original sterilization site and the length of the remaining tubal segments, the following types of anastomoses may be performed: (1) isthmic-isthmic; (2) isthmic-ampullary; (3) ampullary-ampullary; (4) ampullary-infundibular; (5) intramural-isthmic; (6) intramural-ampullary. A schematic of steps in each type of anastomosis is presented. The most favorable[15] and technically simple[16,17] is the joining of segments where there is no great discrepancy in the lumen diameter.

Isthmic–Isthmic Anastomosis

The diameter of the tubal lumen in this region varies from 0.4 to 1.0 mm, and the muscular layer is fairly thick and well defined. Initially, the occluded segments are inspected under magnification. We recommend a circumferential serosal incision using a monopolar needle electrode in the approximate area of the junction of scar tissue and normal tube (Fig. 1). This promotes slight retraction of the serosal edges. Iris scissors are used to excise the scarred portion through the line of serosal incision. The cut segments, especially the proximal segment, should then be carefully inspected under high magnification for evidence of abnormalities. Pathology in the proximal tubal stump (salpingitis isthmica nodosa, endometriosis, hydrosalpinx, chronic salpingitis) may be observed in approximately 13% of patients.[1] Small hydrosalpinx of the occluded isthmus may also occur, particularly when the previous sterilization procedure involved the use of catgut ligatures.[17] If necessary, small sections are further excised until a normal architecture of muscularis and endosalpinges are seen under magnification.

The bleeding points should be controlled using bipolar cautery microforceps or a pinpoint monopolar electrode. Overzealous attempts at coagulation, however, must be

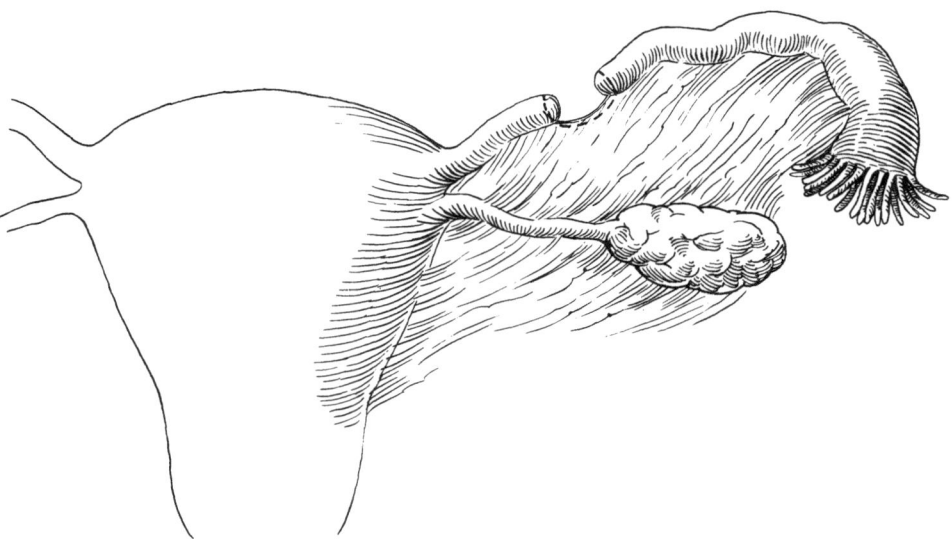

Figure 1. Initial preparation for isthmic–isthmic anastomosis. The dotted line shows the course of serosal incision with needle microelectrode.

avoided. Gomel[1] suggests mild compression of the tube between two fingers to aid in controlling the bleeding. In order to prevent distortion of the endosalpingeal architecture, small mucosal bleeders should not be coagulated. These bleeders usually stop oozing spontaneously.

Transfundal or transcervical perfusion allows the surgeon to establish the presence of patency and normal lumen in the proximal segment. Transfimbrial perfusion, using a perfusion cannula, determines the free flow through the distal segment. The mesosalpinx between these two segments is now incised in a linear fashion with a needle electrode (Fig. 1). If bleeding is encountered, coagulation or or a 6-0 tie on the bleeding points may be used.

Approximating interrupted 6-0 sutures are now placed between the edges of the mesosalpinx to bring the tubal segments into close proximity and to avoid the use of instruments for this purpose (Fig. 2). Additional moistened packs are employed to immobilize the structures. Anastomosis is carried out in two layers. In this segment of the tube, four sutures of 8-0 Vicryl® placed at 6, 3, 9, and 12 o'clock of tubal circumferences in this sequence are sufficient. We recommend that the needle transverse about one-

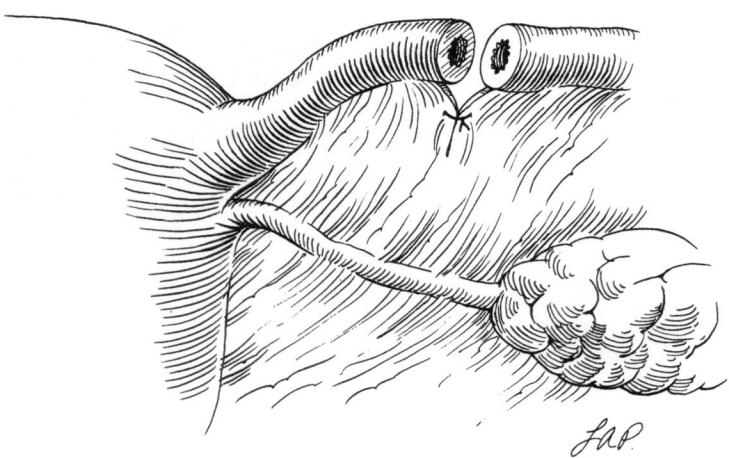

Figure 2. Approximation of tubal segments using a 6-0 suture in the mesosalpinx.

half of the muscle coat and emerge at the edge of, but not through, the mucosa (Fig. 3). For technical ease, the first suture should be placed at 6 o'clock; otherwise, one encounters difficulties in mobilizing and rotating the structures. The sutures are tied in such a fashion that the knots are laid

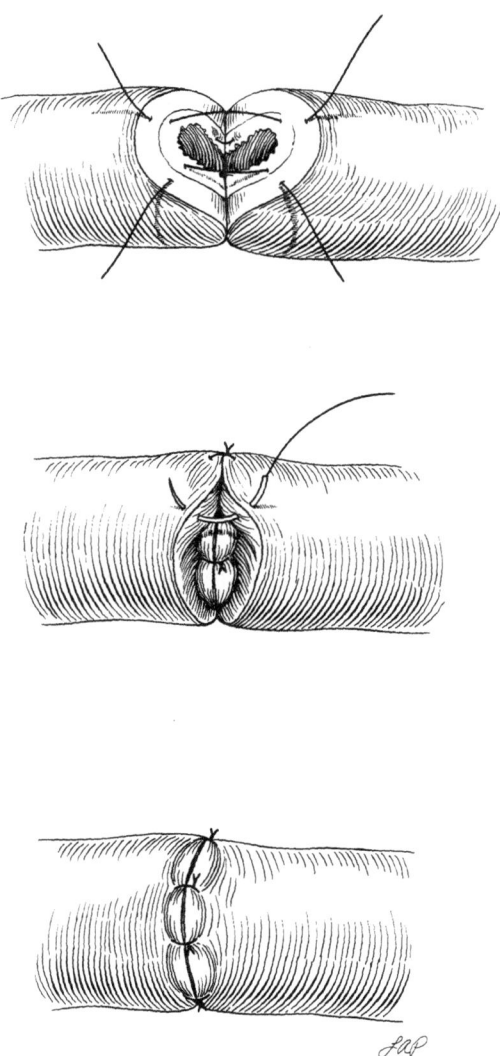

Figure 3. Isthmic–isthmic anastomosis. The placement of sutures through muscularis and mucosa is followed by approximation of serosal edges.

distal to the mucosa (Fig. 3). It is technically preferable to tie each suture as soon as it is placed. Leaving sutures untied until the end of the procedure may cause a hopeless tangle of suture material.

The second layer is placed through the serosal edges. Usually six or eight 7-0 or 8-0 Vicryl® sutures are necessary to obtain a clean suture line (Fig. 3). Finally, any remaining defect in the mesosalpinx should be repaired with interrupted sutures. The lumen and the layers of the transected segment of the Fallopian tube are easily and well defined under magnification. Thus, the need for splints is abolished when working in the isthmic portion.

Transfundal perfusion should be performed to prove the patency of the reconstructed oviduct. The anastomosis in this segment is usually watertight following the repair. Throughout the procedure, all exposed structures must be kept constantly moist. Following removal of the packs, the pelvic cavity should be irrigated thoroughly with dextran 70. Before routine closure of the abdomen, we leave 150 cc of this solution in the pelvic cavity.

Ampullary–Isthmic Anastomosis

The technical challenge of anastomosis between the isthmic and ampullary portions of the tube is the vast discrepancy between the endosalpingeal lumens: 0.6–1.0 mm in the isthmic portion; 4–5 mm in the ampullary portion. The initial preparation of the segments, transsection and visual inspection of the proximal segment, is as previously described. The preparation of the ampullary portion, however, is totally different. In this segment, the muscular layer is very thin and poorly defined, and the mucosa consists of many luxuriant folds that tend to prolapse into the lumen when incised. The task of attempting to sew unequal lumens is compounded by the obstruction of view with the mucosal folds. This results in a technically difficult and frustrating process.

Several methods have been described to approach this problem properly. In their earlier publications, Gomel and McComb[18] suggested a technique for enlarging the caliber of the proximal segment by resecting it at the angle with the mesenteric edge remaining longer. A 2-mm slit is then made at the antimesenteric edge of the proximal isthmic segment, and the little corners thus formed are partially excised. This technique allows for more exact approximation of discrepant lumens.

Winston[17] has described the technique of plicating the cut end of the ampullary segment with 8-0 nylon sutures in order to reduce its luminal size. Winston[17] has, however, suggested a superior technique to tailor the opening of the ampullary stump to the size of the proximal lumen, and his technique has now been widely adopted.[1,18,19] Briefly, it consists of placing a curved 1-mm-diameter grooved probe through the fimbria into the ampulla (Fig. 4). The blind ampullary end stretches with gentle pressure over the blunt tip of the probe. A button of peritoneum is excised over this tip, exposing the muscularis (Fig. 5). Muscularis

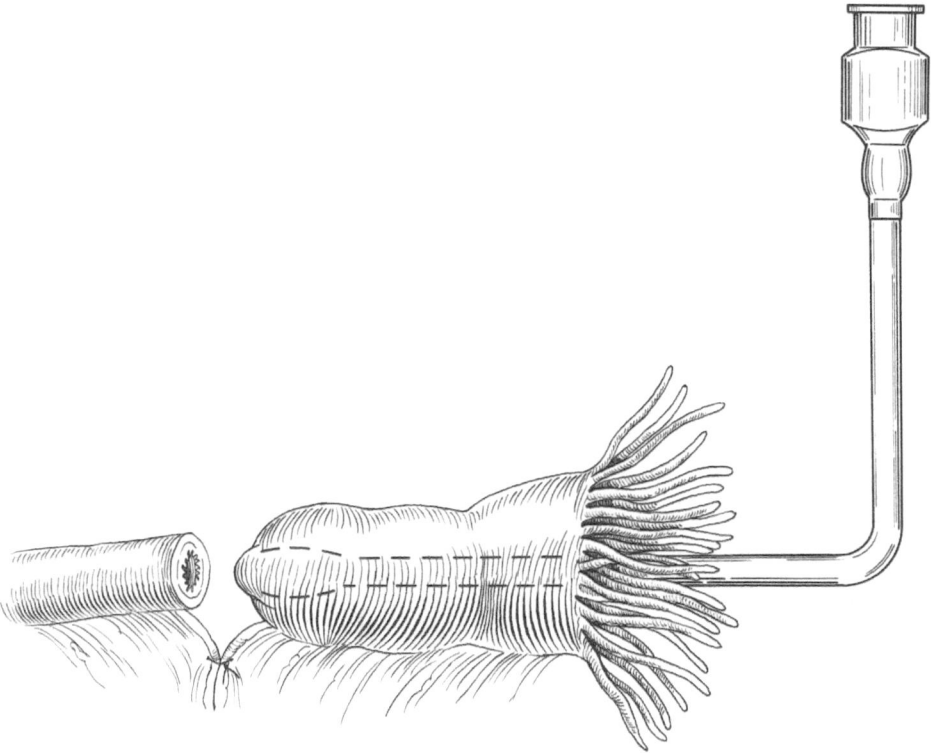

Figure 4. Isthmic–ampullary anastomosis. Preparation of the ampullary segment. The blind end of this segment is stretched over the blunt tip of a perfusion cannula.

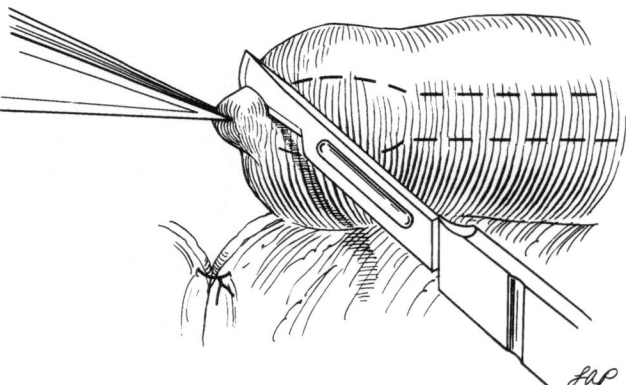

Figure 5. Isthmic–ampullary anastomosis. Preparation of ampullary segment. A button of peritoneum is excised over the blunt tip of a perfusion cannula, allowing subsequent incision of the muscularis and mucosa to create an opening corresponding to the diameter of the isthmic segment.

and mucosa are now cut directly over the tip of the probe, and the size of opening so created can be made to correspond to the diameter of the previously prepared isthmic portion. We have utilized Stangel's perfusion cannula for the same purpose. Approximating mesosalpinx sutures must now be placed to allow performance of two-layer anastomosis without undue tension between the tubal segments.

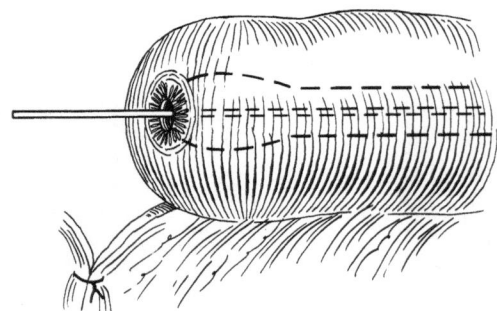

Figure 6. Isthmic–ampullary anastomosis. Placement of a temporary nylon 0 splint. The splint is inserted through the perfusion cannula. Subsequently, the cannula can be withdrawn, leaving the splint in the lumen.

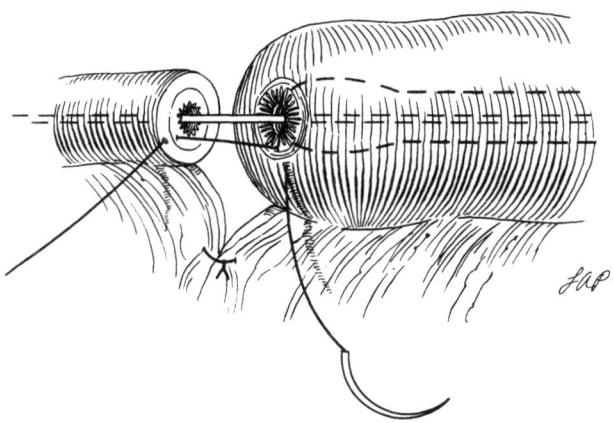

Figure 7. Isthmic–ampullary anastomosis. Placement of sutures over temporary nylon 0 splint. The perfusion cannula is left in the ampullary segment for stabilization.

A temporary nylon 0 or 1 splint can be placed to define the lumens more precisely. We usually feed the suture through the perfusion cannula to avoid unnecessary trauma to the endosalpinx (Fig. 6). The two-layer anastomosis can now be carried out with this approach (Fig. 7). If the opening in the ampullary portion is small, prolapse of the ampullary mucosal folds, which may obstruct the view, is less likely to occur.

Ampullary–Ampullary Anastomosis

Although the lumens in this region of the Fallopian tube are compatable and quite large, difficulty may be encountered in an exact two-layer approximation because of a thin muscle coat and abundant mucosal folds. Two-layer anastomosis always appears advantageous, but because of these technical difficulties, Winston[17] has suggested performing ampullary anastomosis in one layer, incorporating the serosa and muscle in a multiple interrupted sutures (Fig. 8). When, however, two-layer anastomosis is attempted, a helpful maneuver consists of inserting jeweler's forceps in closed position into the lumen prior to the placement of the mucosal suture (Fig. 9). When the tips of the forceps are allowed to separate, the true lumen, under stretch, can be identified.[19] Following additional serosal approximation and repair of the mesosalpinx, the remainder of the procedure is performed as described.

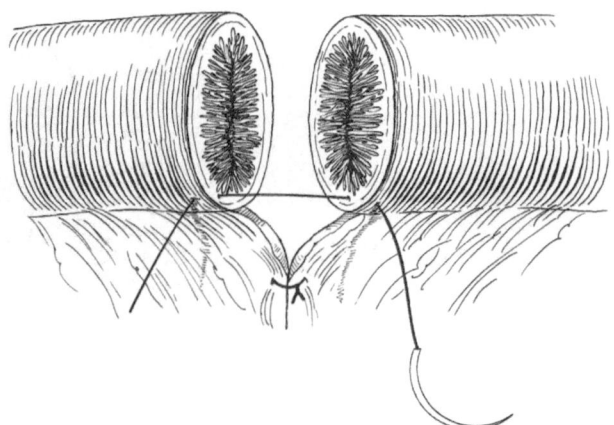

Figure 8. Ampullary–ampullary anastomosis. Technique of one-layer closure. The mesosalpinx suture is placed for close approximation of tubal segments. The first anastomosis suture is placed at 6 o'clock of the tubal circumference.

Tubo-Cornual Anastomosis

This procedure is applicable when the previous sterilization procedure has destroyed or removed the oviduct near the uterine cornu. Winston[20] has pioneered the technique, which is now widely adopted, of joining the remaining tubal segment directly to the intramural portion of the uterine cornu, which has a diameter of about 0.4 mm. Initially, the cornual segment is prepared by scalpel excision of tissue

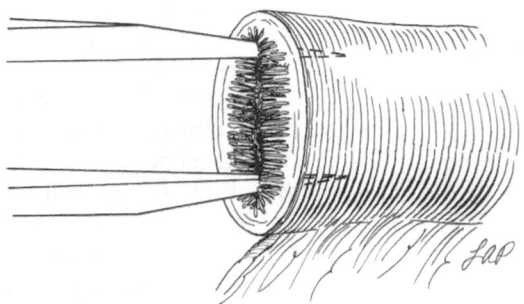

Figure 9. Ampullary–ampullary anastomosis. Identification of tubal lumen for a two-layer anastomosis. Jeweler's forceps were inserted into the lumen in closed position. Allowing the forceps to open permits visualization of the lumen under stretch.

(Fig. 10) under high magnification until the scar is removed and the orifice of the intramural portion becomes clearly visible. Since this excision involves myometrial tissue, the bleeding can be brisk, and we have found it helpful to inject the area with a solution of vasopressin (Pitressin®) in saline. Major bleeders should be coagulated, but it is nearly impossible to induce an absolute hemostasis. Bleeding, however, will be ultimately controlled when anastomosis is laid. Transfundal perfusion allows the documentation of patency of the prepared segment. We use a solution of indigo carmine in dextran 70. Others[19] recommend using clear solution, since the blue dye may obscure the view, but Winston[20] finds the blue staining of the circular muscles surrounding the four primary epithelial folds of the intramural tube helpful.

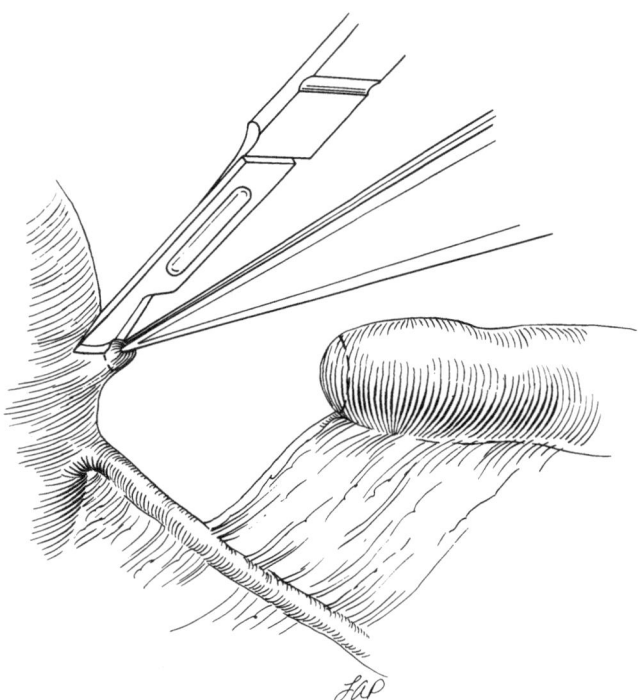

Figure 10. Tubo-cornual anastomosis. Preparation of cornual segment by excision of tissue slices until the scar is removed and the orifice of the intramural segment of the tube becomes visible.

Preparation of the distal segment, whether isthmic or ampullary, is performed as previously described. Again, in the ampullary portion, tailoring a small orifice under the guidance of a probe or a perfusion cannula is helpful. Although the placement of a temporary splint may seem advantageous, it may be technically difficult. The intramural portion is characterized by convolutions and abrupt changes of direction.[21] Forcing even a fine nylon 0 splint into the uterine cavity may lead to formation of a false tract. If use of the splint appears absolutely necessary for technical reasons, we suggest the following approach. After preparation of a distal segment, 0 Prolene® suture is fed through the perfusion cannula which is then removed. Subsequently and most importantly, the mesosalpinx of this segment is sutured to the myometrium and serosa under the cornual region to bring the lumens into very close contact without tension (Fig. 11). Moistened packs are used to stabilize the field, and a nylon splint protruding from the distal segment

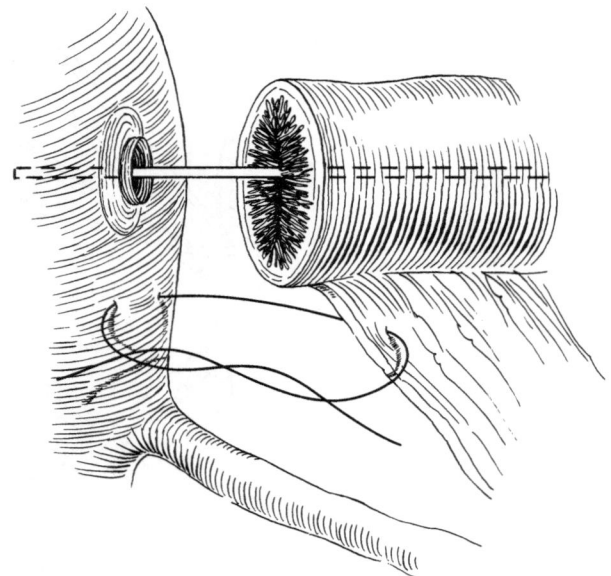

Figure 11. Tubo-cornual anastomosis. Temporary nylon 0 splint *in situ*. Mesosalpinx-to-uterine-serosa suture is placed. The tying of this suture allows for close contact of tubal lumens without tension.

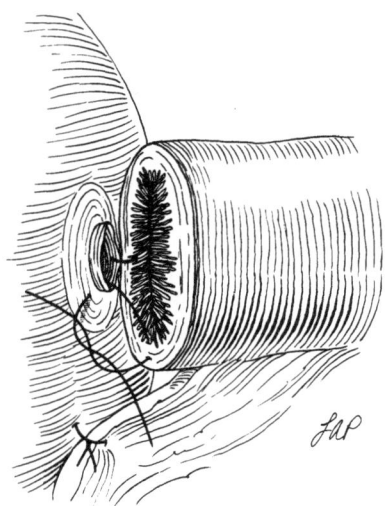

Figure 12. Tubo-cornual anastomosis. Placement of sutures through the muscularis (first layer).

is gently inserted into the cornual opening for the distance of no more than 2–3 mm. No force should be used to insert it deeper or into the uterine cavity.

Two-layer anastomosis is now carried out, placing the sutures of the first layer through the muscularis, beginning with the distal segment. In this fashion, suturing the intramural portion becomes technically easier, as in this region the needle travels from the inside out rather from the outside in (Fig. 12). The controversy still remains whether the sutures should be placed through the lumen or whether piercing the mucosa should be avoided. Usually four sutures placed at 6, 3, 9, and 12 o'clock (in this order) are sufficient for approximation of the first layer. The anastomosis is completed by suturing the serosa of the distal tubal segment to the uterine serosa.

PROBLEMS AND CONTROVERSIES

Tubal Splints

Intraluminal tubal splinting appears to be deleterious to tubal anastomosis on the basis of animal experiments.[22] Adhesions and fibrosis resulted in a decrease in subsequent fertility in rabbits when splints were left for 1 week following anastomosis. It appears that the longer the splints remain *in situ,* the lower the fertility rate of the animal.[23] Gomel[1] recommends the use of a 0.4-mm Prolene® rod as a splint for tubo-cornual anastomosis: the rod is fed into the uterine cavity and left *in situ* for 1 or 2 days. He stresses, however, that if difficulty is encountered during the insertion, the splint be abandoned.

Other authors[19] strongly recommend against the use of any splinting devices in human sterilization reversal. Since there is no doubt that indwelling splints may cause epithelial damage, fibrosis, and infection,[17] we feel that their use should be avoided. If it appears, however, that a splint is technically essential for excellent approximation of lumens, it should be utilized only for the duration of the performance of anastomosis and removed as soon as it is accomplished. Winston[17] has stated that leaving splints in place for a prolonged period of time is unnecessary, since anastomosis stability is achieved within 30–60 min of the completion of surgery as fibrin is laid down at the joint.

Placement of Sutures Some authors recommend placing the sutures through the mucosa, i.e., through the lumen, during the placement of the first layer.[19] Others[1,15,25] approximate only submucosal and muscular layers, avoiding penetration of the lumen. In Winston's experience[15] with animal experiments, the joints were not as histologically satisfactory with mucosal wall suture. Apparently, ectopic islands of epithelium can be "dragged" into the muscle layer, and although it did not effect the subsequent fertility of the experimental animal, it could theoretically increase the chance for ectopic gestation in humans. Under adequate magnification, an excellent approximation can be accomplished in most cases with suturing techniques that avoid piercing of the endosalpinx.

Suturing Material Monofilament 6-0, 9-0, or 10-0 nylon has been used by some authors[9,17,19,24,25] as the least reactive suture material. Others[1] have recommended 8-0 polyglycolic sutures (Vicryl®) on 130-μm, 4-mm tapered atraloc needles.

Type 10-0 nylon has been compared with 8-0 Vicryl® sutures in the experimental animal.[26] In 6 months' follow-up, there was no inflammatory response in the Vicryl® group, whereas the presence of giant cells was noted in association with nylon sutures despite their fine caliber. Monofilament 9-0 Dexon® (polyglycolic acid) sutures, in our experiments,[11] have been shown to restore fertility and cause no tissue reaction in rabbit anastomosis. Vicryl®, however, has been shown to have a higher tensile strength than Dexon® from day 0 to day 35 postoperatively.[26] Vicryl® appears to be completely absorbed within 90 days after the operation,[27] whereas Dexon® persists until the 120th day. The outcome of anastomosis does not, however, appear to be significantly different regardless of the suture material used.

POSTOPERATIVE FOLLOW-UP AND PLANNING OF PREGNANCY

Unprotected coitus to attempt conception can be allowed following the postoperative recovery. In the past, some authors[28] recommended the use of contraception for an arbitrarily chosen period of 3 months. We agree with Gomel,[1] who allows his patients to attempt pregnancy after the first menstrual period following the reanastomosis procedure. In his series, 11% of patients conceived during the first trial cycle. However, the mean time interval between surgery and occurrence of pregnancy was overall 10.2 months.

CAUSES OF FAILURE IN STERILIZATION REVERSAL

The Fallopian tube is an organ with complex and still not completely understood functions (see Chapter 2). In considering the reversal of previous surgical sterilization, one tends to assume that the remaining tubal segments will be normal and healthy. However, despite meticulous techniques of anastomosis, the desired pregnancy will not occur in all patients. Achieving documentable patency of the oviduct does not imply that tubal function will return.

The factors that may affect the outcome of the microsurgical sterilization reversal are as follows:

1. Unrecognized pathology of the remaining tubal segment. In the largest reported series of microsurgical reversals,[1] the incidence of pathological changes in the proximal tubal stump was 12.7%. A recent scanning electron microscopy study[29] of the tubal biopsy specimens of 26 patients undergoing reversal showed that half of these patients had

REVERSAL OF FEMALE STERILIZATION | **155**

anomalies of tubal mucosa. These included loss of mucosal folds, deciliation, and polyposis. Significantly, these pathological conditions increase in incidence the longer the time interval from the original sterilization procedure. Poststerilization polyps of Fallopian tubes vary in size from 40 to 635 μm[29]; thus, preoperative hysterosalpingography will not be diagnostic. They can, however, easily be seen under the operating microscope at a magnification of $\times$20 to $\times$40. The use of high magnification to examine the tubal segments may lead to recognition of a multitude of pathological changes that might be excised even at the expense of the existing significantly shortened tubes. Otherwise, fibrosis, scarring, and possible secondary occlusion at or around the anastomosis site may occur.

2. The length of the anastomosed tube. In a rabbit, more than 47% of the total tubal length is necessary for restoration of fertility.[30] Similar observations have been made in the human female.[1,7] Furthermore, when the anastomosed tube is abnormally short, a lengthy delay may ensue before occurrence of pregnancy. "Shortened tube syndrome" exists and appears to cause a significant reduction in fertility.[31]

3. Coexistent pelvic pathology. Leiomyomata, endometriosis, and pelvic adhesions can be coexistent with the poststerilization status and impair the prognosis for restoration of fertility. The principle of microsurgery is to minimize tissue trauma. Any additional amount of dissection in the removal of coexistent pathology may impair the outcome, possibly by formation of adhesions. It has also been pointed out that there is a direct correlation between the nature and extent of adhesions and the prognosis for the restoration of fertility.[31,32]

4. Formation of adhesions as a result of laparotomy. Surgeons have always tried to design a prophylactic regimen for prevention of postoperative adhesions. The only true prophylactic method in microsurgery is the gentleness in manipulation of tissues and prevention of drying of serosal surfaces.[31] In addition, use of a monopolar needle electrode for careful dissection of adhesions under magnification, identifi-

cation and cautery of bleeding points, and meticulous approximation of cut surfaces will aid in this prevention.

5. Altered tubo-ovarian spatial relationship. Cohen and Katz[33] pointed out the relationship between elongated ovarian ligaments and the fimbria ovaria in infertile women, especially in cases of markedly shortened tubes. Plication of these ligaments, if elongated, to beneficially effect contact of the fimbria and the ovary has been suggested.[31,33]

6. Late reproductive age of the patient—a self-explanatory point.

SUMMARY

Sterilization procedures currently available are intended to be irreversible. Although some authors recommended less destructive procedures for the younger woman, the implication of the operation and the surgical responsibility are to make it fail-proof. A significant number of sterilized women request reversal of such procedures for a multiplicity of reasons. It is only logical that the principles of microsurgery be applied to the reconstruction of the oviduct. One must minimize both tissue trauma and the possible desiccation of exposed serosal surfaces as well as maintaining meticulous control of bleeding. Precise excision of adhesions, tubal scar tissue, and/or coexistent pathology of the tubal segment followed by an excellent approximation of tissue planes using fine nonreactive sutures under adequate magnification should allow the desired result. It now appears obvious that utilization of these principles has nearly tripled the term pregnancy rate that had previously been achieved with conventional surgery.

REFERENCES

1. Gomel V: Microsurgerical reversal of female sterilization: A reappraisal. *Fertil Steril* 33:587, 1980.
2. Gomel V: Profile of women requesting reversal of sterilization. *Fertil Steril* 30:39, 1978.
3. Winston RML: Why 103 women asked for reversal of sterilization. *Br Med J* 2:305, 1977.
4. Siegler AM, Kontopoulos V: Reversal of tubal sterilization: Implications, techniques and results, in Sciarra JJ, Zatuchni GI, Speidel JJ (eds): *Reversal of Sterilization.* New York, Harper & Row, 1977, p 134.
5. Rosenfeld DL, Garcia CRL: Laparoscopy prior to tubal reanastomosis. *J Reprod Med* 17:247, 1976.

6. Gomel V: Laparoscopy prior to tubal surgery for infertility. *J Reprod Med* 18:251, 1977.

7. Silber SJ, Cohen R: Microsurgical reversal of female sterilization: The role of tubal length. *Fertil Steril* 33:598, 1980.

8. Berger GS: Tubal reconstruction after surgical sterilization: Microsurgery in perspective, in Sciarra JJ, Zatuchni GI, Speidel JJ (eds): *Reversal of Sterilization*. New York, Harper & Row, 1977, p 170.

9. Diamond E: A comparison of gross and microsurgical techniques for repair of cornual occlusion in infertility: A retrospective study, 1968–1978. *Fertil Steril* 32:370, 1979.

10. Stangel JJ, Reyniak JV, Stone ML: Conservative management of tubal pregnancy. *Obstet Gynecol* 48:241, 1976.

11. Stangel JJ, Settles HE, Reyniak JV, et al: Microsurgical anastomosis of the rabbit oviduct using monofilament polyglycolic acid suture. *Fertil Steril* 30:210, 1978.

12. Golub S, Schaefer C: Structural alteration in canine fibrin produced by colloid plasma expanders. *Surg Gynecol Obstet* 127:783, 1968.

13. Neuwirth RS, Khalaf SM: Effects of thirty-two percent dextran 70 on peritoneal adhesion formation. *Am J Obstet Gynecol* 121:420, 1975.

14. Utian WH, Goldfarb JM, Starks GC: Role of dextran 70 in microtubal surgery. *Fertil Steril* 31:79, 1979.

15. Winston RML: Reversal of sterilization: Microsurgery of the fallopian tube, in Sciarra JJ, Zatuchni GI, Speidel JJ (eds): *Reversal of Sterilization*. New York, Harper & Row, 1977, p. 184.

16. Hodari AA, Vibhasirix S, Isaac AY: Reconstructive tubal surgery for midtubal obstruction. *Fertil Steril* 28:620, 1977.

17. Winston RML: Tubal anastomosis for reversal of sterilization in 45 women, in Brosens I, Winston RML (eds): *Reversibility of Female Sterilization*. London, Academic Press, New York, Grune & Stratton, 1978, p 55.

18. Gomel V, McComb P: Microsurgery in gynecology, in Silber SJ (ed): *Microsurgery*. Baltimore, Williams & Wilkins, 1979, p 143.

19. Silber SJ, Cohen R: Microsurgical reversal of female sterilization: Techniques and comparison to vasectomy reversal, in Silber SJ (ed): *Microsurgery*. Baltimore, Williams & Wilkins, 1979, p 185.

20. Winston RML: Microsurgical tubocornual anastomosis for reversal of sterilization. *Lancet* 1:284, 1977.

21. Sweeney WJ: The interstitial portion of the uterine tube: Its gross anatomy, course and length. *Obstet Gynecol* 19:1, 1962.

22. Winston RML: Microsurgical reanastomosis of the rabbit oviduct and its functional and pathological sequelae. *Br J Obstet Gynecol* 82:513, 1975.

23. MacKay KV, Khoo SK: Reactions in the rabbit fallopian tube after plastic reconstruction. II. Histopathology. *Fertil Steril* 23:207, 1972.

24. Siegler AM, Kontopoulos V: An analysis of macrosurgical and microsurgical techniques in the management of the tuboperitoneal factor in infertility. *Fertil Steril* 32:377, 1979.

25. Cantor B, Riggal FC: The choice of sterilization procedure according to its potential reversibility with microsurgery. *Fertil Steril* 31:9, 1979.

26. Smith DC: Data presented at the Microsurgery Seminar, Third International Congress of Gynecologic Endoscopy, San Francisco, December, 1977.

27. Craig PH, Williams JA, Davis KW, et al: A biological comparison of polyglycolic and polyglycolic acid synthetic absorbable sutures. *Surg Gynecol Obstet* 141:1, 1975.
28. Williams GEJ: Fallopian tube surgery for reversal of sterilization. *Br Med J* 1:599, 1973.
29. Vasquez G, Winston RML, Boeckx W, et al: Tubal lesions subsequent to sterilization and their relation to fertility after attempts at reversal. *Am J Obstet Gynecol* 138:86, 1980.
30. McComb P, Gomel V: The influence of fallopian tube length on fertility in the rabbit. *Fertil Steril* 31:673, 1979.
31. Gomel V: Causes of failed reconstructive tubal microsurgery. *J Reprod Med* 24:239, 1980.
32. Caspi H, Halperin Y, Bukovsky I: The importance of periadnexal adhesions in tubal reconstructive surgery for infertility. *Fertil Steril* 31:296, 1979.
33. Cohen BM, Katz M: The significance of the convoluted oviduct in the infertile woman. *J Reprod Med* 21:31, 1978.

8 Microsurgical Management of Distal Tube Disease

Sami S. David

Department of Obstetrics and Gynecology
Mount Sinai School of Medicine
New York, New York 10029

Infertility secondary to tubal factors in a plurality of patients may be the result of *distal tubal disease*. This category includes patients who have undergone gynecologic operations such as ovarian cystectomy, myomectomy, or wedge resection, those who have experienced pelvic inflammatory disease, and those who have developed advanced endometriosis with adhesion formation and tubal damage. The surgical management of distal tubal disease is termed fimbrioplasty, but this general terminology encompasses the more precise nomenclature suggested by the Federation of International Gynecology and Obstetrics in 1977 of *salpingolysis, deagglutination,* or *salpingoneostomy*. The application of the principles of microsurgery to surgery for distal tubal disease can increase the success of this surgical management as measured by the achievement of term pregnancy.

GENERAL PRINCIPLES

Despite the rapid development of new, more refined instrumentation, the fact remains that the infertility specialist's most important tools are the surgeon's fingers coupled with the ability and desire to achieve a meticulously executed surgical procedure that restores the pelvic anatomy to normality. Similarly, another important adjunct to infertility surgery is time sufficient to accomplish the goal of reconstruction. The time set aside for reconstructive surgery should be directly related to the degree of adhesions and Fallopian tube damage. A simple salpingolysis or deagglutination may require 1½–2 hr, whereas the repair of bilateral hydrosalpinges with extensive adhesions or severe endometriosis may require 3–5 hr.

The physical and mental state of the surgeon are also crucial factors that directly bear on the surgical outcome, but they are seldom stressed in the literature dealing with microsurgery for infertility. A surgeon who has been awake all night with a patient in labor or has overindulged in alcohol, caffeine, or late-night entertainment may not exhibit the steadiness of hand or the patience and concentration required to achieve optimal surgical results. This should not be construed as a condemnation of "the pursuit of happiness" but rather a gentle reminder of the surgeon's responsibility to deliver the best medical care that can be humanly achieved. Microsurgery requires not only special skill and refinement of surgical technique but also the proper mental attitude—a philosophy—and the acceptance of the responsibility that the first attempt at reconstruction must be made under optimum conditions.

Preoperative Laparoscopy. Many infertility specialists, including the author, prefer to perform the preoperative laparoscopy as a separate procedure from the therapeutic laparotomy. This allows the surgeon to present the patient and her husband with data sufficient to understand the extent of the disease and the prognosis and to make an informed decision based on the laparoscopic findings. Moreover, the separation of the two operations minimizes the risk of introducing infection via chromotubations or inadvertent surgery on a patient with either a low-grade chronic pelvic infection or endometritis.

INSTRUMENTATION

Throughout the past and present literature on infertility surgery, one principle remains universally accepted—that is, the need for minimal instrumentation and avoidance of trauma to the pelvic structures. Successful tuboplasty requires the proper use of either magnifying loupes or an operating microscope which enables the surgeon to delineate more accurately the natural planes of dissection and to identify the minute vessels that are so abundant throughout the mesosalpinx, tubal serosa, and tubal fimbria. Proper illumination is an essential which may be achieved through the built-in light source of the microscope or a head light. The surgeon should use his fingers as much as possible in handling the tube, but when this is not possible, atraumatic forceps, such as the jeweler's, DeBakey, or "diamond-jaw" variety, may be utilized. The tubal serosa and fimbria, however, should not be manipulated with these instruments in order to prevent tissue damage and subsequent adhesion formation. Preferably, forceps should be used to identify and grasp adhesions, and then these adhesions are employed to manipulate and mobilize the pelvic structures.

The needle holder may be of the conventional variety, but it must be lightweight with narrow fine jaws. When fine suture, 8-0 or 9-0, is employed, needle holders with spring handles such as the Castroviejo type are recommended. Much has been written concerning the size and type of suture material that will yield the best surgical results. Authorities uniformly reject the use of chromic catgut and silk suture. Reddick and co-workers[1] compared the tissue response to polyglycolic acid, Dexon® (Davis & Geck), with that of polyglactic acid, Vicryl® (Ethicon), and reached two important conclusions. First, there was less tissue inflammatory reaction and fibrosis in the uterus with the Vicryl® than with the Dexon®. Second, necroscopy in rats revealed that most adhesions form at the surgical knots.

Two varieties of dissecting scissors should be available. The first is a fine iris scissors for close work on the tubes, and the other is a 7-in. Struli scissors which may be employed for both blunt and sharp dissection. The longer Struli scissors is most helpful for the lysis of adhesions deep within the pelvis. Probing of the tube itself must be performed with great care. Instruments for this task are obtained from the ophthalmologist in the form of graded lachrymal duct probes or custom-made pliable nylon or Teflon® probes. A self-retaining retractor is customarily utilized in abdominal surgery. The O'Connor–O'Sullivan retractor is satisfactory for most patients. Caution should be taken, however, to avoid femoral nerve compression in asthenic women, for Meldrum[2] relates a higher incidence of femoral nerve compression damage with the O'Connor-O'Sullivan retractor. If the tuboplasty is expected to last longer than 3–5 hr, it might be advisable to use the Balfour retractor with its shallow blades.

Bipolar coagulation utilizing micro-Mallis forceps is essential for complete hemostasis with minimal tissue damage. The current must be set at the lowest level required to coagulate the small bleeding points as they are encountered. Prior instruction and experience in the use of bipolar coagulation is essential to minimize tissue damage that might result from repeated incorrectly performed coagulations. The tissue between the coagulating forceps tips should include the small bleeding vessel but minimal normal tissue. The forceps tips short-circuit if they touch, but, conversely, if the tips are too far apart, either no coagulation will take place or excessive tissue necrosis will occur. Therefore, a 1- to 2-mm spark gap is required for proper coagulation.

Tissue irrigation with heparinized Ringer's lactate delivered in gentle pulsations from a syringe with a plastic catheter tip allows identification and isolation of the bleeding vessel and keeps surrounding tissues moist and free of clotting blood. Unipolar needle coagulation is acceptable, but certain precautions must be observed. The needle must be very fine and the current set at the lowest level required to prevent lateral and deep thermal damage. Sanfilippo and co-workers[3] compared the hemostatic effects of Avitene®, a topical thrombin, and Gelfoam® and found neither agent superior to bipolar coagulation.

Syringes are used to lavage the surgical site; this permits more accurate identification of minute bleeding points for pinpoint coagulation. A solution of lactated Ringer's containing 5000 units of heparin per liter, which also prevents the peritoneal surfaces from drying, is suggested. Blandau[4] found that lavage with saline alone resulted in edema and the formation of a plasma membrane over Fallopian tubes. Another solution that may be employed for lavage is 6% dextran 70 (Macrodex®). The simplest method utilizes a 50-cc syringe with a 16- or 14-gauge plastic tip to deliver the solution accurately.

SUGGESTED PRE- AND POSTOPERATIVE MEDICATION

It is suggested that the patient receive dexamethasone (Decadron®, Merck, Sharp & Dohme), 20 mg, and promethazine HCl (Phenergan®, Wyeth), 25 mg, intramuscularly in separate syringes approximately 3 hr prior to surgery; the same dose is repeated postoperatively every 4 hr for ten doses according to the protocol advanced by Replogle et al.[5] Ampicillin, 500 mg, or cefazolin sodium (Kefzol®, Eli Lilly & Company), 500 mg, may be given intramuscularly 1 hr prior to surgery and continued 36-48 hr postoperatively. This protocol has been advocated by many surgeons in this subspeciality and reaffirmed most recently by Garcia and Mastroianni.[6]

ENTRANCE INTO THE ABDOMEN

The Pfannenstiel incision is employed whenever possible for both its cosmetic virtues and its ability to aid in early and more comfortable ambulation. It should be emphasized that just as the fertility surgeon must necessarily be meticulous when operating within the abdomen, he must also be meticulous when entering the abdomen. Therefore, the same principles of minimizing blood loss, extreme care in hemostasis, and dissection along proper anatomical planes must be followed. A rapid, bloody entry through the abdominal wall with small bleeders oozing into the abdominal cavity will not only compromise the quality of the tubal surgery but lead to greater risk of postoperative intraabdominal adhesions, wound infection, and hematoma.

The surgeon must request a complete glove rinsing with fresh sterile saline. The moist lap pad technique of removing powder from the gloves is not entirely adequate to prevent the formation of foreign body granulomas.[7] The intestines should be packed with moist pads. The degree of serosal damage to the intestines can be minimized by the use of Silastic® sheets or nonwoven cotton pads.[8] Similarly, a thorough rinsing of the laparotomy pads will lessen the risk of adhesions and granuloma formation from lint and fabric particles.

SALPINGOLYSIS

A simple bilateral hydrosalpinx or clubbed tubes without some degree of periadnexal adhesion is a rare finding. In most cases, periovarian or peritubal adhesions must be removed prior to the fimbrioplasty. The requirement of atraumatic technique in microsurgery raises the issue of how to mobilize the uterus. Several techniques are acceptable. A Babcock clamp or similar atraumatic instrument can be used to grasp the utero–ovarian ligament on the side on which the adhesions are being lysed. Another technique involves grasping the round ligament with Babcock clamps or placing a ligature at the round ligament proximate to its insertion into the uterus. Tension is placed on these attachments to elevate the uterus out of the cul-de-sac; the adnexae are then accessible to surgical repair. A third, but far less acceptable technique, is to place a suture through the uterine fundus and use this suture to elevate the uterus to an anterior position and make the tubes and ovaries more accessible. This method, however, may lead to bleeding or shredding of uterine muscle and subsequent adhesion formation.

The reconstructive procedure involves not only lysis but removal of all adhesions. This includes both filmy and dense adhesions along the serosal surface of the tube and the ovarian surface as well as adhesions on nearby bowel and uterus. The cul-de-sac must be given special scrutiny, for this surface area may be one of the crucial sites of ovum transport from one ovary to the contralateral functioning tube. Indeed, if there has been extensive damage to the cul-de-sac from endometriosis, prior inflammation, or surgery, every effort must be exerted to create a new cul-de-sac free from factors that may lead to new adhesion formation.

A magnifying loupe facilitates the identification of anatomical planes and improves the accuracy of dissection. During the dissection, small vessels must be identified prior to their transection to minimize spillage of even minute amounts of blood into the peritoneal cavity. In the surgeon's attempt to perform reconstructive surgery in a "bloodless" manner, however, caution must be exercised to minimize tissue necrosis. It is, therefore, desirable to coagulate small vessels within the adhesions as they are encountered by either a unipolar microelectrode with pinpoint accuracy or with micro-Mallis bipolar coagulation. The author personally prefers the bipolar technique, because it provides the security that only the tissue grasped within the jaws of the microcautery will be coagulated and lessens the risk of deep or lateral thermal injury to normal tissue. Gauze sponges

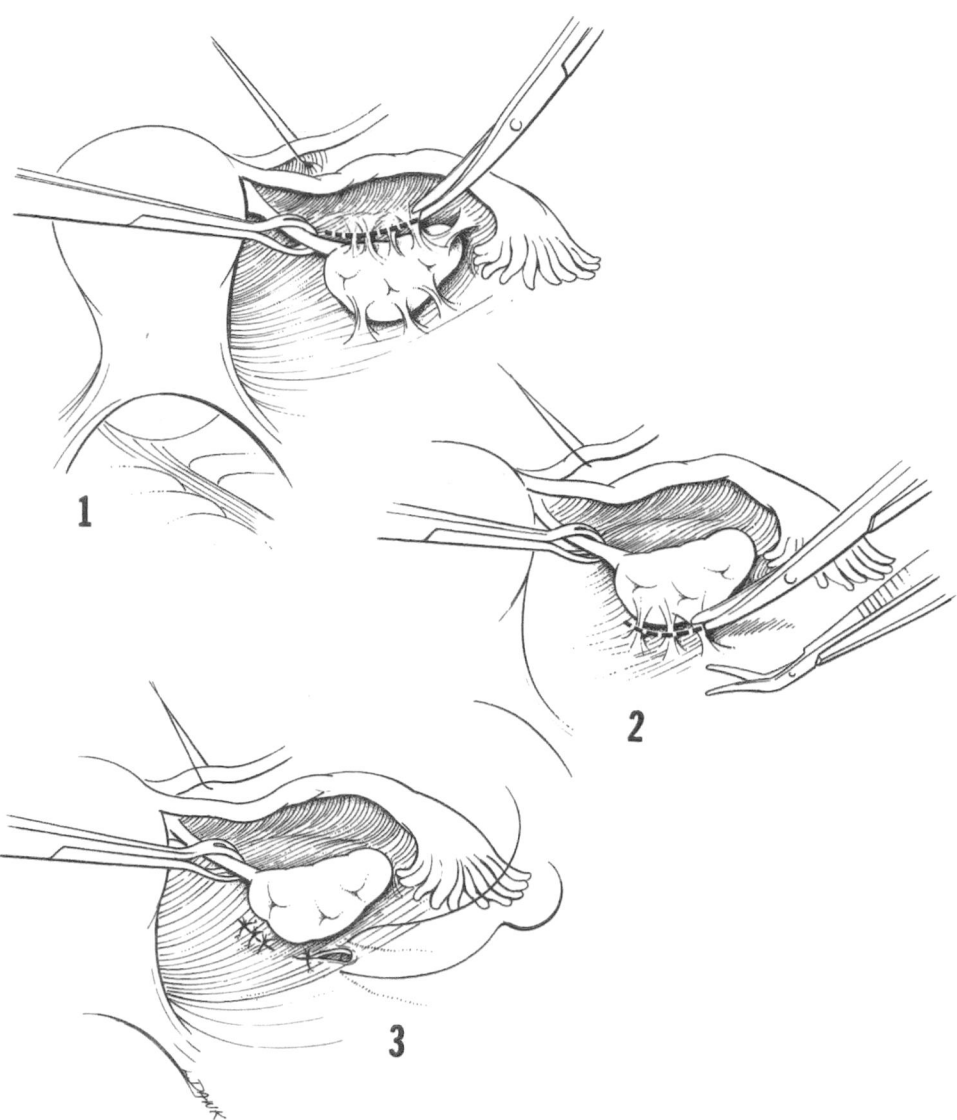

Figure 1. Lysis of adhesions. (1) Either the ipsilateral utero-ovarian ligament is grasped with a Babcock or Williams clamp or a suture is passed beneath the round ligament to elevate the uterus and adnexae. (2) Adhesions are placed on tension and removed precisely at the point of their attachment to peritoneum by sharp dissection. (3) If a defect is created in the peritoneal surface, it is repaired at that time by interrupted 6-0 Vicryl® with care taken to avoid distortion of the normal anatomy.

must not be used. Irrigation with sterile Ringer's lactate or dextran 70 keeps the structures moist and permits identification of oozing or bleeding sites that require coagulation.

Wherever possible, the adhesions should be removed by sharp dissection under direct vision (Fig. 1). Blunt dissection of adhesions can result in incomplete removal and, more importantly, may leave irregular, raw peritoneal surfaces, leading to the redevelopment of adhesions. Raw surfaces and denuded areas are reperitonealized as they are encountered or created so that these sites will not be overlooked prior to abdominal closure. The decision to reperitonealize in a continuous fashion or with interrupted sutures depends on the site to be reperitonealized. Obviously, the goal of reconstructive tubal surgery is to restore the pelvic anatomy to normality. If reperitonealization must be performed on or near the tubal serosa, then interrupted sutures of 6-0 or 8-0 Vicryl® tied with the technique of burying the knot are preferred. If reperitonealization involves the pelvic side wall, broad ligament, cul-de-sac, or bowel, then a continuous suturing technique may be employed without fear of distorting the pelvic anatomy. If the peritoneal defect is not on tension, 6-0 Vicryl® is suggested. On the other hand, if the tissues place the suture line on tension, then a 3-0 Vicryl® is employed.

Preparation for Fimbrioplastic Procedures

It is only after lysis of adhesions, complete and total mobilization of tubes and ovaries, and repair of the cul-de-sac, that the actual fimbrioplastic procedure begins. The posterior cul-de-sac may be packed with long uterine-packing gauze soaked in Ringer's solution or Macrodex®. Ideally, a small Teflon® platform can then be placed atop the packing filling the cul-de-sac. The uterus, tubes, and ovaries then lie on this platform now elevated, fully accessible, and within a comfortable working distance of the surgeon's fine microsurgical instruments.

The ovaries must be given careful attention. It is not sufficient to remove the ovaries from their adhesive attachments to tubes, broad ligaments, or other pelvic structures; the surfaces of the ovaries must be inspected for filmy, translucent adhesions which can be overlooked by the less meticulous surgeon. These "cellophanelike" adhesions or "shaggy" adhesions can be a source of ovum entrapment and resultant infertility.

CLASSIFICATION OF TUBAL DISEASE

Two groups have addressed the problem of developing a uniform method of classification of tubal disease. Adherence to a classification allows the physician a more precise method of retrospective analysis of past experience in tubal surgery and permits him to offer the patient a more reliable prospective estimate of the chances for a successful result. Such a classification system also helps the physician utilize the correct terminology for tubal surgery as suggested by the Federation of International Gynecology and Obstetrics in 1977.

In an early article, Bronson and Wallach[9] referred to an "adhesion score" that correlated to the achievement of successful pregnancy following lysis of adhesions. More recently, Hulka and co-workers[10] offered a detailed and practical method of classification (Fig. 2). The extent of adnexal adhesions is divided into four categories[10]:

Stage I: Minimal adhesions, most of the ovary is visible, and tube is patent.

Stage II: Over 50% of the ovarian surface is free with distal occlusion but preservation of rugae.

Stage III: Less than 50% of the ovarian surface is free with distal occlusion and destruction of rugae.

Stage IV: No ovarian surface is visible with bilateral hydrosalpinx.

The types of adhesions are also distinguished:

Type A: Filmy and avascular.

Type B: Dense and vascular.

Adnexa should be described separately, and the surgery should be classified according to the condition of the more normal side.

Recently, however, Caspi and co-workers[11] published a classification system that is slightly simpler in concept and thus perhaps more readily acceptable and utilized. They basically divide all patients with tubal factors into two major classifications: *Group A* consists of patients with one or

MANAGEMENT OF DISTAL TUBE DISEASE | **169**

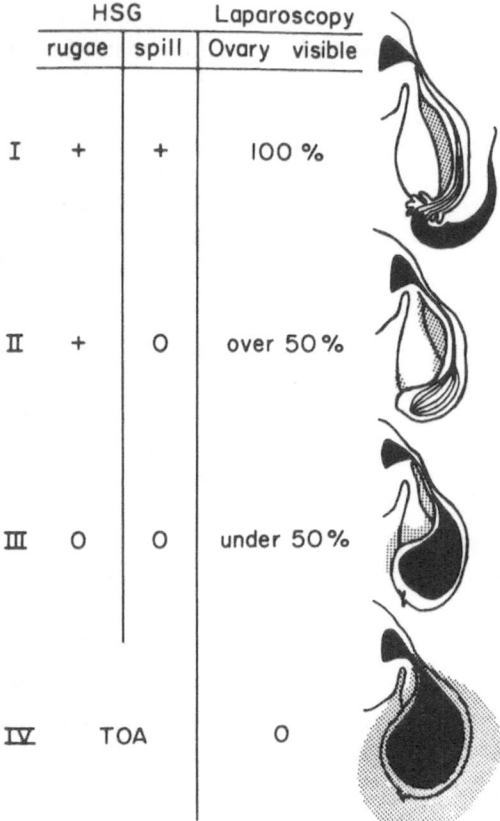

Figure 2. Classification of adnexal adhesions. From Hulka and co-workers.[10] Reprinted with the permission of the publisher, the American Fertility Society.

both tubes patent and *Group B* represents patients in whom both tubes are occluded. The adnexal adhesions are then classified as Grade I or II, filmy adhesions with minimal or extensive involvement, respectively, and Grade III or IV, dense adhesions with minimal or extensive involvement, respectively.

Either method of classification is quite satisfactory. The statistics of Caspi et al.[11] reflect a distinct relationship between grade of adhesion and pregnancy rates. A similar relationship is expressed in the results of Hulka and co-workers.[10] Clearly, as in oncology, a classification system is required to permit valid comparison of pregnancy statistics with treatment methods and to allow a rational prospective prognosis. It is urged that the infertility microsurgeon choose and consistently employ one method for the purposes of evaluating the success of his current techniques as well as forming a prognostic index.

FIMBRIOPLASTY

According to the accepted nomenclature, fimbrioplasty includes procedures such as removal of fimbrial agglutination, resection of perifimbrial constrictive bands, and incisions through the occluded distal tube to recover fimbriae. Fimbrioplasty, which involves preservation of fimbria and tubal rugae, is to be distinguished from a salpingoneostomy. Pregnancy rates following a fimbrioplasty are more favorable than those following a salpingoneostomy, because healthy fimbriae play an important role in ovum pickup and transport.

Fimbrial Agglutination

The processes involved in the identification and removal of fimbrial agglutination are basically simple, and a single-step procedure may be successful in the presence of minimal fimbrial adhesions. At the time of the laparoscopy, a narrow 3-mm smooth probe is inserted at a second puncture site above the symphysis pubis. The fimbriae are identified, and the secondary probe is inserted into the ostium. The fimbriae are probed and teased apart with great caution to prevent rupture and subsequent hemorrhage from fimbrial bridges. If more severe agglutination is present, the smooth narrow probe will frequently hook through one or several fimbrial bridges. This degree of agglutination is further documented by direct observation of the distal tube during chromopertubation. When agglutination is present, the distal ends of the tubes will distend with dye prior to spillage. It would be unwise to attempt deagglutination through the laparoscope for fear of hemorrhage or further damage through the formation of more fimbrial adhesions. Some patients with mild fimbrial agglutination may achieve a pregnancy following hysterosalpingogram or laparoscopy with chromotubation because their tubal disease is minimal. If pregnancy does not ensue within a reasonable time following the laparoscopy, then the surgeon is justified in advising a laparotomy.

At the time of laparotomy, the fimbrial bridges are identified by holding the fimbria in the gloved hand. The delicate fimbrial components are teased with narrow non-conductive probes such as glass or Teflon® rods (Fig. 3). Once isolated, these fimbrial bridges are either removed by fine-needle cautery or cauterized by micro-Mallis-type bipo-

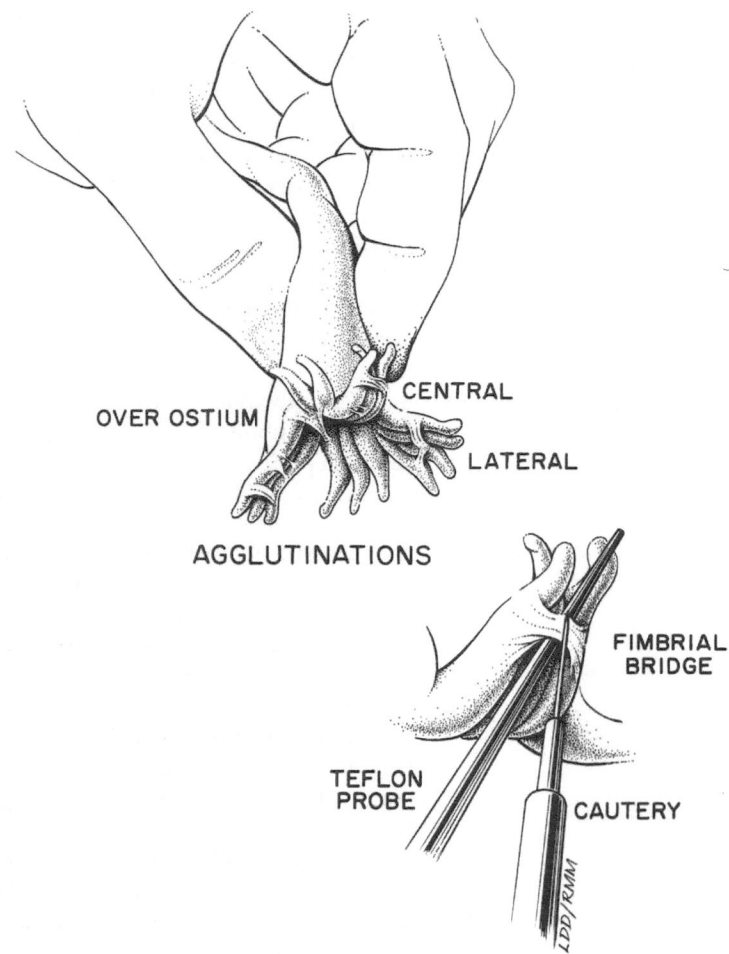

Figure 3. Deagglutination. With the tube held between the surgeon's fingers, a Teflon® probe is passed into the tubal osteum. Fimbrial bridges representing central or lateral agglutination are identified and isolated. The Teflon® probe is scored so that the unipolar microneedle cautery can easily coagulate and cut the sites of agglutination.

lar cautery and separated by a scalpel. Postoperative pregnancy rates as high as 50–70% may be expected.

Constrictive Rings of Adhesions

Constrictive rings of adhesions surrounding the fimbria can interfere with ovum pickup and transport. The typical appearance at laparoscopy or laparotomy in these cases is of a healthy Fallopian tube with "sparse" or "clubbed" fimbria. During chromotubation, the distal end of the tube dilates before the dye spills out into the pelvic cavity. Management of the constrictive bands of adhesion is similar to tubal deagglutination. The adhesions are isolated and cut with an electrosurgical needle along several sites to free the fimbria. The most effective technique utilizes a Teflon® probe to separate the adhesive band from the fimbria; a cutting current is then applied to the isolated adhesive band. An alternative approach involves transection of the full thickness of the tubal wall starting from the fimbrial osteum to beyond the sites of constriction, eversion of the edges, and fixation of the endosalpinx to the serosa with 6-0 Vicryl® sutures in interrupted fashion.

Occluded Distal Tubes

The third category of tubal disease included under the major heading of fimbrioplasty is the severely phimotic or totally occluded tube. Only 10–20% of hydrosalpinges will have fimbria with only little or no damage; the customary finding is flattened or absent fimbria and rugae. In the severely phimotic tube, the thin sheets of adhesions overlying the fimbria are put on tension by grasping these adhesions, not the tubal serosa, with very fine serrated or smooth forceps. Magnification, Teflon® or glass probes, and fine iris scissors are utilized systematically to isolate adhesions and remove them from the surface of the fimbriae. The need for everting and suturing the edges is infrequent.

The site of entry into the tubal lumen in cases of total occlusion may usually be identified as the center of a stellate white or pale area. The lumen is entered with a small puncture employing a #11 scalpel blade. A fine hemostat is then inserted into the lumen, and the fimbrial adhesions are stretched over the hemostat. Magnification aids in the identification of adhesions and the choice of the least vascular lines of dissection. The fimbrial osteum is enlarged sufficiently to allow eversion of the edges, creating a cuff approximately 1 cm wide. The edges are sutured at

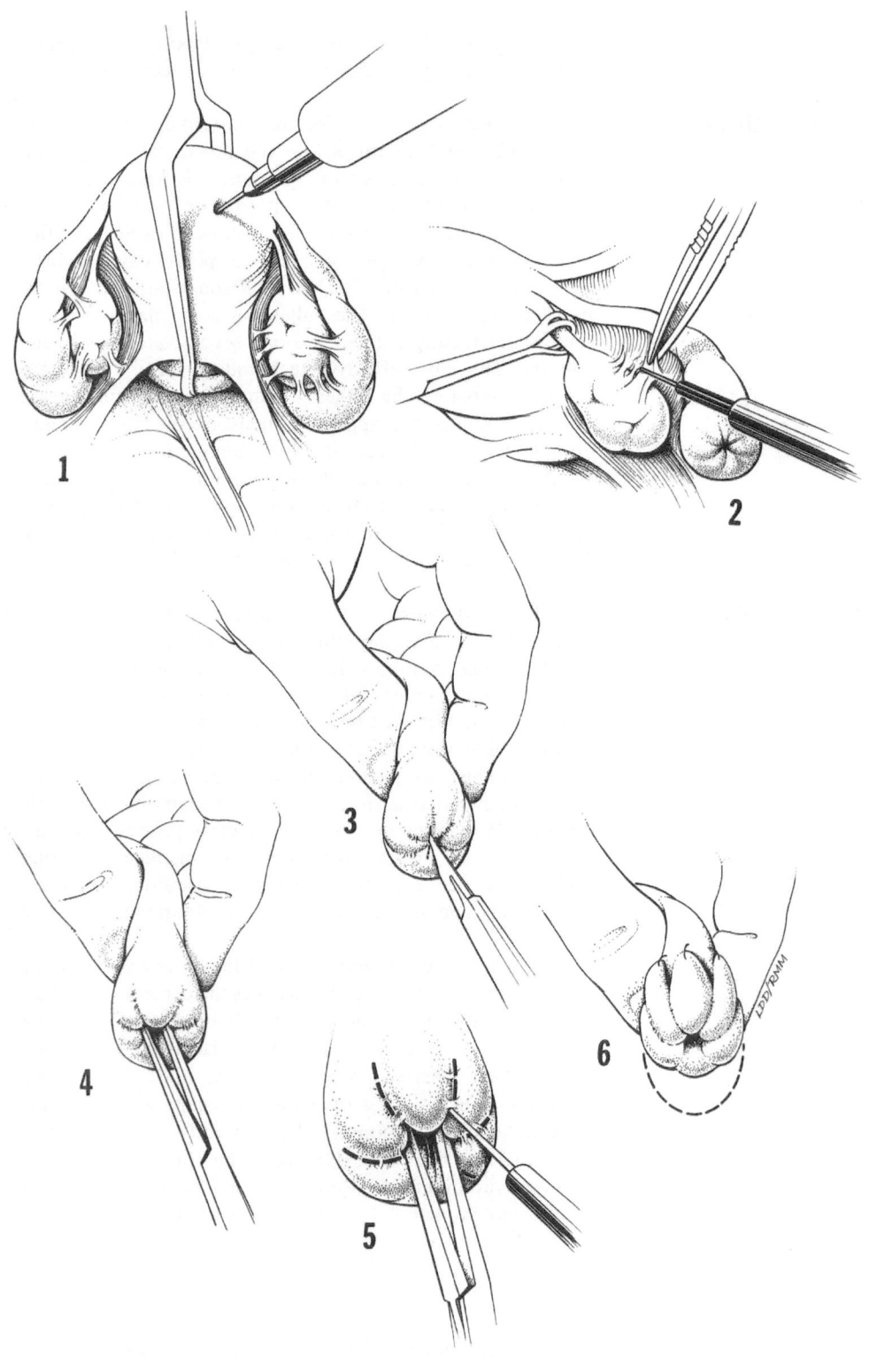

several sites to the surrounding tubal serosal surface taking care not to distort or "kink" the distal segment. The suture must be 6-0 or finer, and all knots must be buried beneath the edge of the cuff (see Fig. 4).

SALPINGONEOSTOMY

Salpingoneostomy is not unlike fimbrioplasty for complete distal occlusion. The accepted nomenclature, however, defines this operation as the creation of a new tubal osteum in the absence of identifiable fimbriae.

All peritubal and periovarian adhesions must be removed and all raw surfaces reperitonealized, as in the fimbrioplastic technique, prior to the final step of creating a tubal osteum [Fig. 4 (2)]. The distal site of tubal occlusion may be identified as the site of the stellate scar tissue or the pucker site. Magnification with loupes or microscope facilitates the identification of the appropriate site of entry into the hydrosalpinx. The tube may then be entered by either a fine, electrosurgical needle or fine, pointed scalpel [Fig. 4 (3)]. The distal salpinx is placed on tension with a fine hemostat or two fine forceps (these may be jeweler's forceps) [Fig. 4 (4)]. The osteum is widened by sharp dis-

Figure 4. Salpingoneostomy. (1) Distal tubal occlusion is confirmed by employing a Buxton or similar clamp and utero-tubal lavage with dilute indigo carmine. If there is any spillage of the dye, the site of dye egress will represent the area of severe phimosis. There will be no egress of dye if both tubes are hydrosalpinges. (2) The tube and ovary are completely mobilized by removal of all adhesions with either a unipolar microneedle cutting cautery or a bipolar microcautery. (3) With the tube held in the surgeon's hand, the central site of tubal closure is identified, and entrance into the hydrosalpinx is accomplished by a scalpel. (4) A fine hemostat is inserted into the tubal lumen, and the tubal osteum is stretched gently to avoid shredding or tearing the tissues. (5) The thinnest, least vascular tissue planes are identified with the use of a hemostat or a Teflon® probe and cut with unipolar cautery or bipolar cautery and scalpel. This process is continued until the fimbria are uncovered and freed from the distal adhesions. (6) The distal edges of the uncovered fimbria are everted and sutured to the tubal serosa with 6-0 Vicryl®. Prior to placing these sutures, the surgeon should be certain that the cuff is neither so broad as to distort the tube nor so shallow as to increase the risk of recurrent occlusion.

section along avascular planes [Fig. 4 (5)]. A cuff 1–2 cm in width is created merely by everting the edges with two atraumatic forceps or with the fingers.

An alternative, simple technique may be employed to create a large cuff. A fine skin hook is inserted into the tubal lumen for a distance of 2–3 cm. The point is passed through the entire thickness of the tubal wall by counterpressure against the point of the skin hook with fingers or forceps. This anchoring site is used as a fulcrum, and it is then simple to evert the edges and create a wide cuff. The skin hook may be used to manipulate and mobilize the tube for easier suturing. The cuff edges are secured to the tubal serosa with 6-0 to 8-0 Vicryl®, and the surgeon must be certain to bury the knot [Fig. 4 (6)].

When a new tubal osteum is created without evidence of the presence of healthy fimbria, the question arises whether the tubes will remain open and normal function return. Grant[12] advocated the use of early postoperative hydropertubations and reported an improvement in pregnancy rates from 16% in the nontreated group to 41% in the treated patients. Postoperative hydrotubations, however, carry the risk of introducing bacteria into the recently operated raw surfaces, leading to postoperative infection and recurrent tubal closure.

A number of investigators have studied the use of Silastic® hoods in salpingoneostomy. Rock et al.,[13] Buxon and Mastroianni,[14] Garcia,[15] Lamb and Moskovitz,[16] and recently Garcia and Mastroianni[6] have all advocated the use of hoods to prevent tubal closure and thereby promote fimbrial regeneration. On the hand, De Cherney and Kase[17] reported on pregnancies in four of nine women following microsurgical correction of hydrosalpinges compared to two pregnancies in nine women who underwent a two-stage tuboplasty involving Silastic® hoods. There was, however, no grading of the severity of the hydrosalpinx or adhesions. Certainly, the issue remains in controversy. It seems advisable to select the technique for each patient individually and to reserve the use of the Silastic® hood for the hydrosalpinx without healthy fimbria.

The application of the Silastic® hood, when it is determined to be appropriate, requires meticulous care. Both tubes must be completely repaired and patent with bilateral cuff salpingoneostomies. Hemostasis and reperitonealization must be complete. The distal ends of the tubes must be sufficiently free and mobile to allow placement of the hood. Prolene®, a nonabsorbable monofilament suture of 5-0 strength, is placed at three sites along the rim of the new osteum [Fig. 5 (1)]. *At no point must the silastic hood be touched by the gloved fingers or come in contact with gauze.* The surgeons must wash their gloves and instruments in a fresh saline bath to remove all tissue debris and blood clots. The hood is removed from its sterile, dust-proof container with atraumatic blunt forceps to prevent tearing or puncture of the Silastic® material and placed into a hood retractor [Fig. 5 (2)]. Three anchoring Prolene® sutures are passed through the apex of the hood with Keith needles. Care must be exercised not to entangle the six Prolene® strands. The hood is then gently lowered into position as the hood retractor guides the hood's intratubal conical portion into the distal Fallopian tube without traumatizing the endosalpinx [Fig. 5 (3)]. This may be accomplished by maintaining tension on the six Prolene® strands, thus straightening the distal end of the Fallopian tube and facilitating simple hood insertion. The Prolene® strands are tied snugly but not too tightly, for this will shred or deform the hood. The hood retractor is then carefully removed. The Prolene® is knotted several times and the strands cut to approximately ½ inch to facilitate in their identification and recovery at repeat laparotomy. Three more Prolene® 5-0 sutures are placed at the base of the hood, incorporating the hood and tubal serosa and muscularis [Fig. 5 (4)], snugly tied, and the ends cut to ½ inch.

After the application of the hoods, a uterine suspension is performed employing a modification of the Olehausen technique using #1 Vicryl® to bring the round ligament to the anterior abdominal wall. The suspension allows the tubes to remain out of the cul-de-sac where cellular debris could collect and promote adhesion formation. Prior to closure of the abdominal peritoneum, a solution of 250 cc saline containing 20 mg dexamethasone and 25 mg promethazine is instilled.

It is generally acknowledged that a midampullary salpingoneostomy has a very poor prognosis for future

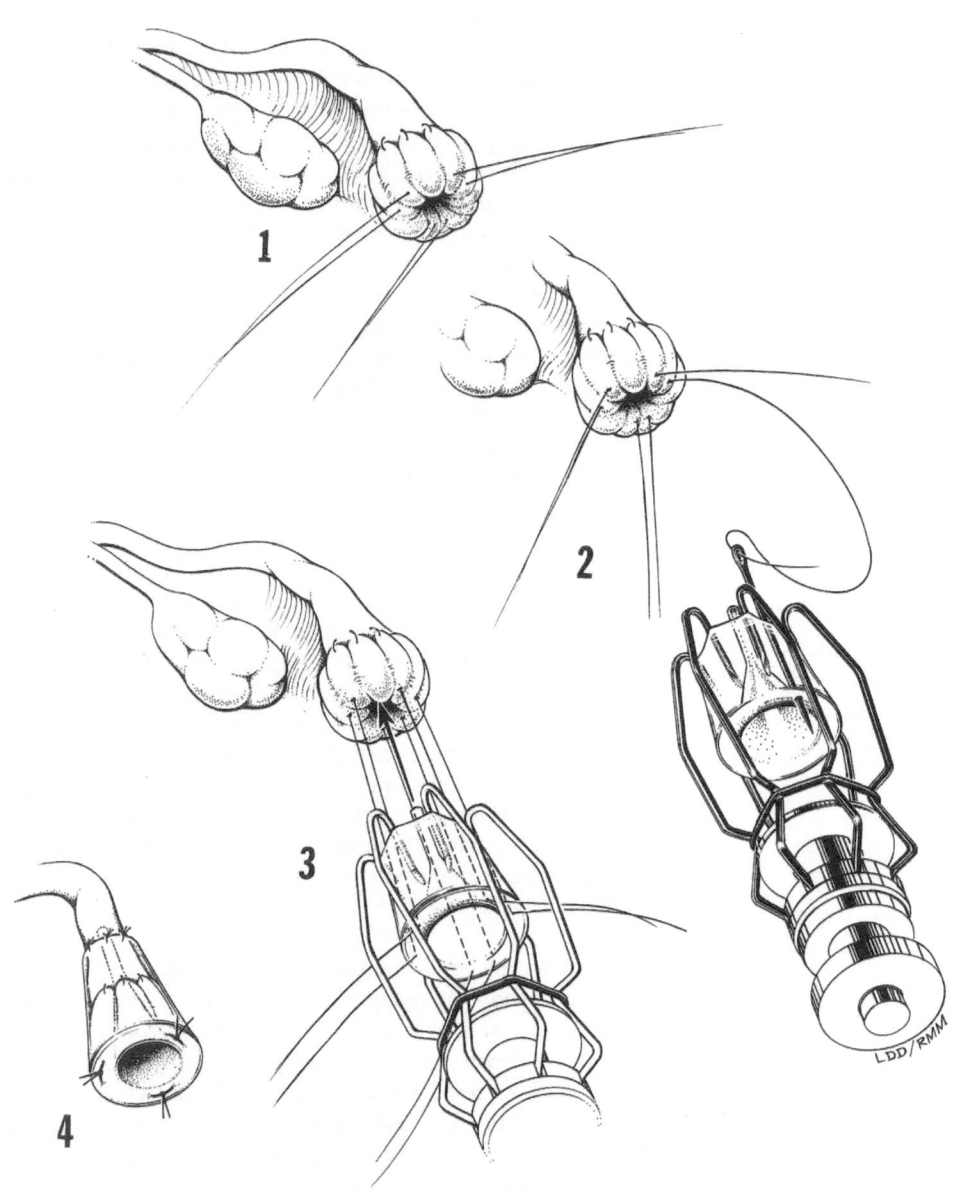

1

2

3

4

LDD/RMM

fertility. This assumption, however, has been recently challenged. Metz and Mastroianni,[18] utilizing animal models, resected the fimbriae and observed that ova were retrieved from washings of the uterus and tubes. They concluded that ova may enter the Fallopian tube through fistulae, and indeed, fimbriae were not essential for ovum pickup. Similarly, Novy[19] reported on the successful microsurgical reversal of Kroener fimbriectomy sterilization. Four of nine patients undergoing salpingoneostomy following the fimbriectomy procedure achieved pregnancy. The tubal patency rate of 83% and intrauterine pregnancy rate of 44% compare quite favorably to the pregnancy statistics relating to fimbrioplastic procedures. In general, the pregnancy rate following salpingoneostomy is approximately one-half of the tubal patency rate. Presumably, the lack of pregnancy despite tubal patency may be explained by recurrence of adhesions or by the alteration of tubal function secondary to the initial disease process. The ability of the tube to pick up the ovum and transport it at the correct pace may be disrupted by intratubal pathology.

COEXISTENT PROXIMAL AND DISTAL TUBAL OCCLUSION

If diagnostic laparoscopy reveals the presence of bilateral hydrosalpinx coexistent with bilateral cornual occlusion, the patient should be discouraged from proceeding to reconstructive laparotomy. The reported success rates following reparative surgery in these cases are uniformly poor.

Figure 5. Salpingoneostomy with application of Silastic® hoods. (1) After salpingoneostomy and the creation of an ample cuff, the fimbria and endosalpinx are noted to be severely damaged. Complete hemostasis and total removal of all adhesions should have been previously accomplished, and tubal patency established by utero–tubal lavage. Sutures of 5-0 Prolene® are then placed at three sites along the newly formed cuff. (2) The Prolene® strands are attached to straight Keith needles. The Silastic® hood has been previously placed within the hood retractor with extreme care. The Prolene® strands are passed through the apex of the hood with care to avoid entanglement of the strands or touching or contamination of the hood. (3) The surgeon then lowers the hood into position while the assistant keeps the strands and tube on tension. (4) The hood is tied in place by the three apical sutures, and three additional Prolene® sutures are placed through the base of the hood and tubal serosa and muscularis to further secure the prosthesis.

Siegler, in an extensive review,[20] suggested that tuboplasty is contraindicated with bipolar occlusion.

FACTORS LEADING TO CONCEPTION FAILURE AFTER TUBOPLASTY

One of the major causes for failure to conceive following reconstructive surgery is the recurrence or new formation of adhesions (See Chapter 11). The most effective tools to prevent formation of adhesions are careful reperitonealization, gentle handling of tissues, and meticulous hemostasis. Without strict adherence to these techniques, adhesions will form despite the use of dextran, corticosteroids, antihistamines, fibrinolysin, or antiinflammatory agents. Recurrence of adhesions is more common following reconstructive surgery to remove dense and vascular adhesions and resection of endometriosis, even with meticulous surgical technique.

If the patient has undiagnosed endometritis or chronic salpingitis, postoperative adhesions may form with disastrous effect. It is suggested that patients with evidence of old pelvic infection submit to a preoperative endometrial biopsy. Cervical cultures are to be routinely performed 1 week prior to the laparotomy, and a careful pelvic examination should be done by the principal surgeon the day before surgery. These precautions will help the surgeon identify the patient at risk for a flare-up of an old infection.

Another major factor for postoperative pregnancy failure is the irreversible damage to the endosalpinx caused by pelvic inflammatory disease. The patient with an inflammatory hydrosalpinx has at one time experienced endosalpingitis. This infection could lead to intratubal adhesions that create a honeycomb effect and may interfere with ovum pickup or transport and predispose the patient to tubal pregnancy. If these intratubal adhesions are accessible during surgery, their removal may improve the chances for a successful pregnancy. Endosalpingitis can alter the number or function of the ciliary cells, and according to Brosens and De Graef,[21] there is a direct relationship between a reduction in the numbers of ciliary cells in the fimbria and a poor prognosis for future pregnancy. Gomel[22] hypothesized that cellular alteration of the endothelium after endosalpingitis may be the reason why 53% of salpingostomy patients with patent tubes did not achieve a pregnancy. He also alludes to a possible process of tubal endothelium regeneration which may explain why 60% of his patients who achieved pregnancy following salpingostomy did so only *after* the first postoperative year.

Iatrogenic distortion of the Fallopian tube may result in failure to conceive. Repair of tubal serosal defects should, therefore, be performed with interrupted 6-0 to 8-0 sutures. The use of a continuous stitch may cause the serosal scar to shrink and distort or "kink" the tube.

Failure to create adequate fimbrial–ovarian mobility may lead to decreased pregnancy rates. The patent fimbria that is adherent to the ovary must be freed from the ovary. The distal tube must be mobile so that it can not only sweep across the surface of the ovary but also reach the cul-de-sac to achieve proper ovum pickup. Without this freedom of motion, tubal patency alone will not achieve a reasonable degree of success. Recently, two studies were reported lending credence to the efficacy of microsurgical tubal reconstruction. Diamond[23] found significantly higher pregnancy rates using the microsurgical approach. Unfortunately, the staging of adhesions was not undertaken.

In an eloquent extensive appraisal of microsurgical technique, Siegler and Kontopoulos[24] concluded that microsurgery improved the term pregnancy results among patients undergoing anastomosis, salpingoneostomy, and fimbrioplasty (See Chapter 5).

The results following microsurgical repair of bilateral hydrosalpinx seem to indicate term pregnancy rates of 30–40%. Recently, De Cherney and Kase[17] reported a term pregnancy rate of 44% with no ectopic pregnancies. The results of this study are most impressive; however, the number of patients (9) is small. In a larger series, Gomel[25] reported a 30% term pregnancy rate with 10% ectopic pregnancies among 72 patients. Garcia and Mastroianni[6] report a 40% pregnancy rate with the use of Silastic® hoods with a 6–8% ectopic pregnancy rate in an extensive clinical experience.

CONCLUSIONS   The conclusions that may be drawn from reported results of studies on the management of distal tube disease are irrefutable. The gentle handling of the pelvic organ, the preservation or creation of smooth peritoneal surfaces, the accurate and meticulous removal of adhesions, and meticulous hemostasis are the primary advances that have been made in the field of infertility surgery. The use of loupes or an operating microscope merely grants the surgeon the ability to observe the pelvic structure at closer range. Certainly, not every surgeon who wears loupes or employs the microscope can call himself or herself a "microsurgeon" without the careful tissue handling and hundreds of hours of teaching and practice involved in the learning and performance of tubal reconstructive surgery.

REFERENCES

1. Riddick DH, De Grazia CT, Maenza RM: Comparison of polyglactic and polyglycolic acid sutures in reproductive tissue. *Fertil Steril* 28:1220, 1977.
2. Meldrum D: Femoral nerve compression injury and tubal microsurgery. *Fertil Steril* 32:345, 1979.
3. Sanfilippo JS, Barrows GH, Yussman MA: Comparison of avitene, topical thrombin, and Gelfoam as sole hemostatic agent in tuboplasties. *Fertil Steril* 33:311, 1980.
4. Blandau RJ: Comparative aspects of tubal anatomy and physiology as they relate to reconstructive procedures. *J Reprod Med* 21:7, 1978.
5. Replogle RL, Johnson R, Gross R: Prevention of post-operative intestinal adhesions with combined promethazine and dexmethasone therapy. *Ann Surg* 163:580, 1966.
6. Garcia CR, Mastroianni L: Microsurgery for treatment of adnexal disease. *Fertil Steril* 34:413, 1980.
7. Yoffe H, Beyth Y, Reinhartz T., et al: Foreign body gramulomas in peritubal and periovarian adhesions: A possible cause for unsuccessful reconstructive surgery in infertility. *Fertil Steril* 33:277, 1980.
8. Swolin K, Bendz A, Larsson B, et al: Traumatization of the abdominal serosa. A comparison between non-woven and cotton abdominal swabs. *Acta Chir Scand* 140:203, 1974.
9. Bronson RA, Wallach EE: Lysis of periadnexal adhesions for correction of infertility. *Fertil Steril* 28:613, 1977.
10. Hulka J, Omran K, Berger G: Classification of adnexal adhesions: A proposal and evaluation of its prognostic value. *Fertil Steril* 30:661, 1978.
11. Caspi E, Halperin Y, Bukovsky I: The importance of periadnexal adhesions in tubal reconstructive surgery for infertility. *Fertil Steril* 31:296, 1979.
12. Grant A: Infertility surgery of the oviduct. *Fertil Steril* 22:496, 1971.
13. Rock J, Mulligan WJ, Easterday CL: Polyethylene in tuboplasty. *Obstet Gynecol* 3:21, 1954.
14. Buxton CL, Mastroianni L: Surgical treatment of infertility. *Obstet Gynecol* 20:844, 1962.
15. Garcia CR: Surgical reconstruction of the oviduct in the infertile pa-

tient, in Behrman SJ, Kistner RW (eds): *Progress in Infertility*. Boston, Little, Brown, 1968, p 255.

16. Lamb EJ, Moskovitz W: Tuboplasty for infertility: A review of 100 cases. *Int J Fertil* 17:53, 1972.

17. De Cherney, AH, Kase NG: A comparison of treatments for bilateral fimbrial occlusion. *Fertil Steril [Suppl]* 33:240, 1980.

18. Metz K, Mastroianni L: Dispensability of fimbriae: Ovum pickup by tubal fistulas in the rabbit. *Fertil Steril* 32:329, 1979.

19. Novy M: Reversal of Kroener fimbriectomy sterilization. *Am J Obstet Gynecol* 137:198, 1980.

20. Siegler A: Surgical treatment for tuboperitoneal causes of infertility since 1967. *Fertil Steril* 28:1019, 1977.

21. Brosens IA, De Graef R: Microbiospy of the Fallopian tube as a method for clinical investigation of tubal function in infertility. *Int J Fertil* 20:55, 1975.

22. Gomel V: Causes of failed reconstructive tubal microsurgery. *J Reprod Med* 24:239, 1980.

23. Diamond E: Lysis of post-operative pelvic adhesions in infertility. *Fertil Steril* 31:287, 1979.

24. Siegler AM, Kontopoulos V: An analysis of macrosurgical and microsurgical techniques in the management of the tuboperitoneal factor in infertility. *Fertil Steril* 32:377, 1979.

25. Gomel V: Microsurgery of the oviduct for infertility, in: *Infertility Surgery, Syllabus Courses IV*. Presented at the 36th Annual meeting of the American Fertility Society, Houston, March 18–22, 1980.

9 Uterotubal Implantation

John A. Rock

Department of Gynecology and Obstetrics
Division of Reproductive Endocrinology
Reproductive Surgery
The Johns Hopkins Hospital
Baltimore, Maryland 21205

In the past, proximal obstruction (intramural or isthmic obstruction) has been considered an indication for uterotubal implantation. However, with the development of microsurgical techniques for cornual–isthmic anastomosis that produce pregnancy success rates reported in excess of 60%,[1] uterotubal implantation is now primarily reserved for patients with intramural obstruction. Furthermore, patients are candidates for uterotubal implantation using the posterior fundal incision technique when one encounters a short oviduct the mobilization of which is difficult without distortion of the tubo-ovarian relationship. Although uterotubal implantation is considered a rather gross technique, the reproductive surgeon should approach this procedure with the same attitude as when performing a tubal anastomosis. Gentle handling of tissues with fine instruments to avoid serosal trauma, the use of a delicate electrocautery needle for precise hemostasis, and the use of fine nonreactive suture will decrease postoperative adhesion formation. The use of minimal magnification ($\times 1.7-\times 2.5$) assists in the placement of sutures and in obtaining accurate tissue approximation as well as complete hemostasis. Using these precepts, the surgeon should minimize iatrogenic adhesion formation, which should improve surgical results and subsequent pregnancy success.

This chapter will describe the techniques of uterotubal implantation in patients with intramural obstruction or shortened oviducts. Specifically, this section will review the current status of uterotubal implantation in light of the development of microsurgical techniques for tubo-tubal anastomosis.

UTEROTUBAL JUNCTION

The length of the intramural portion of the oviduct may range from 1.5 to 2.5 cm.[2] Its pathway is characterized by convolutions and abrupt changes in direction. The lumen follows a straight course through the uterine wall to the muscular layer and then angles sharply into the vascular layer.[3] Thus, any attempt to pass a probe into the uterus most often results in false passage.

The uterotubal junction may serve as a mechanical barrier and a site of sperm reserve in some species.[4] The importance of intrinsic motility in sperm transport through the uterotubal junction is unclear. Motile sperm may be transported more efficiently than dead sperm; however, dead sperm do pass through the junction[5] in the gilt. These observations suggest that contractions or fluid currents may play some role in sperm transport. Furthermore, the competence of the uterotubal junction varies with the hormonal environment in several species.[6] Unfortunately, conflicting results in different species limit the application of these animal observations to the human.

If the uterotubal junction is removed in rabbits, sperm migration, fertilization, and ovum transport culminate in implantation of a fertilized ovum at a decreased frequency.[7] However, Winston[1] has reported intrauterine pregnancies in 11 of 16 patients after microsurgical tubocornual anastomosis (ampullary intramural). Furthermore, pregnancy does occur in patients following uterotubal implantation where the uterotubal junction is removed. Thus, pregnancy is possible if the uterotubal junction is absent or destroyed.

DIAGNOSTIC TECHNIQUES

Proximal occlusion with abnormal fimbria and distal fimbrial obstruction are contraindications of uterotubal implantation. Patients with dense pelvic or adnexal adhesions with fixation of the ovary to the broad ligament and/or pelvic side wall have a poor prognosis for conception after uterotubal implantation.[8,9] It is therefore essential that a careful and accurate laparoscopic assessment of the pelvis be performed to aid in patient selection.

Each patient with proximal obstruction receives a complete infertility evaluation including documentation of ovulatory status, postcoital test, and an analysis of the husband's semen. Prior to uterotubal implantation, an evaluation of the intramural block should consist of two diagnostic tests, hysterosalpingography and laparoscopy. Errors in technique and mistaken interpretation of results of hysterosalpingography can account for inaccurate diagnoses by this technique. False-positive laparoscopy findings of cornual obstruction may be expected in 3% of patients (J. A. Rock, unpublished data, 1980). In the author's opinion, hysterosalpingography is easy to perform with minimal risk to the patient and is superior to laparoscopy in the diagnosis of intrauterine or endometrial lesions. Therefore, hysterosalpingography and laparoscopy should be looked on not as alternative but rather as complementary diagnostic procedures.

SURGICAL TECHNIQUES

General Considerations

One should make every attempt to maintain tuboovarian spatial relationships and to preserve as much Fallopian tube as possible. Although the minimum length of Fallopian tube necessary for conception has not been determined, preliminary results suggest that pregnancy rates following tubal reanastomosis are highest where 4–5 cm of Fallopian tube are preserved[10] (R. M. L. Winston, personal communication, 1980).

There are three principal types of uterine incisions for the creation of a stoma for tubal implantation (Fig. 1). Bonney[11] advocated sharp excision of a cornual wedge prior to implantation, whereas Holden and Sovak[12] used a reamer to make a cornual opening prior to implantation. There have been numerous modifications of these techniques, including the transverse fundal incision which enables the surgeon to visualize clearly the position of the implanted tube as it is sutured into place.[13] Most recently, Von Csaba et al.[14] and Peterson et al.[15] reported uterotubal implantation through a posterior fundal incision between the utero-ovarian liga-

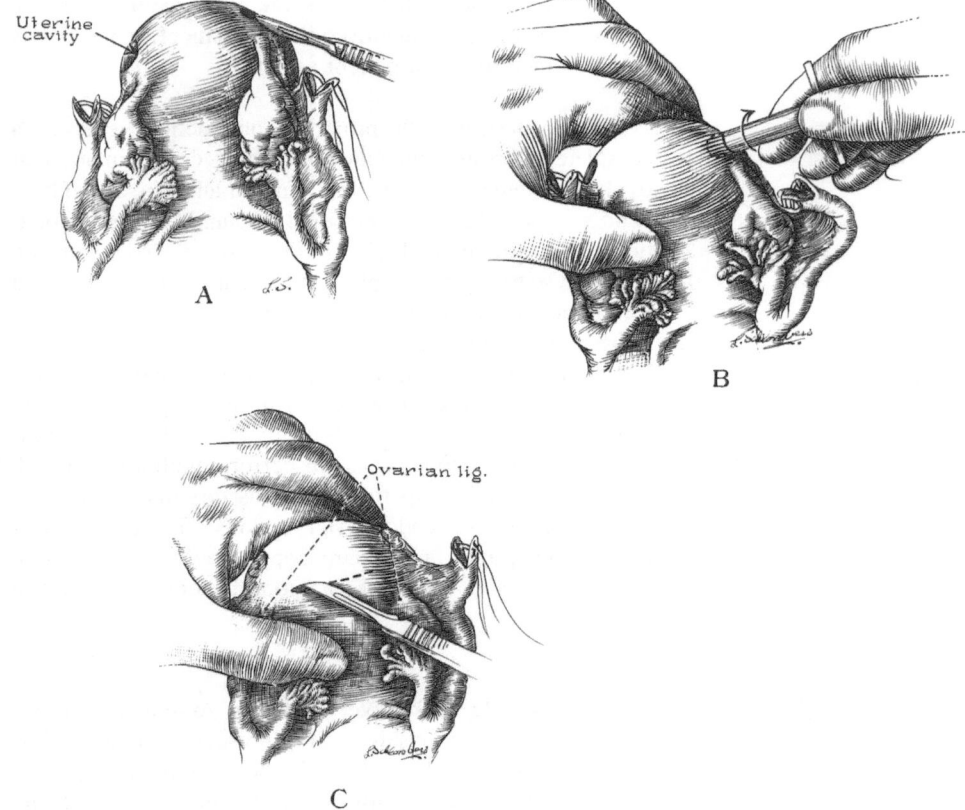

Figure 1. Uterine incisions for implantation techniques. (A) Sharp cornual wedge excision; (B) reamer; (C) posterior fundal technique. (From Jones and Rock,[26] reprinted with permission of the publisher.)

ments. Peterson et al.[15] advocated the transverse fundal approach to overcome difficulties with mobilization of a shortened tube, where cornual implantation might distort the normal utero-ovarian relationships. Furthermore, this procedure is purported to take advantage of any sphincteric action of the uterotubal junction which is removed with cornual implantation.

There is controversy as to whether the isthmic or ampullary portion of the Fallopian tube should be inserted into the uterus. Palmer[16] reported a series of 118 patients who underwent uterotubal implantation, 25 of whom received an isthmic implantation. When compared to the 93 ampullary implantations, a 10% difference was noted in the term pregnancy rate. Unfortunately, variation in technique, histological diagnosis, and the extent of disease were not taken into consideration in these comparisons. The author reviewed 52 patients following uterotubal implantation, 17 of whom received an ampullary implantation.[9] The term pregnancy rate was 10% higher in this group than among 35 patients who received isthmic implantation. The highest pregnancy rate was observed in patients who received ampullary implantation with the reamer technique. This improved pregnancy rate resulted in part from the lower reobstruction rate of these patients. Consideration must be given to the fact that fewer patients with chronic salpingitis had ampullary implantation; therefore, these observations must be stated with reservation. As larger numbers of patients accumulate, comparisons of homogeneous groups may allow us to resolve this controversy.

In light of our observation that the reobstruction rate in our series of patients was markedly decreased when the wider lumen had been implanted into the uterus, it has been our practice to sacrifice the isthmus when implanting the tube into the cornua. The posterior fundal incision technique, in our experience, has been useful in patients with excessively short tubes. Thus, the ampulla is implanted into the posterior uterus.

Cornual Uterotubal Implantation

A generous transverse abdominal incision in most instances will provide excellent exposure. However, we prefer to leave the muscles attached to the fascia so that the muscles may be partially split if further exposure is indicated. The lateral abdominal walls are then wrapped with Sof-Wick® (Johnson & Johnson) low-lint laparotomy pads. Filmy adhesions may then be lysed with fine-needle electrocautery and removed. Once both tubes are completely mobilized, one should again test for tubal patency. If proximal obstruction is noted, one should incise the tube approximately 0.5 cm from the cornua and attempt to pass a 2-0 nylon suture into the uterus. On occasion, this may pass freely into the uterus, demonstrating the fickleness of our present methods to document proximal obstruction. If this occurs, it is our practice to insert approximately 20 in. of 2-0 nylon into the uterus and pass the nylon distally through

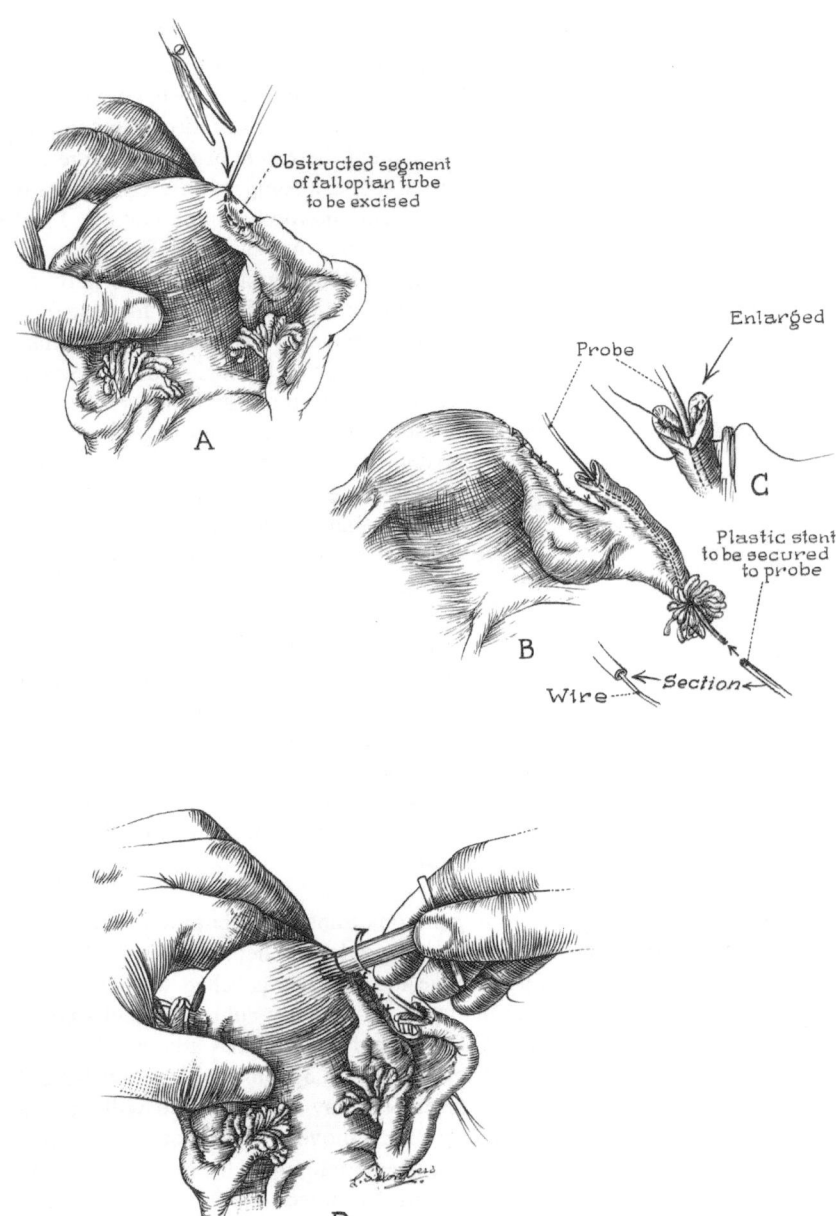

Figure 2. Ampullary–uterotubal implantation. (A) The obstructed proximal segment of Fallopian tube is excised. If an ampullary implantation is desired, sufficient isthmus must be sacrificed. (B) A fine lachrymal duct probe to which a Teflon® ring prosthesis (0.028–0.68 ID) is attached is placed through the fimbriated portion of the Fallopian tube and brought through the lumen of the tube. (C) The end of the oviduct to be implanted into the uterus is split longitudinally for a distance of 0.5 cm. A 5-0 polygalactic suture is then placed through the edge of each end. (D) A 7-mm reamer is used to remove the interstitial portion of the Fallopian tube. Small monofilament nylon suture may be placed at the ring for easy extraction of the splint at a later date. A #28 wire guide within the Teflon® splint lends rigidity and serves to prevent expulsion. (E) A fine hemostat is inserted through the uterine defect on the opposite side, and the tip of the Teflon® splint is grasped and brought through the uterine cavity so that the ring rests at the midportion of the cavity. A needle director over which a Ferguson needle

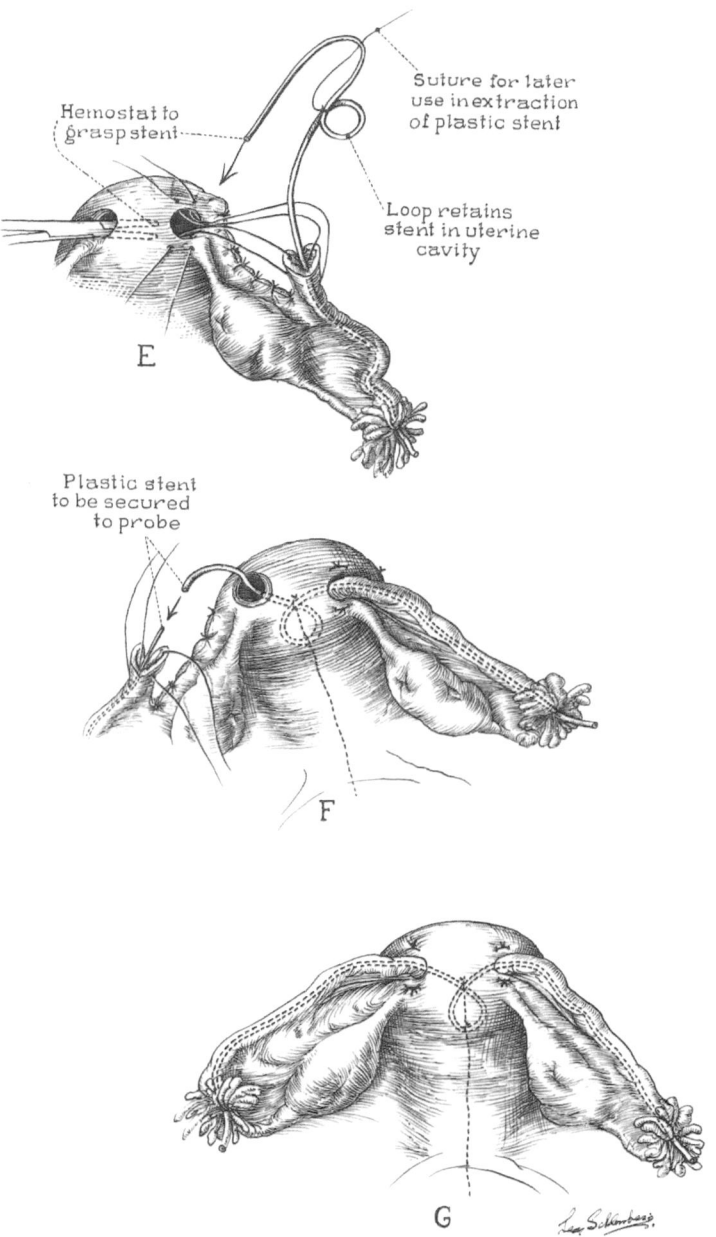

Hemostat to
grasp stent

Suture for later
use in extraction
of plastic stent

Loop retains
stent in uterine
cavity

E

Plastic stent
to be secured
to probe

F

G

may be guided may be introduced into the uterine defect so that two sutures are brought out through the anterior uterine wall, whereas the other two sutures are brought out through the posterior uterine wall. These sutures are tied securely as the tube is inserted into the uterine cavity. The oviductal serosa may be sutured to the adjacent uterine serosa with interrupted 7-0 nonreactive absorbable suture. (F) The small lachrymal duct probe is then gently inserted into the fimbrial portion of the distal segment of the oviduct on the opposite side. The stent is attached to the probe and pulled through the lumen, and the polygalactic sutures are then placed through the longitudinally split oviduct and brought out through the anterior and posterior uterine walls and tied securely. On occasion, a few 6-0 polyglactic sutures are necessary to approximate the mesosalpinx. (G) The Teflon® splint is in place with both ampullary portions of the oviduct implanted into the uterine cavity. (From Jones and Rock,[26] reprinted with permission of the publisher.)

the fimbriated portion of the tube, over which a two-layer isthmic anastomosis is performed. If, however, obstruction is noted, one may then shave portions of the Fallopian tube until the intramural portion of the oviduct is encountered (Fig. 2A). If this is obstructed, one should then proceed with the techniques for cornual uterotubal implantation.

Preparation of the Distal Oviduct

Our results following uterotubal implantation have suggested that the reobstruction rate is lower and the pregnancy rate higher if the ampullary portion of the Fallopian tube is implanted into the uterus. Therefore, it has been our practice to sacrifice approximately 2 cm of Fallopian tube to reveal an ampullary lumen for uterotubal implantation.

We have preferred using a Teflon® ring splint to maintain established patency (Fig. 3). A small monofilament nylon suture may be placed at the ring for easy extraction at a later date. A #28 wire guide within the Teflon® splint lends rigidity and serves to prevent expulsion. A fine lachrymal duct probe to which a Teflon® ring prosthesis is

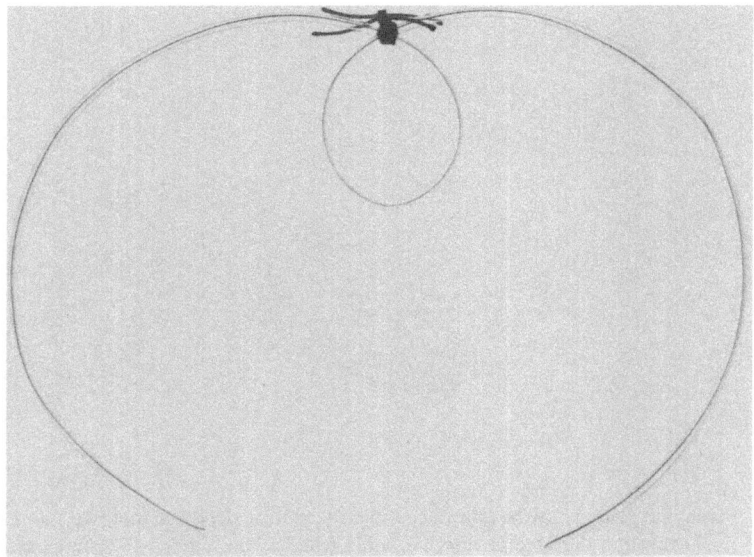

Figure 3. Teflon® ring prosthesis with #28 wire guide. Size range: internal diameter, 0.027–0.053 cm; external diameter, 0.047–0.077 cm. (From Jones and Rock,[26] reprinted with permission of the publisher.)

attached is passed through the fimbriated portion of the oviduct. The probe is then retracted, bringing the Teflon® through the lumen of the tube (Fig. 2B). The Teflon® must be carefully selected, so that the smallest diameter is utilized. With an ampullary implantation, this consideration is often moot, as the lumen is quite large. The end of the oviduct to be implanted into the uterus is then split longitudinally for a distance of 0.5 cm (Fig. 2C). This is required with an ampullary implantation so as to minimize the possibility of tearing the anterior and posterior portions of the Fallopian tube as each is sutured to the wall of the uterus. By slightly bivalving the tube, one can separate the ends easily and still avoid tension.

Once the end of the oviduct is bivalved by a longitudinal split, a suture of 5-0 nonreactive absorbable suture is then placed through the edge of each end (Fig. 2C).

Uterine Incision

A uterine stoma is created with the use of a 7-mm reamer (cork borer). When the intramural portion of the Fallopian tube is removed, the uterus should be grasped with the left hand so that the thumb stabilizes the posterior wall of the uterus (Fig. 2D). The reamer then may be precisely guided toward the uterine cavity while excising the intramural portion of the tube as the core.

Tubal Implantation

A fine hemostat is inserted through the uterine defect on the opposite side, and the tip of the Teflon® splint is grasped and brought through the uterine cavity so that the ring rests at the midportion of the cavity (Fig. 2E). The opposite oviduct is then prepared to be brought through the splint (Fig. 2F). A grooved needle director over which a Ferguson needle may be guided is introduced into the uterine defect so that two sutures are brought out through the anterior uterine wall and the additional two sutures through the posterior uterine wall. These sutures are tied securely as the tube is inserted into the uterine cavity (Fig. 2G). The oviductal serosa may be sutured to the adjacent uterine serosa with several interrupted sutures of 7-0 nonreactive absorbable suture.

Posterior Fundal Uterotubal Implantation

When the tubes are shortened (3–4 cm), we prefer a posterior fundal uterotubal implantation. The tube is mobilized to perform a posterior implantation. The Fallo-

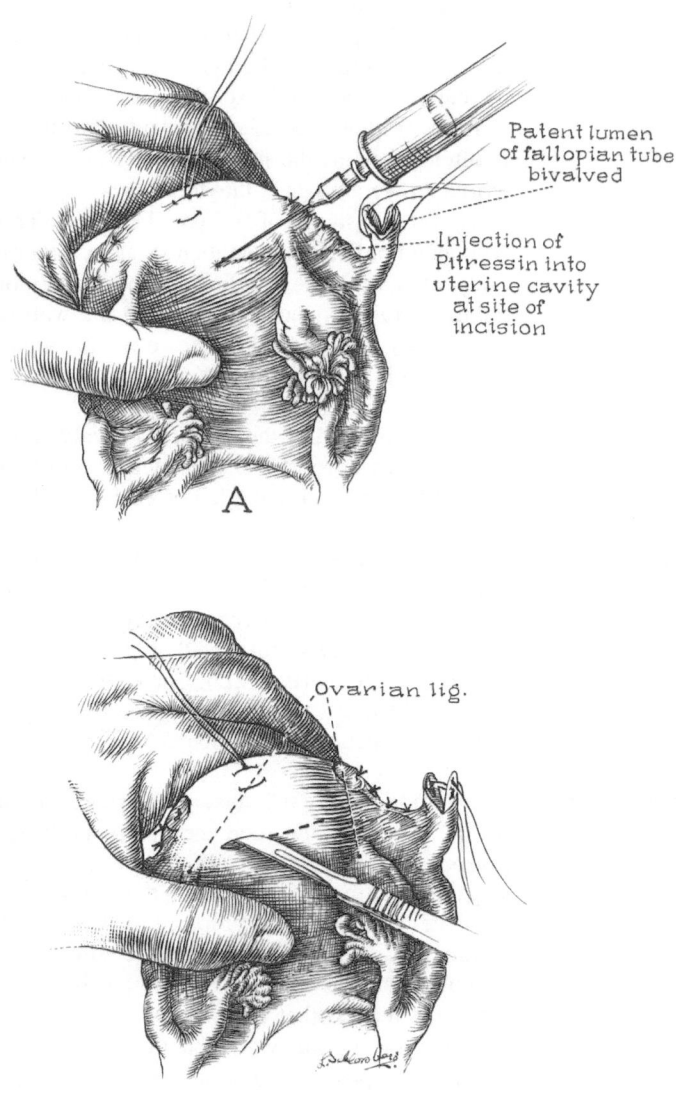

Patent lumen of fallopian tube bivalved

Injection of Pitressin into uterine cavity at site of incision

A

Ovarian lig.

B

Figure 4. Posterior fundal uterotubal implantation. (A) Sufficient isthmus is sacrificed to reveal an ampullary lumen. The tube is then split longitudinally, and a suture of 5-0 polygalactic suture is placed through the edge of each end. The posterior uterine fundus is then injected with a dilute solution of Vasopressin (Pitressin®) (1 : 20 saline dilution) or approximately 1 U/cc. (B) A posterior fundal incision exposes the posterior uterine cavity, and the ampullary portions of the Fallopian tubes are then

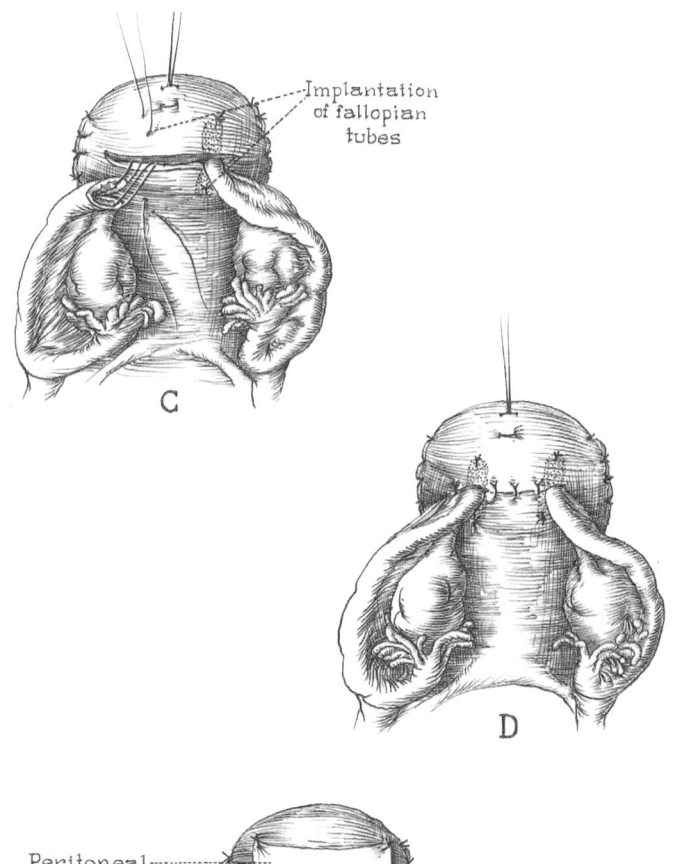

Implantation of fallopian tubes

C

D

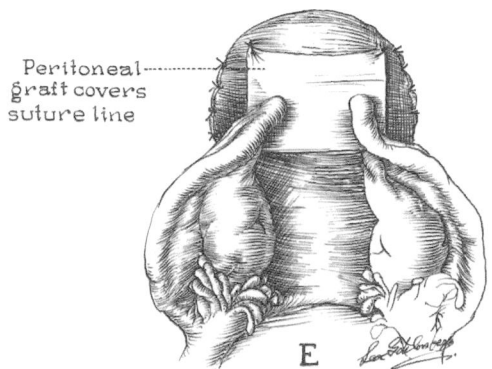

Peritoneal graft covers suture line

E

inserted into the uterine cavity. (C) The Vicryl® sutures are brought out superior and inferior to the transverse incision and tied securely. (D) Myometrium of the uterus is closed in two layers, the first consisting of interrupted 3-0 nonreactive absorbable suture, and the second of a serosal approximation. (E) A peritoneal graft taken from the anterior abdominal wall may then be placed over the incision to minimize adhesion formation.

pian tube is prepared in a similar manner as described for a cornual implantation. The posterior fundus is injected with a dilute solution of vasopressin (Pitressin®) (1 : 20 saline dilution) (Fig. 4A). A posterior fundal incision, approximately 4 cm, is placed between the utero-ovarian ligaments, thus exposing the posterior uterine cavity (Fig. 4B). The ampullary portions of the Fallopian tube are then inserted into the uterine cavity, and the nonreactive absorbable suture is brought out through the uterus, superior and inferior to the transverse incision, and tied securely (Fig. 4C). The myometrium between the Fallopian tubes is then closed in two layers, the first consisting of interrupted 3-0 nonreactive absorbable suture, and the second of a serosal approximation using interrupted sutures of 6-0 nonreactive absorbable suture (Fig. 4D). A peritoneal graft is then taken from the anterior abdominal wall and placed over the incision to minimize adhesion formation (Fig. 4E).

POSTOPERATIVE THERAPY

All patients receive prophylactic antibiotics to minimize the possibility of an acute flare of postoperative salpingitis. We have not used steroids or antihistamines postoperatively, although during the procedure the peritoneal cavity is lavaged with copius amounts of lactate Ringer's solution containing 1 g of hydrocortisone and 5000 units of heparin per liter. The Teflon® splint is left in place for 4 months and then removed through the cervix with a Novak curet. A postoperative hysterosalpingogram is performed 2 months after splint removal. A second-look laparoscopy is performed if the patient has not conceived within the subsequent 13 ovulatory cycles.

COMPLICATIONS

Complications following uterotubal implantation among 52 patients with proximal obstruction are summarized in Table I. The most common complication observed was postmenstrual irregular spotting. In most instances, this will resolve without therapy and appears to be associated with the presence of the intrauterine Teflon® splint. On occasion, however, progestin therapy may be necessary to prevent this irregular shedding of endometrial tissue. Two patients developed excessive menstrual bleeding, which resolved on oral contraceptive therapy while the splint was in place. One patient had a flare of chronic pelvic

Table I
Complications following Uterotubal Implantation
(52 Patients)

Difficult prosthesis removal	0
Irregular bleeding (spotting)	18 (35%)
Hypermenorrhea	2 (4%)
Endometriosis caused by retrograde menstruation	0
Cornual repture of an intrauterine pregnancy	0
Escape of prosthesis into peritoneal cavity	0
Ectopic gestation	2 (4%)
Flare of chronic pelvic inflammatory disease	1 (2%)

inflammatory disease 1 week postoperatively and was treated with intravenous antibiotic therapy. This patient conceived approximately 4 months postoperatively and delivered a term infant. Two patients (4%) developed ectopic pregnancies in the ampullary portion of the Fallopian tube. This ectopic pregnancy rate is similar to that reported by Grant[17] and Wirtz.[18]

We have advised our patients to accept a delivery by cesarean section. There were no ruptures of the uterus as a result of the weakening of the uterine wall at the cornua in any of our patients following cornual uterotubal implantation.

Shirodkar[8] advocated the use of a pseudopregnancy regimen during the first 4 postoperative months following uterotubal implantation. He felt that this prevented endometriosis caused by menstrual blood spilling through the shortened tube. Endometriosis has not been observed as a complication of uterotubal implantation in our series.

FAILURE OF UTEROTUBAL IMPLANTATION

A life table analysis of pregnancy success following uterotubal implantation reveals that the maximum cumulative rate of pregnancy is achieved approximately 48 months after surgery (Fig. 5). A few pregnancies occur after that time. In fact, a majority of the pregnancies occur within the first 18 months following surgery. Therefore, the strict definition of failure would include the failure to conceive after 48 months provided the patient has had regular ovulatory cycles and an adequate male factor. It has been our recent

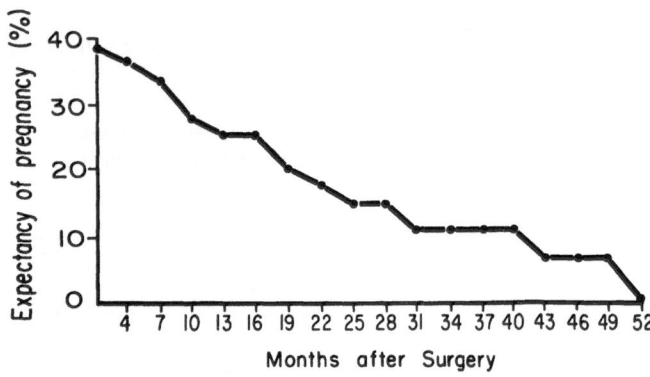

Figure 5. Life table analysis. Expectancy of pregnancy in 52 patients treated with uterotubal implantation. (From Rock et al.,[9] reprinted with permission of the publisher.)

practice to perform diagnostic laparoscopy after 13 ovulatory cycles if the patient has not conceived. This allows us the opportunity to lyse adhesions and to directly visualize patency with insufflation of indigo carmine dye.

If the patient does not conceive, this may be attributable to a variety of factors, which may be divided into two categories, postoperative obstruction and technical errors (Table II). Tubal obstruction may occur because of adenomyosis and/or fibrosis as a result of an inflammatory reaction to the splint. Furthermore, a flare of chronic pelvic inflammatory disease or a postoperative ascending salpingitis may result in subsequent proximal and/or distal fimbrial obstruction. In our experience with the ampullary im-

Table II
Etiology of Failure of Techniques of Uterotubal Implantation

Postoperative obstruction
  Tubal obstruction caused by adenomyosis and/or fibrosis.
  Flare of chronic pelvic inflammatory disease with subsequent proximal and/or distal obstruction.
Technical errors
  Hematoma formation with explusion of the implanted tube.
  Escape of the prosthesis into the peritoneal cavity with subsequent adhesion formation.
  Proximal oviduct malposition so that the lumen is buried in the uterine mucosa or extends too far into the cavity.
  Lack of microsurgical atraumatic techniques.

plantation, obstruction is rare. With the use of prophylactic antibiotics, salpingitis should rarely be observed.

Technical errors may result in failure of uterotubal implantation. If careful hemostasis is not achieved, hematoma formation may result in the expulsion of the implanted tube. Furthermore, if careful attention is not directed toward prosthesis placement within the uterine cavity, it may be subsequently expelled into the abdominal cavity, resulting in peritoneal reaction and adhesion formation. Proximal oviduct malposition may result if the sutures through the tips of the ampulla are tied so as to bury the tubal ostia in the uterine mucosa. Furthermore, if the sutures are brought too close to the midline of the uterus, the oviduct may extend too far into the uterine cavity. Finally, and perhaps more importantly, the lack of microsurgical atraumatic techniques may result in postoperative adhesion formation.

In our most recent series of 18 patients following uterotubal implantation, all patients had documented tubal patency. In four patients, post-uterotubal-implantation laparoscopy revealed normal appearing oviducts with free spill of dye into the peritoneal cavity. In one patient, filmy adhesions noted about the shaft of the tube and the ovary were lysed during laparoscopy. In patients who have not conceived as of this date, no obvious technical errors have been demonstrated.

RESULTS AND DISCUSSION

Successful pregnancy following uterotubal implantation is thought to depend on the operative technique, the extent of adhesion formation, tubal pathology, and pre- and postoperative management. In addition, the postoperative tubo-ovarian relationship and the length of the oviduct may also have a bearing on pregnancy success. Comparison of results is difficult because of the lack of large homogeneous patient groups having the same basic etiology for proximal obstruction. Furthermore, confusion in comparisons is created by the optional use of different splinting techniques and postoperative therapy regimens. As a result, it is difficult to establish the advantage of a particular technique by a simple comparison of pregnancy success rates.

Results must be stated in terms of the nature and extent of pathological change. Shirodkar[8] graded the extent of disease and correlated subsequent pregnancy success. He noted pregnancy success to be approximately 40% in patients with occlusion at the cornua, extending not beyond the first 2 inches of tube, leaving two-thirds of the tube for implantation. Pregnancy success dropped off markedly once the fimbriated ends of the tube were involved with adhesions. This has also been our experience. The patients with minimal or no peritubular adhesions and without involvement of the fimbriated portion of the Fallopian tube were found to have the best chance for pregnancy. Once the fimbriated ends of the Fallopian tube were involved or fixation of the adnexal structures was noted, the pregnancy success rate dropped to less than 10% (Table III).

Proximal cornual obstruction may result from an episode of acute salpingitis or, less often, from salpingitis isthmica nodosa (Fig. 6A–D). Intramural occlusion is also observed when sterilization is accomplished by aggressive monopolar electrocautery (Fig. 6E,F).

The histological confirmation of the clinical diagnosis of intramural obstruction is not always verified by the pathologist's report of the excised isthmic or intramural portion of the Fallopian tube. Grant[17] reported histological observations on 67 excised specimens, 87% of which were of inflammatory origin. Mucosal or interstitial involvement was found in 49 of 67 specimens. Grant suggested that obstruction in a number of instances was related to a flaplike block and, in his view, did not represent tubal spasm. Ar-

Table III
Pregnancy Outcome and Tubal Patency following Uterotubal Implantation[a]

Extent of disease	Pregnancy outcome		Patency on hysterogram	
	No. of patients	No. pregnant	No. of patients	No. with patent tubes
Mild: Minimal or no peritubular adhesions	29	11 (38%)	15	8 (53%)
Moderate: Substantial peritubular and periovarian adhesions without fixation	10	3 (30%)	5	5 (100%)
Severe: Dense pelvic or adnexal adhesions with fixation of ovary	13	1 (8%)	9	3 (33%)

[a] Adapted from Rock et al.[9]

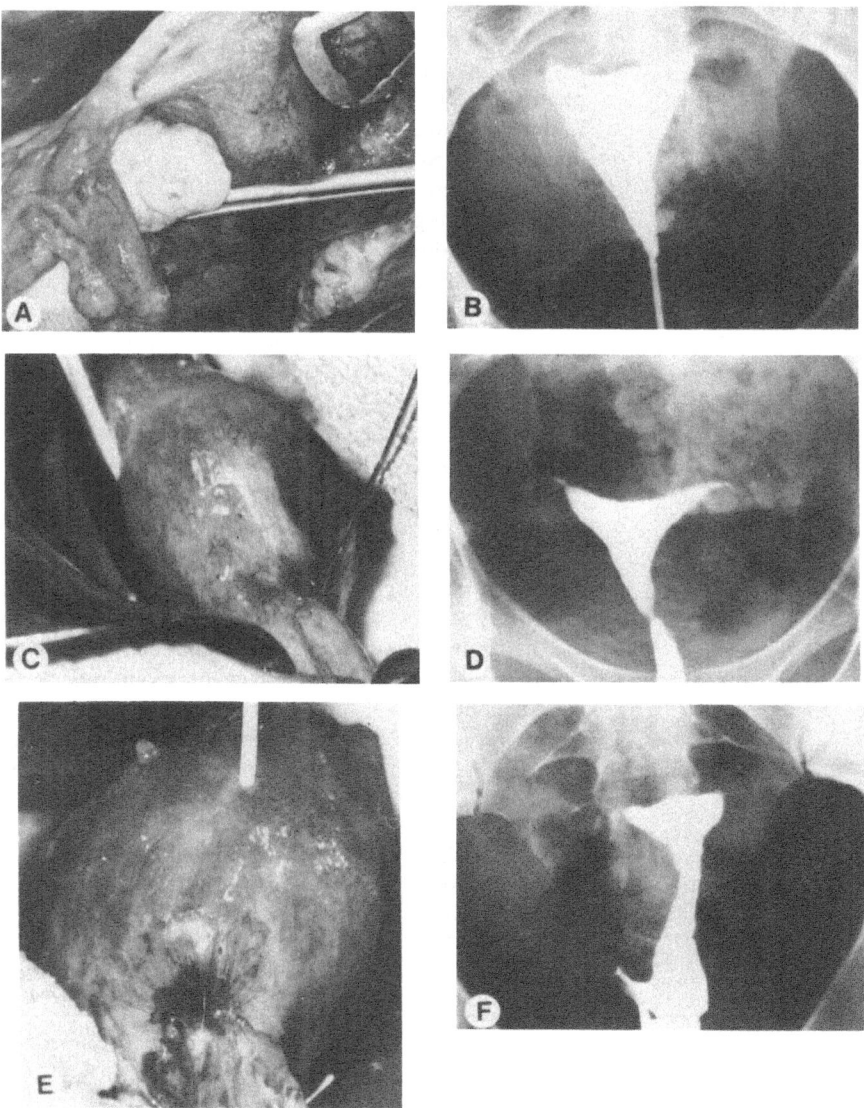

Figure 6. Gross and hysterographic findings in proximal occlusion. (A) Intramural occlusion may result from chronic pelvic inflammatory disease. (B) Often, these thickened and fibrotic oviducts have associated peritubal and periovarian adhesions. A small portion of the intramural oviduct is identified by hysterosalpingography. (C) Salpingitis isthmica nodosa grossly appears as nodular thickening of one or both oviducts. (D) Severe constriction may result in complete tubal occlusion. Radiologically, a punctate accumulation of contrast medium in the isthmico–cornual region is noted. (E) Previous aggressive monopolar electrocautery has resulted in complete destruction of the proximal oviduct. Grossly superficial endometriosis may be noted at the cornua. (F) The oviduct is virtually destroyed with a thickened fibrotic consistency. No intramural tube is noted on hysterogram. (From Jones and Rock,[26] reprinted with permission of the publisher.)

ronet and co-authors[19] reported 37 specimens from 42 patients who underwent tubal implantation. They indicated that 57% of specimens were of noninflammatory origin; 57% of these patients conceived following uterotubal implantation. Thirty-eight percent of the specimens were inflammatory, and only 13% of these patients conceived postoperatively. Rock and co-authors[9] reported evidence of chronic salpingitis in 21 patients (40%), 5 of whom (24%) conceived. Pregnancy success was higher in patients with salpingitis isthmica nodosa or intramural block resulting from a sterilization procedure. Moore-White[20] reported a pregnancy rate of 31% among patients with pure cornual obstruction. Thus, patients with chronic pelvic inflammatory disease are less likely to conceive following uterotubal implantation; this may be related to the high incidence of associated pelvic adhesion formation and fimbrial involvement at the time of uterotubal implantation.

Although postoperative patency rates have been reported in the 70–90% range, the term pregnancy rate has been disappointingly low (0–48%, Tables IV and V).[21–24] Pregnancy success following uterotubal implantation using the sharp cornual wedge technique and the reamer technique has been difficult to gauge from previous reports, as the patient population is not clearly defined as to age, race, parity, duration of infertility, and extent of adhesion formation. Furthermore, only two reports take into consideration

Table IV
Pregnancy Outcome following Uterotubal Implantation
(Sharp Cornual Wedge Excision Technique)

Author (year)	No. of patients	Pregnancy rate	Term delivery	Technique
Shirodkar (1960)[8]	25	25%	0	Fundal incision splint
Siegler (1969)[21]	12	8%	0	Splint
Young et al. (1970)[22]	11	9%	9%	Ring splint
Horne et al. (1973)[23]	11	64%	46%	Ring splint
Palmer (1977)[16]	118	44%	38%	No splint
Ampullary	93	42%	33%	
Isthmic	25	46%	43%	
Rock et al. (1979)[9]	26	16%	8%	Ring splint
Ampullary	20	15%	10%	
Isthmic	6	17%	0	

Table V
Pregnancy Outcome following Uterotubal Implantation (Reamer Technique)

Author (year)	No. of patients	Pregnancy rate	Term delivery	Technique
Shirodkar (1960)[8]	140	35%	0	Ring splint
Hanton et al. (1964)[24]	22	48%	48%	No splint
Arronet et al. (1969)[19]	37	43%	43%	Ring splint
Grant (1971)[17]	73	34%	26%	Splint (cervical removal)
Rock (unpublished data)	33	41%	23%	Ring splint
Isthmic	15	27%	13%	
Ampullary	18	64%	36%	

the segment of Fallopian tube implanted into the uterus. Palmer[16] divided his patients into groups depending on whether the ampullary or isthmic portion of the Fallopian tube was implanted into the uterus; however, splints were not used. Rock and co-authors[9] similarly divided patients into ampullary and isthmic categories, and splints were used. Palmer demonstrated that an isthmic implantation was associated with a 10% increase in pregnancy rate, whereas Rock (unpublished data, 1980) demonstrated than an ampullary implantation was associated with a 10% increase in pregnancy rate (Table V).

Since the report of improved pregnancy success following uterotubal implantation of the ampullary portion of the Fallopian tube using the reamer technique (J. A. Rock, unpublished data, 1980), this technique has been used ex-

Table VI
Ampullary–Uterotubal Implantation
Using the Reamer Technique
in 18 Patients with Proximal Obstruction

Number of patients	18
Patients pregnant	10 (56%)
Patients with living children	7 (39%)
Patients with ectopic pregnancy	1 (.05%)
Total patients	12
Living child	8 (66%)
Abortion	3 (25%)
Ectopic	1 (8%)

clusively at The Johns Hopkins Hospital. Of the 18 patients so treated, 10 patients conceived, with term pregnancies resulting in 7 (Table VI). Pregnancy success was noted to be higher in patients with salpingitis isthmica nodosa or intramural obstruction resulting from previous electrocauterization. Of note is the observation that the single ectopic pregnancy occurred in a patient with intramural block as a result of chronic salpingitis (Table VII). We hope that, with careful patient selection, the accumulation of a large patient group may demonstrate the efficacy of this particular type of technique for uterotubal implantation.

Most recently, Von Csaba et al.[14] and Peterson et al.[15] have reported uterotubal implantation through a postuterofundal incision between the uteroovarian ligaments. Von Csaba et al. reported that 3 of 9 patients with a proximal obstruction caused by pelvic inflammatory disease conceived, for a pregnancy rate of 33%. Peterson and coauthors reported a 50% pregnancy rate and a 77% tubal patency rate in 16 patients with obstruction after previous sterilization. We have found this technique particularly useful in patients who have had excessively shortened Fallopian tubes as a consequence of vigorous electrocauterization for sterilization. The tube may be easily implanted into the posterior uterus without distorting the tuboovarian relationships.

Over the past decade, there has been a decline in the number of uterotubal implantations performed in our institution. Diamond[25] has reported a comparison of macro- and microsurgical techniques for the repair of cornual occlusion

Table VII

Histological Diagnosis and Pregnancy Success among 18 Patients Undergoing Ampullary–Uterotubal Implantation

Diagnosis	No. of patients	Patients pregnant	Intrauterine pregnancy
Chronic salpingitis	4	2[a]	1 (25%)
Previous sterilization (electrocautery)	9	5	5 (56%)
Salpingitis isthmica nodosa	5	3	3 (60%)
Totals	18	10	9

[a] One patient with an ampullary ectopic pregnancy.

in infertility, demonstrating a 4.7-fold improvement in term pregnancy rate using microsurgery for anastomosing the transected ampulla or isthmus to the intramural portion of the tube. With the development of these new microsurgical techniques, uterotubal implantation may be reserved for patients with intramural obstruction.

REFERENCES

1. Winston RML: Microsurgical tubocornual anastomosis for reversal of sterilization. *Lancet* 1:284, 1977.
2. Sweeney WJ: The interstitial posture of the uterine tube: Its gross anatomy, course and length. *Obstet Gynecol* 19:3, 1962.
3. Rocker I: The anatomy of the uterotubal junction area. *Proc R Soc Med* 57:707, 1964.
4. Rigby JP: The persistence of spermatozoa at the uterotubal junction of the sow. *J Reprod Fertil* 11:153, 1966.
5. Baker RD, Degen AA: Transport of live and dead boar spermatozoa within the reproductive tract of gilts. *J Reprod Fertil* 28:369, 1972.
6. Rowson LEA: The movement of radio-opaque material in the bovine uterine tract. *Br Vet J* 111:334, 1955.
7. David A, Brackett BG, Gardia CR: Effect of microsurgical removal of the rabbit uterotubal junction. *Fertil Steril* 20:250, 1969.
8. Shirodkar VN: *Contributions to Obstetrics and Gynecology*. London, Livingstone, 1960, p 65.
9. Rock JA, Katayama, PK, Martin EJ, et al: Pregnancy outcome following uterotubal implantation: A comparison of the reamer and sharp cornual wedge excision techniques. *Fertil Steril* 31:6, 1979.
10. Gomel V: Causes of failed reconstructive tubal microsurgery. *J Reprod Med* 24:242, 1980.
11. Bonney V: The fruits of conservatism. *J Obstet Gynaecol Br Commonw* 44:1, 1937.
12. Holden FC, Sovak FW: Reconstruction of the oviducts: An improved technique with report of cases. *Am J Obstet Gynecol* 24:684, 1932.
13. Shirodkar VN: Further experiences in tuboplasty. *Aust NZ J Obstet Gynaecol* 5:1, 1965.
14. Von Csaba I, Keller G, Magy P, et al: Chirurgische Behandbing der Weiblichen Steriletat Tubenimplantation. *Zentralbl Gynaekol* 96:490, 1974.
15. Peterson EP, Musich JR, Berhman SJ: Uterotubal implantation and obstetrics outcome after previous sterilization. *Am J Obstet Gynecol* 128:662, 1977.
16. Palmer R: Presented to the *ad hoc* committee on tubal surgery, Thirty-Third Annual Meeting of the American Fertility Society, Miami, Fla., 1977.
17. Grant A: Infertility surgery of the oviduct. *Fertil Steril* 22:496, 1971.
18. Wirtz JW: Experience with a method for implantation of the Fallopian tubes into the uterus. *Aust NZ J Obstet Gynaecol* 5:7, 1965.
19. Arronet GJ, Eduljee SY, O'Brien JR: A nine-year survey of Fallopian tube dysfunction in human infertility: Diagnosis and therapy. *Fertil Steril* 20:903, 1969.
20. Moore-White M: Evaluation of tuboplastic operations: Classification of tubal disease. *Int J Fertil* 5:237, 1960.

21. Siegler AM: Salpingoplasty: Classification and report of 115 operations. *Obstet Gynecol* 34:339, 1969.
22. Young PE, Egan JE, Barlow JJ, et al: Reconstructive surgery for infertility at the Boston Hospital for Women. *Am J Obstet Gynecol* 108:1092, 1970.
23. Horne HW, Clyman M, Debrovner C, et al: The prevention of postoperative pelvic adhesions following conservative operative treatment for human infertility. *Int J Fertil* 18:109, 1973.
24. Hanton EM, Pratt JJ, Banner EA: Tubal plastic surgery at the Mayo Clinic. *Am J Obstet Gynecol* 89:934, 1964.
25. Diamond E: A comparison of gross and microsurgical techniques for repair of cornual occlusion in infertility: A retrospective study, 1968–1978. *Fertil Steril* 32:370, 1979.
26. Jones HW Jr, Rock JA: *Reparative and Constructive Surgery of the Female Generative Tract*. Baltimore, Williams & Wilkins, 1981, Chapter 7.

10 Conservative Techniques for the Management of Tubal Pregnancies

John J. Stangel

Department of Obstetrics and Gynecology
Section of Reproductive Endocrinology and Infertility
New York Medical College
Westchester County Medical Center
Valhalla, New York 10595

and

J. Victor Reyniak

Department of Obstetrics and Gynecology
Division of Reproductive Endocrinology
Mount Sinai School of Medicine
New York, New York 10029

The techniques for and approach to reconstructive tubal surgery have changed greatly in the past 10 years. The utilization of optic magnification, atraumatic techniques, and finer, less reactive sutures has doubled the pregnancy rates subsequent to certain procedures. We have now reached a time when it is appropriate to reevaluate the surgical management of tubal pregnancies. Based on existing data and current surgical techniques, conservative tubal surgery, rather than the usual salpingectomy, should be considered for the woman with an unruptured tubal pregnancy who still desires to bear children.

Following the removal of one tube, women have a marked reduction in fertility; the incidence of intrauterine gestation has been variously reported as 26%,[1] 38%,[2] and 48.1%.[3] In 1953, a salpingotomy procedure was described[4] that allowed the removal of the tubal conceptus without sacrificing the oviduct. That initial report has been followed by subsequent reports of favorable results with various conservative surgical techniques.[5-16] This chapter summarizes conservative surgical techniques for the management of tubal gestation.

TECHNIQUES

The basic principle of the conservative surgical approach to ectopic gestation is to remove the conceptus and maximally preserve the Fallopian tube that contained it. The choice of the technique employed depends on the patient, the location of the gestation, and the surgical experience of the operator.

Patient Selection

The appropriate patient candidate should be of reproductive age, surgically stable, with an unruptured tubal gestation or tubal abortion and the desire for further childbearing. Women who either do not desire further pregnancy or are beyond the optimal reproductive age are not candidates for conservative tubal surgery. In those patients, salpingectomy is the procedure of choice. The presence of an ectopic gestation should be confirmed by laparoscopy in all patients.

Procedures

There are three basic conservative procedures. In the first procedure, a linear incision is made in the tube and the conceptus removed. This is the salpingotomy first described by Stromme.[4] The second procedure consists of removing the tubal segment containing the ectopic pregnancy and performing a microsurgical tubal anastomosis under the same anesthesia. This is defined as "segmental tubal resection with anastomosis." The third mode of conservative surgical treatment is a segmental resection of the oviduct portion containing the pregnancy without anastomosis at the time of initial surgery, the "segmental tubal resection without anastomosis."

Salpingotomy Technique

The most common location of extrauterine gestation (Fig. 1)[17] is the ampulla, and the salpingotomy procedure is most applicable to ampullary pregnancies. The abdomen is entered in the conventional manner. The tube containing the gestation is raised and isolated from the surrounding area by packing the abdomen with well-moistened laparotomy pads. An incision is made with a needle electrode and a minimal cutting current in the tube on the antemesenteric border directly over the pregnancy; the tube is opened, and the conceptus is gently removed with forceps and suction. Care must be exercised to remove all of the gestational tissue from the tube. Any tissue remaining will be sloughed later and could possibly result in a delayed postoperative hemorrhage.[18]

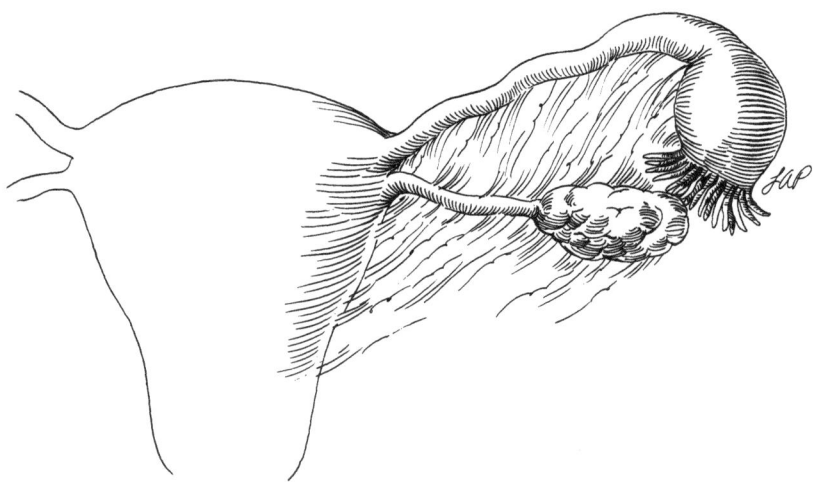

Figure 1. In the unruptured ampullary tubal pregnancy, salpingotomy represents the most applicable conservative approach.

Hemostasis is accomplished by electrocoagulation with a needle electrode and minimal coagulation current and/or hemostatic sutures of 6-0 polyglycolic acid (Dexon®) or nylon suture. We have found that injecting a dilute vasopressin (Pitressin®) solution into the wall of the tube causes marked localized vasoconstriction, reduces generalized oozing to a minimum, and facilitates isolation of discrete bleeding areas. Four units of Pitressin® are diluted in 20 ml of saline; 3 ml of this solution are drawn into a 5-ml syringe with a 25-gauge needle and are injected into the tubal wall as needed. The solution must not be injected intravenously; therefore, the surgeon must aspirate with the syringe prior to each injection.

The tubal incision may be sutured or left open for secondary closure. We feel that suturing is associated with less tubal scarring and, therefore, use a two-layer closure of the tubal incision with an 8-0 polyglycolic suture (Fig. 2). This procedure can be used for isthmic as well as ampullary ectopic pregnancies. In our opinion, however, segmental resection with anastomosis offers a different and perhaps more advantageous surgical approach to the isthmic ectopic pregnancy.

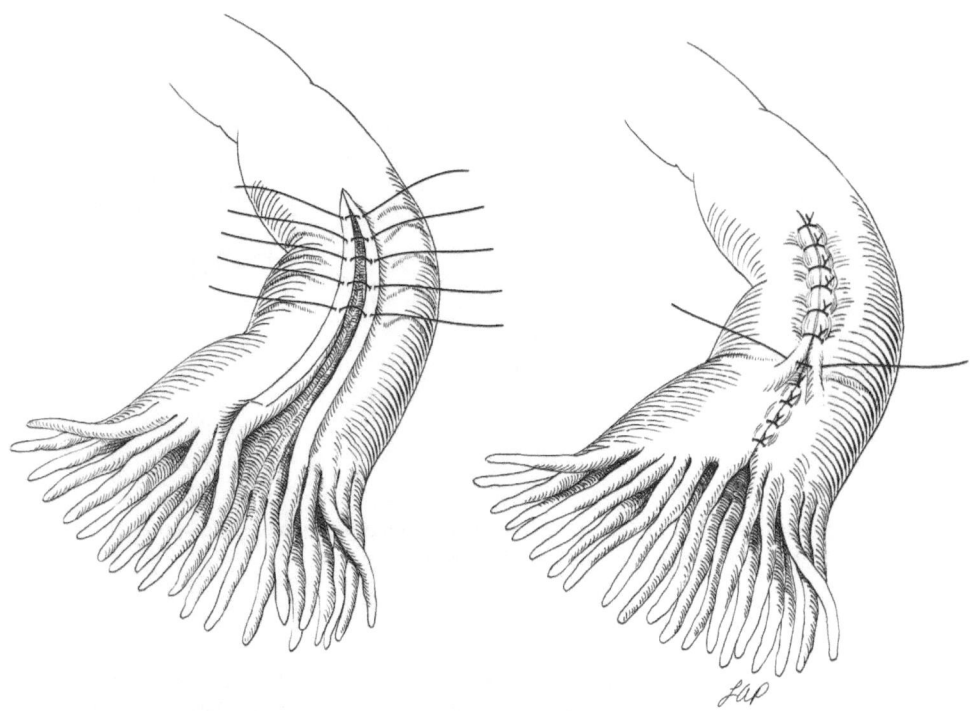

Figure 2. A two-layer closure of salpingotomy incision in the ampullary portion of the tube is the technique of choice.

Segmental Resection with Anastomosis Technique

This procedure is most applicable for isthmic pregnancies (Fig. 3). Following laparoscopy, a laparotomy is performed. The tube containing the gestation is raised and isolated by packing the abdomen with well-moistened laparotomy pads. Babcock clamps or stabilization mini-clamps are placed on either side of and immediately next to the ectopic pregnancy. A 6-0 Vicryl® or Dexon® suture is placed through the mesosalpinx, entering beneath one clamp and exiting beneath the second. This suture is not tied until after the excision of the tubal segment. The portion of the tube containing the pregnancy is excised between the Babcock clamps. A linear incision is then made at the junction between the mesosalpinx and the tube segment, separating it from the underlying tissue (Fig. 4). The 6-0 suture is then tied.

Bleeding vessels are identified and electrocoagulated using bipolar diathermy under constant irrigation. The ends

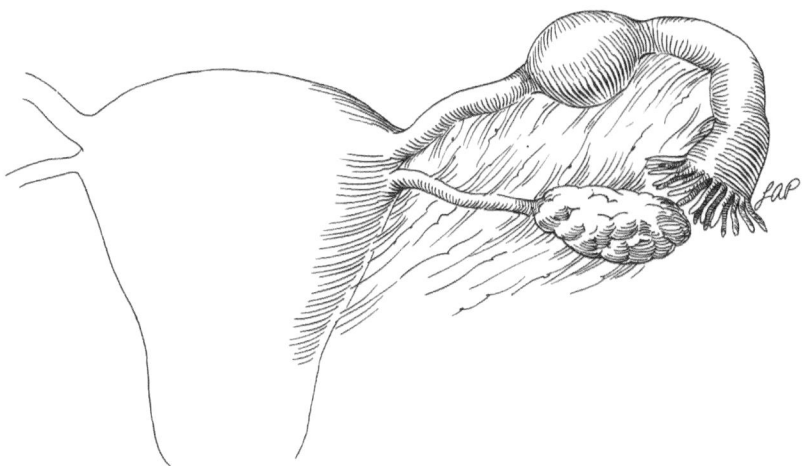

Figure 3. In the unruptured isthmic tubal pregnancy, a segmental resection with anastomosis represents the most applicable conservative approach.

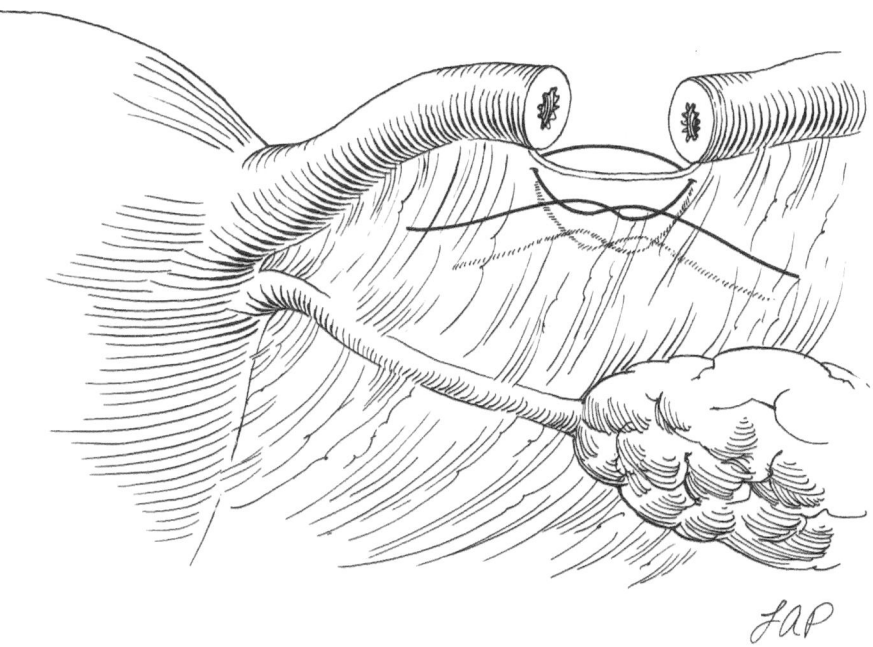

Figure 4. The isthmic portion of the tube containing ectopic pregnancy has been excised. The 6-0 suture placed through the mesosalpinx can now be tied, allowing for approximation of tubal segments.

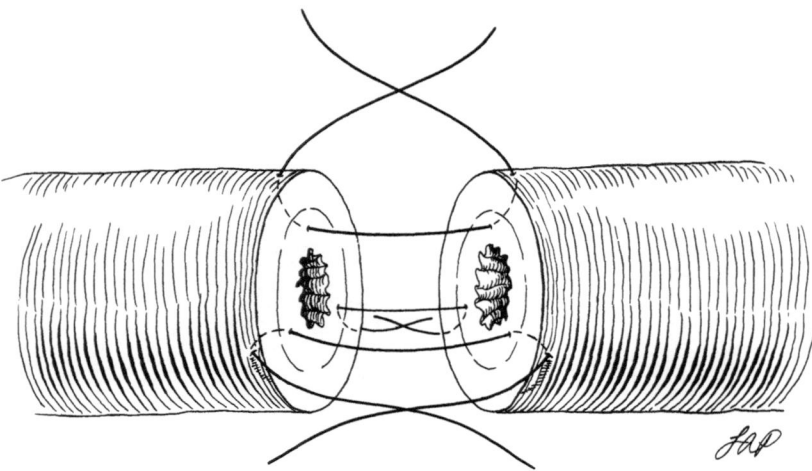

Figure 5. Technique of anastomosis. 8-0 sutures have been placed through the serosa and muscularis at 8, 12, and 4 o'clock positions around the circumference of the tube.

of the oviduct are visualized by an operating microscope with a 300-mm lens. The anastomosis of the Fallopian tube is accomplished with three sutures of 8-0 Dexon® suture. These sutures are placed through the serosa and muscularis at 8, 12, and 4 o'clock positions around the circumference of the tube (Fig. 5), carefully avoiding the endosalpinx. After these sutures are tied, additional interrupted 8-0 sutures are used to approximate the serosa and provide a smooth covering over the anastomosis site. At the completion of the anastomosis, patency is confirmed by transfundal tubal perfusion.

Segmental tubal resection with end-to-end anastomosis appears to be a more logical therapy than salpingotomy for isthmic pregnancies. The site of ectopic pregnancy represents an area of preexisting tubal pathology. Damage done by a tubal gestation to the narrow lumen of the isthmus can worsen the scarring in this area, making recurrent ectopic pregnancy more likely. Salpingotomy leaves this area of scarring extant. In contrast, excision and anastomosis allows the removal of the site of pathology and minimizes the probability of recurrent tubal pregnancy.

Segmental Resection without Anastomosis Technique

The previously described procedure may be minimally modified to provide segmental resection without anastomosis. A 2-0 nylon suture can be passed through the mesosalpinx on either side of the tubal gestation and each ligature tied around the Fallopian tube. The Fallopian tube is thus suture-ligated with 2-0 nylon on either side of the ectopic pregnancy. The tubal segment between the two sutures is then excised, and its bleeding areas, as well as the mesosalpinx defect, are oversewn with 3-0 Dexon®. The laparotomy is then completed in the conventional manner. If the contralateral tube appears functional, the patient is allowed to attempt to conceive. If pregnancy does not occur within 1 year, a microsurgical anastomosis can be performed as with reversal of tubal sterilization.

Segmental resection without anastomosis is especially useful for the patient who is not sufficiently stable either medically or surgically at the time of initial surgery to be a candidate for more complex procedures. Moreover, segmental resection without anastomosis takes less time to perform than a salpingectomy, and it requires neither special instrumentation nor tubal surgery experience.

GENERAL COMMENTS

Timing of Anastomosis

The question arises whether tubal anastomosis should be performed at the time of laparotomy for the removal of the ectopic pregnancy or at a later date when the procedure can be done as elective surgery. At present, we have observed 100% patency rate in 11 patients following the anastomosis at the time of the initial laparotomy. If an anastomosis accomplished with a single laparotomy results in tubal patency and intrauterine pregnancy, there is no need to subject the patient to additional risk of a two-stage procedure. On the other hand, if circumstances are less than ideal at the time of the initial laparotomy (i.e., the patient is not surgically stable, or the surgeon is inexperienced in reconstructive tubal techniques), the surgery may be done in two stages.

Use of Magnification

Both salpingotomy and tubal anastomosis can be accomplished without optical magnification because the tissues are enlarged and edematous. The ability of the patient to become pregnant, however, will depend, at least in part, on the quality of the tubal repair. It is our opinion that magnification—loupes or, preferably, the operating microscope—allows a more accurate anatomic reconstruction. Whether the surgeon elects to use magnification or not, it is still mandatory to observe the general principles of microsurgical techniques. The tissues must always be handdled only when necessary and then gently; they must constantly be irrigated and moistened. Sponging should be reduced to a minimum by substituting suction and irrigation. Finally, the finest, least reactive suture available must be utilized for the tubal repair. Chromic and plain gut sutures should be avoided, and nylon or polyglycolic sutures should be substituted.

Ruptured Tubal Pregnancy

The previously discussed procedures are recommended for unruptured tubal pregnancies. They may also be used for ruptured tubal gestations, but only if the patient is stable at the time of surgery. We have reported an anastomosis performed at the time of ruptured isthmic tubal pregnancy. The patient had a unicornuate uterus and subsequently experienced intrauterine gestation.[19] If the patient is not stable, however, and the blood loss is significant, a rapid segmental tubal resection is indicated. The basic principle to be emphasized is the preservation of a maximum amount of normal appearing tube. The segments of the tube left *in situ* must be ligated with a permanent suture to minimize the chances of tubal fistula formation and a recurrent ectopic pregnancy. As long as tubal segments remain, it is theoretically possible to construct one functional tube by a composite anastomosis using sections of oviduct from each side. Shapiro and Hanig[20] have reported a pregnancy 18 months after surgery to join a left fimbrial pedicle graft to a right proximal fallopian tube segment.

Tubal Abortions

A tubal abortion results when an ampullary pregnancy is spontaneously extruded from the tube through the fimbria. Often the surgeon may convert a distal ampullary gestation to a tubal abortion by expressing and extruding the products of conception from the end of the tube. The result is an iatrogenic tubal abortion. Whether the process is spontaneous or iatrogenic, the surgeon faces the same problem. Frequently, there is continued bleeding from the implantation site. First, care must be taken to remove all gestational

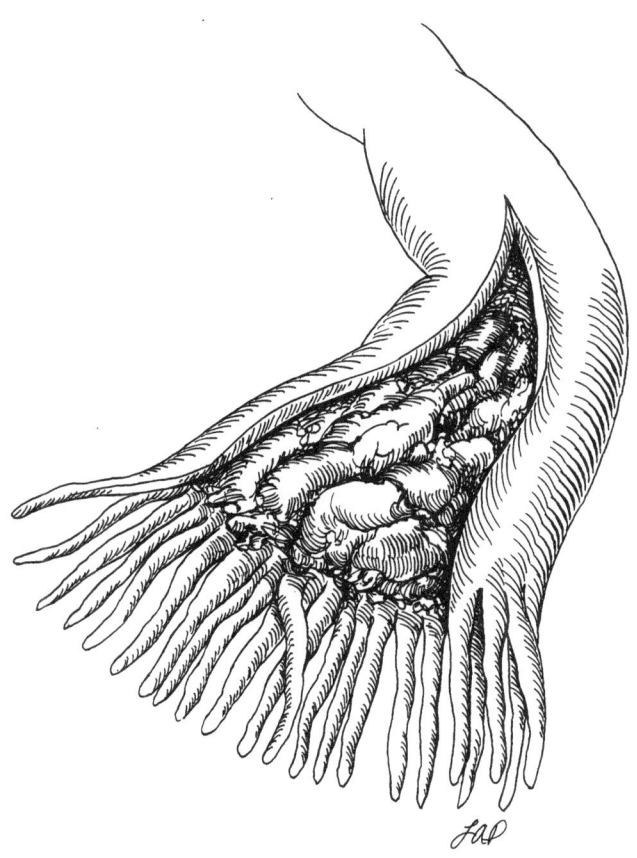

Figure 6. A tubal abortion managed by salpingotomy incision allows debridement and hemostasis at the implantation site.

tissue from this area. Once this is done, hemostasis must be accomplished either by suture or electrocoagulation. Adequate exposure is necessary to accomplish debridement and hemostasis; this is not difficult if implantation was on the fimbria. On the other hand, if implantation was within the ampulla of the oviduct, a salpingotomylike incision is required to enable the surgeon to lay open the lumen of the tube, debride it properly, and obtain hemostasis. Local infiltration with a Pitressin® solution, as described previously, is very helpful to stop generalized oozing. Specific bleeding vessels then become apparent and can easily be controlled by suture or electrocoagulation (Fig. 6).

SUMMARY   Tubal gestation in a woman who desires further childbearing can and should be safely managed by conservative surgical means. The decision to perform a salpingectomy for an unruptured tubal pregnancy must always be questioned, for although it is still the accepted treatment for tubal pregnancy, it can reduce a patient's subsequent fertility. A number of different techniques are available to preserve the Fallopian tube and the fertility potential of a surgically stable woman with unruptured tubal pregnancy.

An ampullary gestation should be removed by a salpingotomy. The implantation site must be debrided of gestational tissue and hemostasis accomplished. Local infiltration with Pitressin® is helpful. The tubal incision may be closed in two layers or may be allowed to heal by secondary intention; the former is recommended on a theoretical basis.

An isthmic gestation may be treated by either a linear isthmic salpingotomy or a segmental excision of the tube portion containing the pregnancy followed by an end-to-end anastomosis. The excision and anastomosis may be done as either a one- or two-stage procedure.

A tubal abortion is treated as an ampullary pregnancy. Debridement and hemostasis of the implantation site are accomplished with care. If the site is deep within the ampullary lumen, a salpingotomylike incision is made for proper exposure, and the repair is carried out as previously described. The advantages of each have been discussed.

All of these conservative procedures may be performed without magnification, but the optimal restoration of anatomy and function is accomplished with the use of magnification. Whether or not lenses are used, the principles of microsurgical technique must be used in all cases of tubal surgery including conservative surgery for tubal pregnancies. If one is not able to preserve enough tubal tissue to allow oviduct reconstruction, one should at least attempt to preserve any portion of apparently normal Fallopian tube. The tissue may be used at another time to construct a composite Fallopian tube if necessary.

Conservative surgery for tubal pregnancy in the hands of an experienced operator adds only about 15–20 min to the total operating time usually required for an uncomplicated salpingectomy. Blood loss is the same or even less than that of salpingectomy. The postoperative course is usually uncomplicated. These procedures merit more serious consideration by the clinical practitioner and continued investigation by researchers.

REFERENCES

1. Limoni NS, Milmini NV: Tubal pregnancy: Choice of operation and method of treatment. *Acta Obstet Gynecol Scand* 40:327, 1967.
2. Franklin EW III, Ziederman AM, Laemmle P: Tubal ectopic pregnancy: Etiology and obstetric and gynecologic sequelae. *Am J Obstet Gynecol* 117:220, 1973.
3. Schenken JG, Eyal F, Polishok WZ: Fertility after tubal surgery. *Surg Gynecol Obstet* 135:74, 1972.
4. Stromme WB: Salpingotomy for tubal pregnancy. *Obstet Gynecol* 1:472, 1953.
5. Stromme WB: Conservative surgery for ectopic pregnancy. *Obstet Gynecol* 41:215, 1973.
6. Barcklay SDEC: Conservative surgery in tubal ectopic gestation. *Aust NZ J Surg* 31:51, 1961.
7. Bukovsky I, Langer R, Herman A, et al: Conservative surgery for tubal pregnancy. *Obstet Gynecol* 53:709, 1979.
8. Decherney A, Kase N: The conservative surgical management of unruptured ectopic pregnancy. *Obstet Gynecol* 54:451, 1979.
9. Kucera E, Macku F, Novak J, et al: Fertility after operations for extrauterine pregnancy. *Int J Fertil* 14:127, 1969.
10. Ploman L, Wicksell F: Fertility after conservative surgery in tubal pregnancy. *Acta Obstet Gynecol Scand* 39:143, 1960.
11. Rosenblum JM, Dowling RW, Barnes AC: Treatment of tubal pregnancy. *Am J Obstet Gynecol* 80:274, 1960.
12. Skuli V, Pavic Z, Stoilkovic C, et al: Conservative operative treatment of tubal pregnancy. *Fertil Steril* 15:634, 1964.
13. Stangel JJ, Reyniak JV, Stone ML: Conservative surgical management of tubal pregnancy. *Obstet Gynecol* 48:241, 1976.
14. Swohn K: Spontanheilung Mach Querre Sektion der tuba Fallopii. *Acta Obstet Gynecol Scand* 46:219, 1967.
15. Thompkins SP: Preservation of fertility by conservative surgery for ectopic pregnancy. *Fertil Steril* 7:448, 1976.
16. Vehaskav A: The operation of choice for ectopic pregnancy with reference to subsequent fertility. *Acta Obstet Gynecol Scand* 39(Suppl 3):XX, 1960.
17. Pauerstein CJ: *The Fallopian Tube: A Reappraisal*. Philadelphia, Lea & Febiger, 1974, p 99.
18. Kelly RW, Martin SA, Strickler RC: Delayed hemorrhage in conservative surgery for ectopic pregnancy. *Am J Obstet Gynecol* 133:225, 1979.
19. Reyniak JV: Microsurgical repair of ruptured tubal pregnancy. *Fem Patient* 3:102, 1978.
20. Shapiro FS, Hanig RV: Tubal anastomosis of a fimbrial segment pedicle graft. *Fertil Steril* 32:478, 1979.

11 Postoperative Adhesions
Etiology and Prevention

Martin Greenberg and Niels H. Lauersen

Department of Obstetrics and Gynecology
Mount Sinai School of Medicine
New York, New York 10029

Infertility surgeons are keenly aware that attempts at tubal reconstruction have frequently yielded disappointing results, in part because of the presence or development of intraperitoneal adhesions. The prevention and management of these adhesions is a continuing professional challenge, which requires periodic reconsideration. Prophylaxis has been approached from an overwhelming number of aspects. Our present inability to provide adequate prophylaxis may be founded in our insufficient knowledge concerning the development of intraperitoneal adhesions and the lack of uniform patient response to numerous factors.

In the era before abdominal and infertility surgery, these adhesions were considered of little importance and are not mentioned in the principal surgical texts of the 1800s. With the increase in number of surgical procedures, the role of adhesions as a common cause of intestinal obstruction and fertility failure became evident. Surely, as noted by Becker,[1] the most common cause for abdominal adhesions is previous surgical treatment, for he found 90% of 412 cases of obstruction studied had adhesions. Postmortem examinations and the clinical observations of abdominal surgeons led to the awareness of the existence of early fibrinous adhesions of intestinal loops to abdominal viscera within a short interval following surgery, trauma, or inflammation. As early as 1919, Hertzler[2] came to the conclusion that to prevent adhesions is to prevent healing. "This sequence lasts as long as the patient does, or the helpful persistence of the surgeon endures." Most of these adhesions, however, cause no harm, but they still remain high on the etiologic list for infertility surgery failure. There is no greater frustration than to succeed technically in often tedious, difficult, and extremely delicate tuboplastic surgery only to have the results thwarted by adhesions leading to conception failure.

PATHOGENESIS OF PERITONEAL ADHESIONS

The formation of peritoneal adhesions had been explained by the classical concept that serosal damage leads to an outpouring of fibrinogen followed by the formation of a fibrin clot and its organization into a fibrinous adhesion. Fibroblastic invasion and conversion to a fibrous adhesion then occurs. Numerous experiments, however, have demonstrated that this concept is fallacious.[3] It is well documented that the usual mechanism of peritoneal healing is very rapid and without adhesion formation. Large defects often heal as rapidly as small ones. Peritoneal adhesions can be produced experimentally only with great difficulty, highly artificial methods, and severe damage, i.e., crushing bowel, dividing major vessels, introduction of foreign bodies. Paradoxically, it is with the greatest of ease that postoperative adhesions form following pelvic and abdominal surgery. It is readily evident that the classical theory of peritoneal healing leaves much to be desired.

In 1973, Rafferty's[4] electron-microscopic studies showed that new mesothelium originates from subperitoneal connective tissue cells, either fibroblastic or mesenchymal, within 48 hr of peritoneal injury. Healing is achieved by development of a single layer of mesothelial cells within 5 days. Experimentation and clinical experience have shown that inflammation and ischemic tissues are the sine qua non of adhesion formation. In the late 18th century, Von Dembrowski[5] and Franz,[6] and again Ellis in 1962,[7] demonstrated that raw peritoneal defects can heal without the formation of adhesions. They noted, however, that the easiest way to insure fibrous adhesion development was to either patch or suture those defects. Tissue ischemia rather than a loss of mesothelium prevents the absorption of fibrin. The mesodermal derivative peritoneum, unlike cutaneous surface lesions, seems to form adhesions caused by vascular injury.

Trompke and Siegner[8] showed that peritoneal insults result in serosanguinous exudates. Within several hours, the coagulation of these exudates can result in adhesions on the injured peritoneal surface. Jackson[9] demonstrated that the vast majority of fibrinous adhesions are spontaneously lysed within 72 hr and, for the most part, represent a transient phase of the healing mechanism. Some of these adhesions, however, will undergo subsequent organization into fibrinous adhesions. Fibroblastic and capillary infiltration will collagenize and lead to permanent fibrous bands. The classical hypothesis considered the mesothelium as the key to fibrin absorption. This approach led to the meticulous reperitonealization of denuded areas, which Ellis[7] later demonstrated to be erroneous. Serosal defects without underlying vascular injury failed to provide the necessary stimulus for adhesion formation.[10] The outpouring of fibrin, however, after injury or inflammation of abdominal viscera can cause these structures to adhere to one another through formation of fibrinous transient adhesions in as little as 3 hr.

In the late 19th century, researchers found that peritoneal defects in the dog[5,6] could heal without adhesions. Thomas and co-workers[11] noted that the oversewing of serosal defects increased rather than decreased the formation of adhesions. Ellis[7] demonstrated that excision of parietal peritoneum from rats healed without adhesion formation in 52 out of 58 experiments. On the other hand, he found that meticulous repair of peritoneal defects with silk suture resulted in fibrous adhesion formation in 16 of 19 rats. Foreign body response was ruled out as the etiology of the fibrous adhesions by Ellis through an experiment that showed that similar black suture material loosely applied to the parietal peritoneum did not cause fibrous adhesions. Baillie[12] showed that fibrous adhesions to the abdominal wall were accompanied by tiny vessels, and Benzi and Boeri[13] suggested that ischemia was a major etiologic factor in adhesion formation.

The theory that the continuity of the peritoneal endothelium is a major factor in the absorption of the fibrinous exudate and the organization of fibrous adhesions is still widely accepted. The false concept that any damage to the endothelium will necessarily be followed by persistent adhesion formation had formally led most standard surgical texts to recommend the oversewing of denuded serosal defects or the use of peritoneal flaps. *Tissue ischemia*, however, is now recognized as a potent stimulator of adhesion formation; *torsion of pelvic tumors* that undergo *avascular degeneration* may cause them to become engulfed in dense adhesions. Adhesions to raw peritoneal edges occur because of the association of vascular injury and not because of the peritoneal defect itself. Detached free grafts of omentum are to be avoided, for they provoke, rather than prevent, adhesion formation.

There are numerous tissue insults that can lead to adhesions. Drying of tissue appears to be a mild injury as compared to when *drying* is *accompanied by bleeding*. Experimentally, this combination seems to be the most potent precursor of adhesion formation. Fibrin appears to have two sources: (1) exudates, which form the initial bridge between two surfaces; (2) blood clots, which bring the cellular elements leading to the ingrowth of granulation tissue. A relatively innocuous serosal injury, when combined with hemorrhage, can lead to permanent adhesion formation.

The results of experimentation in this field are fairly confusing. There is an acknowledged species difference in peritoneal reactivity to mechanical, chemical, and pharmacological influences. In addition, most likely, there are individual variations in synthesis and remodeling of scar tissue. It is known that thin women are less susceptible to adhesion formation, whereas heavy women, especially if they are of short stature, have a higher risk of postoperative adhesions. This may be related to the increased amount of *surgical time* and degree of *trauma* involved in surgical procedures of the obese. In addition, females run a 4% greater risk than males of adhesion formation. This may be related to the rupture of ovarian follicles with the ensuing hemorrhage.

Among the known causes of adhesions are (1) *infection*, (2) *foreign bodies*, (3) *vascular insufficiency*, and (4) *trauma*. The first three of these causes may be considered as promoting factors. Trauma alone usually will not produce adhesions without the presence of the additional promoting factors. There may be two types of healing: (1) injury to or removal of peritoneum that can lead to fibrinous adhesion formation with eventual spontaneous lysis and dispersion of these adhesions and (2) injury or removal plus promoting factors resulting in fibrinous adhesions that eventually undergo a dense organization by connective tissue, yielding fibrous adhesions. Hertzler wrote, "Fibrous adhesions are the bogey of most surgeons, an essential factor in disease of all abdominal viscera."[2]

Surprisingly, the time-honored methods of serosal repair are still found today in the majority of operating theaters in the face of both clinical and experimental evidence that the classical concepts of peritoneal healing were erroneous. The principle that denuded areas on the posterior abdominal or pelvic floor should be immediately reconstructed by suturing peritoneum must be reevaluated. Modern biological principles dictate that the *closing of peritoneal defects does more harm than good to the patient*. As more accurate information on the formation of adhesions becomes available, a more rational approach to their prophylaxis can be formulated. This prophylaxis is of importance to all surgeons, but it is particularly a necessity to the infertility microsurgeon. Microsurgery in infertility is not simply surgery with magnification; the ultimate success of infertility microsurgery may depend on the avoidance of adhesions, and the application of certain surgical and medical principles may help achieve this goal (Table I).

Table I
Factors That Contribute to
Formation of Adhesions

Ischemia
Drying of serosal surfaces
Excessive suturing
Gut or chromic sutures
Omental patches
Traction of peritoneum
Blood clots retained in the peritoneal cavity
Prolonged operating time
Instrumentation of adnexae

PROPHYLAXIS OF PERITONEAL ADHESIONS

Foreign Body Granulomas

In 1917, Shattock[14] described granuloma formations in silica-contaminated wounds; magnesium silicate was then the material used as a dusting powder for gloves. Schade and Williamson[15] demonstrated that silica also causes degeneration and desclamation of mesothelial cells. Similarly, Fienberg[16] reported wound granulomas caused by talcum powder. The subsequent replacement of talc by starch powder in surgical gloves has reduced granuloma formation but has not eliminated it. Yaffe and co-workers[17] reported on the contamination of the pelvic cavity by corn starch particles at the time of tubal reconstructive surgery and hysterectomies. This deposition may have undesirable effects leading to adhesion formation.

Most lesions caused by corn starch powder contamination are asymptomatic, but Webb and Regan[18] reported on three cases of corn starch granuloma, and one of these patients died after surgery for resection of adhesions. These foreign body granulomas can easily be seen as a hidden nemesis of tubal reconstruction.[19] They produce inflammation and fibrous adhesions in the peritoneal cavity. Starch is usually resorbed in 6 months, but several studies have shown this starch to be present for up to 2 years.[20] Cursory washing of gloves may be the causative factor that results in clumping of the starch particles and delayed absorption.[21]

Particles of other materials are also etiologic causes of foreign body granulomas. These include pieces of gauze from surgical sponges and pieces of the surgical glove material. It can be recommended that the careful and mechanical washing of surgical gloves should be followed by a wiping of these gloves with laparotomy pads prior to introduction of hands into the abdomen; a second wash of the gloves will considerably decrease the glove powder contamination factor.

Suture Material (Synthetic Absorbable Sutures)

Advances in surgery are concurrent with advances in surgical suture materials. Rhoads and co-workers,[22] in 1937, in an extensive review of the chronological history of surgical suture materials, wrote of the advances in the evolution and development of these materials. That review could not cover the use of synthetic absorbable sutures now so important in modern-day surgery and of paramount importance in microsurgical techniques.

Prior to the development of polyglycolic acid sutures (Dexon®) and polyglactin (Vicryl®), catgut suture material was the mainstay of infertility surgery.[23] Catgut was not ideal because its absorption was unpredictable, ranging from 7 days to up to several years, but it was the best available suture material. Although we have a personal preference for Vicryl® (polyglactin) suture, polyglycolic acid (Dexon®) possesses similar working qualities and characteristics. Absorption of both Vicryl® and Dexon® is apparent at 15–30 days postoperative and is completed within 60–90 days. Their tensile strength surpasses that of polyethylene, silk, and catgut sutures of similar size, which allows the surgeon to use finer suture material without sacrificing strength.[24] The fact that these materials show a tissue reactivity far less than catgut suture is of utmost importance in the prevention of adhesions. Katz and Turner[25] stated that the tissue response to Dexon® was a foreign body reaction and not the antigenic reaction of catgut. The inflammation caused by initial trauma decreases as these synthetic sutures are absorbed. Numerous studies show that Vicryl® and Dexon® cause fewer and lesser tissue reactions than do natural absorbable materials. Knot security is essentially equivalent to that with Dacron® polyester and superior to plain and chromic catgut.[26]

In summary, *synthetic absorbable sutures are recommended* as an important step forward in the prevention of peritoneal adhesions because of (1) their low tissue activity, (2) their dependable increased tensile strength allowing the use of finer sutures, and (3) knot security. These synthetic absorbable sutures provide a major advance in the development of suture material and in infertility surgery. The decreased tissue reactivity surely provokes far fewer adhesions than any other available suture material.

In addition to these previously described surgical techniques, certain medical therapies have been proposed for the prevention of adhesions.

Hydrotubation   At the American Fertility Society's convention in 1979, 85 of 108 surgeons polled used hydrotubation. Jarvinen and Nummi[27] reported a 50% pregnancy rate subsequent to conservative treatment for tubal pregnancies with daily hydrotubation, and Bukovsky et al.[28] reported an even higher 70% pregnancy rate. The risk of hydrotubation, however, is peritonitis. Hydrotubation has been done with solutions containing antibiotics, steroids, enzymes, and dextran as commonly used tubal adjuvants, although the results are questionable.

Anticoagulants

Anticoagulants have been extensively utilized to prevent fibrin deposition. Heparin, administered either systemically or intraperitoneally, was shown to be effective in the inhibition of adhesion formation or reformation after lysis. Katz and Cohen[25] instilled 2500 units of heparin with dexamethazone intraperitoneally without complications. The risk of hemorrhage, however, has limited the clinical use of most anticoagulants, and they are ineffective in removing fibrin deposits. Choate and co-workers[30] reported no significant advantage when heparin was used in combination with dextran.

Steroids

Replogle et al.[31] in 1965 and Horne and co-workers[32] in 1973 popularized the prophylactic use of promethazine and dexamethazone in an attempt to prevent postoperative adhesion formation. A surgical procedure within the pelvis and abdomen initiates an inflammatory response, and it was hypothesized that promethazine and dexamethazone could counter this inflammatory response. The problem with these substances is that the clinical use of large doses of corticosteroids leads to an increased incidence of adverse side effects such as wound disruption, infection, gastrointestinal ulcers, and hemorrhage.

Swolin[33] reported a significant reduction of adhesion formation following administration of hydrocortizone at the time of peritoneal closure. Because of the immunosuppressive action of the corticosteroids, antibiotics are usually given concurrently. Although questionably effective and controversial, promethazine and dexamethasone are widely used. The standard regimen of steroid treatment is dexamethasone, 20 mg, and promethazine, 25 mg, at 6 and 3 hr prior to laparotomy, at the time of laparotomy, and then every 4 hr postoperatively for nine doses.

Although this standard regimen has gained wide popularity, it has been not proven effective in controlled studies in the Rhesus monkey.[34]

Crystalloid Solutions

Intraperitoneal saline solutions are commonly used to wash irritants such as blood and tissue fragments from the pelvis. Blandau[35] observed evidence of edema in the formation of plasma membranes of the Fallopian tubes following daily administration of saline solution. Lactated Ringer's solution has been suggested, for it exposes the mesothelium to more physiological amounts of lactate, calcium, and potassium. The utilization of fluids of greater molecular weight, such as dextran 70, for tissue lavage, however, offers significant advantages over the previously used crystalloid solutions.

Hyskon® (32% Dextran 70 in Dextrose)

Several investigators[36-38] reported significant inhibition of formation of adhesions when Hyskon® (32% dextran 70 in dextrose) was administered after peritoneal injury. Holtz et al.[39] using Hyskon® at a dose of 2.5 ml/kg of body weight, found a significant inhibition of re-formation of adhesions after severe peritoneal insult. The inhibition of re-formation after lysis, however, was not significantly different in treated and controlled animals. This is contrary to the results of Mazuji and Fadhli[40] who used 20 ml/kg of body weight of dextran 75.

Dextran

Of the many solutions utilized in attempts to improve mechanical tissue separation during the postoperative period to prevent peritoneal adhesions, *dextran appears to have achieved the greatest success.*

The mechanism of dextran's effects includes the following actions:

1. The siliconizing effect of dextran is antithrombotic. Dextran coats raw serosal surfaces and retards peritoneal abrasions and blood clot adherence.
2. By its nonpolar properties, dextran maintains the negativity of the serosal surface that may cause the repulsion of fibrinogen molecules and decrease or prevent adhesions.
3. Dextran has a mechanical effect. Tissues are held apart by a heavy fluid in the pelvis, a hydroflotation effect. Dextran establishes an osmotic gradient, increasing the content of intraperitoneal fluid and thereby decreasing tissue apposition during the early stages of repair.

4. Dextran modifies the fibrin network and renders it more susceptible to lysis. Plasmin-induced lysis of a fibrin clot formed in the presence of dextran 70 is considerably increased as compared to controls.[41,42] Dextran does not alter the activity of thrombin but changes the kinetics of polymerization of fibrin monomers and yields a decreased clotting time. The change in structure, however, may be caused by the physical chemical properties of dextran rather than a specific biochemical interaction with the clotting system. The increased efficiency of plasmin on such clots is possibly related to the chain structure of the clot. Dextran causes the formation of loosely packed polymerized fibrin monomers so that the interior is more accessible to plasmin, thereby augmenting lysis.

Early experimental animal models demonstrated that low-molecular-weight dextran 40 was successful in decreasing adhesions. In human tubal surgery, however, dextran 40 only minimally prevented adhesion formation; this may be related to its rapid absorption from the peritoneal cavity.[43] On the other hand, 50% of an initial quantity of dextran 70 remained in the peritoneum for as long as 10 days after surgery. It is possible that dextran 70 exerts a far greter beneficial effect than is presently postulated or proven. The increased utilization of "second look" procedures may demonstrate that dextran 70 is the superior liquid for preventing adhesions. In a recent paper, Utian et al.[36] reported that there were significant differences in the fertility rates between dextran- and non-dextran-treated animals as determined by the formation of adhesions. Similarly, Luengo and Van Hall[44] demonstrated that the utilization of Spongostan® and 32% dextran decreased the degree and extent of intraperitoneal adhesions. These substances both prevented the apposition of damaged tissues and appeared to have hemostatic properties.

By these methods, the surgeon can prevent fibrin from accumulating as a peritoneal exudate and can remove a certain quantity of the fibrin that has formed. By the use of dextran, with its separation of raw surfaces, siliconizing, and antithrombotic effects, and other modalities discovered, the surgeon may hope to minimize, if not prevent, peritoneal adhesion formation.

Table II
Current Prophylaxis for the Prevention
of Intraperitoneal Adhesions

Utilize microsurgical technique
    Minimize tissue trauma and initial injury
    Minimize instrumental handling of tissues
    Use pinpoint and meticulous hemostasis
    Use atraumatic dissection wherever possible (needle cautery with minimal
        cutting current)
    Minimize sponging
    Use magnification (loupes or operating microscope)
    Moisten all exposed serosal surfaces by constant irrigation with dextran
        70
Avoid the introduction of foreign bodies into the peritoneal cavity (gauze,
        glove powder, toxic chemicals, bacteria) by careful washing of surgi-
        cal gloves
Avoid ischemia
    Do not reperitonize raw areas (avoid underlying vascular injury)
    Do not use peritoneal graft to patch serosal defects
Carefully remove all blood and clots from the peritoneal cavity
Use dextran 70 (6%) as the only fluid in the peritoneal cavity
    To moisten all sponges and lap pads
    For all irrigation of the peritoneal cavity
    Approximately 150–200 cc instilled into the cul-de-sac at the time of
        peritoneal closure

SUMMARY

The formation of pelvic adhesions can have very adverse effects on microsurgery for the treatment of infertility. Although controversy still exists concerning the prophylaxis of these adhesions, there are certain steps that a microsurgeon should take to help insure the success of his surgery. These include the observance of strict microsurgical technique; the avoidance of ischemia, the introducton of foreign bodies, or the retention of blood clots within the peritoneal cavity; and, finally, the use of high-molecular-weight fluids such as dextran 70 for tissue irrigation and instillation into the peritoneal cavity (Table II).

REFERENCES

1. Becker WF: Acute adhesive ileus; a study of 412 cases with particular reference to the abuse of tube decompression in treatment. *Surg Gynecol Obstet* 95:472, 1952.
2. Hertzler AF: *The Peritoneum*. St. Louis, C. V. Mosby, 1919, Vol. 1.
3. Adam JE: Peritoneal adhesions; an experimental study. *Lancet* 1:663, 1913.
4. Rafferty AT: Regeneration of parietal and visceral peritoneum: An electron microscopic study. *J Anat* 115:375, 1973.
5. Von Dembrowski T: Ueber die Ursachen der peritoneum Adhasionen

nach cirugischen: Eiugriffen mit Rucksieht auf die Frage des Ileus nach Laparotmien. *Arch Klin Chir* 37:745, 1888.

6. Franz K: Uber die Bedeutung der Branschorfe in der Bauchhohle. *Z Geburtshilfe Gynaekol* 47:64, 1902.

7. Ellis H: The cause and prevention of postoperative intraperitoneal adhesions. *Surg Gynecol Obstet* 133:497, 1971.

8. Trompke R, Siegner R: Ein Beitrag zu den Verhutunesmabnahmen postoperativer interaabdomiller Verwachsugen. *Arch Klin Chir* 281:323, 1956.

9. Jackson BB: Observations or intraperitoneal adhesions, an experimental study. *Surgery* 44:507, 1958.

10. Donaldson JK: Study regarding abdominal adhesions and cotton and gauze sponges. *Am J Surg* 39:3711, 1938.

11. Thomas J, Jackson G, Portnoff C, et al: Further experiments on influence of hyaluronidase on formation of intraperitoneal adhesions in the rat. *Proc Soc Exp Biol Med* 74:497, 1950.

12. Baillie M: *The Morbid Anatomy of Some of the Most Important Parts of the Human Body,* 8 ed. London, C M Derby for J Thomas Cox and E Portwine, 1833.

13. Benzie EDE, Boeri G: Das Netz als Schutzorgan. *Berl Klin Wochenschr* 40:773, 1903.

14. Shattock SG: Psuedotuberculoma silicoticum of the lip. *Proc R Soc Med* 10:6, 1917.

15. Schade DS, Williamson JR: The pathogenesis of peritoneal adhesions; an ultrastructural study. *Ann Surg* 167:500, 1968.

16. Fienberg R: Talcum powder granuloma. *Arch Pathol* 24:36, 1937.

17. Yaffe H, Reinhartz CT, Laufer N, et al: Potentially deleterious effects of cornstarch glove powder in tubal reconstructive surgery. *Fertil Steril* 29:699, 1978.

18. Webb DF, Regan J: Starch powder granulomas in the peritoneal cavity. *Arch Surg* 84:282, 1962.

19. Nash DFE: Glove powder peritonitis. *Br Med J* 1:485, 1973.

20. Kent JS, Burn KG, Owen D: A method of removing starch powder from surgeons' gloves. *Ann R Coll Surg Engl* 57:212, 1975.

21. Lee CM, Marchall C, Collins WT, et al: A reappraisal of absorbable glove powder. *Surg Gynecol Obstet* 95:727, 1952.

22. Rhoads JE, Horrenstein HF, Hudson, IF: The decline in the strength of catgut after exposure to living tissues. *Arch Surg* 34:377, 1937.

23. Haxton HA, Clegg JF, Lord M: A comparison of catgut and polyglycolic sutures in human abdominal wounds. *J Abdom Surg* 16:239, 1974.

24. Craig PH, Williams JA, Davis KW, et al: A biological comparison of polyglactin 910 and polyglycolic acid synthetic absorbable sutures. *Surg Gynecol Obstet* 141:1, 1975.

25. Katz AR, Turner RJ: Evaluation of tensile and absorption properties of polyglycolic acid sutures. *Surg Gynecol Obstet* 131:701, 1970.

26. Laufman H, Rubel T: Synthetic absorbable sutures. *Surg Gynecol Obstet* 145:597, 1977.

27. Jarvinen PA, Nummi S: Prevention of intraperitoneal adhesions by dextran, hydrocortisone and chymotrypsin. *Acta Obstet Gynecol Scand* 55:271, 1976.

28. Bukovsky I, Langer R, Herman A, et al: Conservative surgery for tubal pregnancy. *Obstet Gynecol* 53:709, 1979.

230 | CHAPTER 11

29. Cohen EM, Katz M: The significance of the convoluted oviduct in the infertile woman. *J Reprod Med* 21:31, 1978.

30. Choate W, Just-Viera J, Yaegar G: Prevention of experimental adhesions by dextran. *Arch Surg* 88:294, 1964.

31. Replogle RL, Johnson R, Gross RE: Prevention of postoperative intestinal adhesions with combined promethazine and dexamethazone therapy: Experimental and clinical studies. *Ann Surg* 163:580, 1966.

32. Horne HW, Clyman M, Debrovner C, et al: The prevention of postoperative pelvic adhesions following conservative operative treatment for human infertility. *Int J Fertil* 18:109, 1973.

33. Swolin K: Laparoscopy as a tool in female sterility. *J Reprod Med* 19:167, 1977.

34. Seitz HM, Schenker JG, Epstein S, et al: Postoperative intraperitoneal adhesions: A double blind assessment of their prevention in the monkey. *Fertil Steril* 24:935, 1973.

35. Blandau RJ: Comparative aspects of tubal anatomy and physiology as they relate to reconstructive procedures. *J Reprod Med* 21:7, 1978.

36. Utian WH, Goldfand JM, Starks GC: Role of dextran 70 in microtubal surgery. *Fertil Steril* 31:79, 1979.

37. Neuwirth RS, Khalaf SM: Effect of 32% dextran 70 on peritoneal adhesion formation. *Am J Obstet Gynecol* 121:420, 1975.

38. Zerega GS, Hodgen GD: Prevention of postoperative tubal adhesions. *Am J Obstet Gynecol* 136:173, 1980.

39. Holtz G, Baker E, Tsai C: Effect of thirty-two percent dextran 70 on peritoneal adhesion formation and re-formation after lysis. *Fertil Steril* 33:660, 1980.

40. Mazuji M, Fadhli HA: Peritoneal adhesion, prevention with povidone and dextran 75. *Arch Surg* 91:872, 1965.

41. Muzaffar TZ, Youngson GG, Bryce WAJ, et al: Studies on fibrin formation and effects of dextran. *Thromb Diathes Haemorrh* 28:244, 1972.

42. Muzaffar TZ, Stalker AL, Bryce WAJ, et al: Structural alterations of fibrin clots with dextran. *Thromb Diathes Haemorrh* 28:257, 1972.

43. Kapur BML, Gulati SM, Talwar JR: Prevention of peritoneal adhesions by low molecular dextran in the monkey. *Indian J Med Res* 56:1406, 1968.

44. Luengo MD, Van Hall EV: Prevention of peritoneal adhesions with spongostan and dextran 70. *Fertil Steril* 29:447, 1978.

12 Hormonal and Surgical Management of Pelvic Endometriosis

W. P. Dmowski

Division of Reproductive Endocrinology and Infertility
Department of Obstetrics and Gynecology
University of Arkansas for Medical Sciences
Little Rock, Arkansas 72205

Endometriosis is an enigmatic disease of the menstruating female. It affects women and female rhesus monkeys as well as females of other species of primates.[1] It is not observed in men or males of other species, although men may be susceptible to this disease if their hormonal milieu is changed. Two well documented cases exist of men who developed endometriosis of the urinary bladder following prolonged treatment with estrogen for prostatic carcinoma.[2,3]

Endometriosis afflicts women in their reproductive years, limits their fertility, and seriously impairs their health, although it is not life threatening. The first recorded reference to characteristic symptoms of endometriosis might have been made as early as 1600 B.C. in the Egyptian Papyrus Ebers.[4] The first histological description of the endometriotic lesion is credited to Von Rokitansky who described an "adenomyoma" in 1860.[5] However, it was not until the beginning of this century that a detailed study of this disease was performed by Sampson, who coined the name "endometriosis" and who postulated an acceptable theory on its histogenesis.

The exact mechanism for the development of endometriosis is unknown in spite of numerous studies and several postulated theories. Probably the most popular theory on the histogenesis of endometriosis remains the theory of Sampson.[6] It postulates that viable endometrial fragments are "regurgitated" through Fallopian tubes into the peritoneal cavity where they undergo subsequent implantation. Indeed, there is clinical and experimental evidence supporting this theory. Sampson's theory, however, does not satisfactorily explain the origin of endometriotic foci in areas distant from the pelvis or the origin of bladder endometriosis in men.[2,3] Other theories on histogenesis of endometriosis postulate metastatic or metaplastic mechanisms and find evidentiary support.

Both clinical and experimental evidence, however, indicate that viable endometrial fragments may be disseminated from the uterine cavity through Fallopian tubes and into the peritoneal cavity in many women whether or not they have the disease. Similarly, metastatic and metaplastic mechanisms should be operative in all women. It is not known why endometriosis develops in some women and not in others. It is possible that specific predisposing factors that facilitate implantation of regurgitated endometrial fragments or formation of the endometrial tissue *de novo* exist in those who are affected by the disease. Change in the endocrine milieu could be one such factor and appears to be directly involved in two unusual cases of male bladder endometriosis. It is well accepted that the persistence and spread of endometriosis are stimulated by cyclic secretion of ovarian hormones. Its symptoms and findings, however, are variable; no two patients are alike. Severe, incapacitating dysmenorrhea and pelvic pain are often observed with minimal endometriosis, whereas extensive disease is at times symptom-free. The disease interferes with the reproductive function of the patient and is frequently diagnosed at the time of infertility investigation.

The unknown etiology of endometriosis is the limiting factor in the development of an effective treatment. There is no drug available that could prevent endometriosis or selectively destroy ectopic endometrium and cure the disease. Current therapeutic approaches include surgery and hormonal therapy. Both intend to eradicate the ectopic endometrium and improve the patient's chances for conception. The choice of therapy is frequently influenced by physician bias, generally based on his expertise with a specific therapeutic method. Thus, the published results of treatment, especially when combined with the surgical approach, vary significantly and often cannot be duplicated by those less experienced with the technique. The effectiveness of treatment has been judged by a combination of objective and subjective responses including the degree of symptomatic or clinical improvement, laparoscopic evidence, rate of recurrence, and need for subsequent surgery, as well as posttreatment pregnancy rates. Regardless of the method of treatment employed, endometriosis demonstrates tendencies to recur. All modes of therapy usually offer to a patient only a temporary remission and a chance for pregnancy if infertility was the presenting symptom. The only definitive method of treatment that assures permanent cure of the disease and prevents its recurrence requires bilateral oophorectomy.

ENDOMETRIOSIS AND INFERTILITY

The association of endometriosis and infertility is well established. The incidence of infertility in the presence of endometriosis approximates 30–40%.[7] However, infertility in women with proven endometriosis is relative, and conceptions do occur. The direct cause of infertility in patients with endometriosis is unknown; it is likely that several mechanisms that interfere with conception are operative.

When women have extensive pelvic endometriosis, the mechanism of infertility is obvious. In these patients, bilateral ovarian enlargement by multiple endometriomas and severe pelvic adhesive disease distorting the entire pelvic anatomy are the characteristic features. Although endometriosis of the Fallopian tubes, even in the presence of severe disease, is rare, and commonly there is bilateral tubal patency, both Fallopian tubes are frequently surrounded by adhesions with their fimbriated ends separated from the ovaries and opening into peritoneal pockets enclosed by adhesions. These adhesions limit ovarian and tubal mobility and may change ovarian location and distort tubal passage. It is reasonable to assume in these patients that mechanical interference with ovum release and transport is the primary reason for infertility. It should be kept in mind, however, that infertility even in such patients is relative, and conceptions occasionally occur in the presence of extensive endometriosis.

The cause or causes of infertility in women with few small endometriotic implants and otherwise normal pelvic structures is less easily comprehended. Several mechanisms have been suggested. Dyspareunia resulting in coital avoidance or inadequate penile penetration may be a contributory factor.[7] Interference with the ovum transport may be another cause. Although a fertilized or unfertilized ovum has no movement of its own, it has been suggested that it may be chemotactically attracted toward ectopic rather than uterine endometrium.[8]

Recent studies indicate that the peritoneal fluid in women with endometriosis may contain a high concentration of prostaglandins and especially $PGF_{2\alpha}$.[9] It is likely that $PGF_{2\alpha}$, produced by the ectopic endometrial foci and transferred to the peritoneal fluid in which Fallopian tubes as well as the rest of the reproductive system is bathed, is responsible for the characteristic symptoms and the infertility associated with this disease. Increased local concentrations of $PGF_{2\alpha}$ could cause such symptoms as dysmenorrhea, nausea, vomiting, pelvic pain, and dyspareunia. Moreover, increased tubal motility, luteolytic action, as well as other effects of $PGF_{2\alpha}$ on the reproductive system could explain the mechanism of infertility. The antifertility effect, according to this hypothesis, would depend on the concentration of $PGF_{2\alpha}$ in the reproductive system and, therefore, on the amount of the endometriotic tissue, its access to the peritoneal fluid, the volume of the peritoneal fluid, as well as other factors. It is clear that such an antifertility effect would be inconsistent and variable.

Some investigators[10,11] believe that the luteinized unruptured follicle syndrome is the cause of infertility in women with endometriosis. This entity, which cannot be diagnosed by any means other than a direct inspection of the corpus luteum, seems to be observed, however, with at least the same frequency in other disorders associated with infertility.[12] A recent study suggests yet another possible infertility mechanism associated with endometriosis. Weed et al.[13] postulate that an autoimmune response to the absorbed constituents of desquamated ectopic endometrium results in the formation of an antibody that can cause uterine endometrial changes unfavorable to the nidation of the fertilized ovum.

Regardless of its cause, infertility in many patients with endometriosis is corrected by the treatment of this disease.[7] Most conceptions occur immediately after completion of therapy, and the cause-and-effect relationship between treatment of endometriosis and improved fertility can be readily established. For this reason, posttreatment pregnancy rates have been used to evaluate the effectiveness of various therapeutic approaches.

CLASSIFICATION OF ENDOMETRIOSIS

Endometriosis is characterized by extreme variability in the extent of involvement of the pelvic organs. It is generally agreed that the process begins with occasional endometriotic implants that increase in number, form plaques, and gradually give rise to small, medium, or large endometriomas. The disease then gradually spreads from the most common initial location in the cul-de-sac throughout the entire pelvis. The extent of endometriosis, its location, and unilaterality or bilaterality of the involvement should be considered in making the diagnosis and choosing the method of therapy. Uniform classification or staging of endometriosis is also required to evaluate and compare the therapeutic results of different methods of treatment, the posttreatment recurrence, and the pregnancy rates.

Several classifications of endometriosis have been suggested, yet none has become uniformly accepted. A classification of endometriosis should (1) be fairly simple, (2) be reasonably complete, (3) take into consideration the location of the lesions on the outside of the reproductive system, (4) recognize unilateral or bilateral involvement, and (5) have provisions for including the extent and location of pelvic adhesive disease.

One of the earliest and most frequently cited classifications of endometriosis was introduced in 1973 by Acosta et al.[14] One of its major advantages is simplicity in staging endometriosis as mild, moderate, and severe. This classification, however, has several disadvantages; the major disadvantage is the lack of consideration for unilaterality versus bilaterality of the involvement. According to this classification, unilateral endometrioma larger than 2×2 cm would be considered as severe endometriosis, whereas smaller endometriomas involving both ovaries would be classified as a moderate disease. It would, therefore, be reasonable to expect better treatment results in terms of posttreatment pregnancy rates in patients with severe disease than in those with moderate disease, especially if surgery was the treatment of choice. To achieve a more meaningful evaluation of posttreatment pregnancy rates, Dmowski and Cohen[15] classified endometriosis as mild when only small endometriotic implants were present, moderate when, in addition to the above, one ovary was enlarged by endometrioma, and severe when bilateral ovarian endometriomas were present.

Kistner et al.,[16] in 1977, suggested another classification of endometriosis that placed particular attention on its relationship to infertility. This classification, although more elaborate than its predecessors, also suffered from disregard for unilateral versus bilateral involvement. A year later, Buttram[17] suggested a classification designed to take into consideration unilaterality or bilaterality of adnexal involvement. This, probably the most exhaustive and complicated classification, was soon followed by one suggested by a specially appointed committee of the American Fertility Society.[18]

The American Fertility Society (AFS) classification (Fig. 1) is based on a point system and takes into consideration the number, size, and location of endometrial implants, plaques, or endometriomas. It provides evaluation of unilateral and bilateral involvement and recognizes the significance of adhesions, their extent, and location. The number of points for each pathological change (area of endometriosis or adhesions) is then totaled, and the sum indicates the stage of the disease (mild, moderate, severe, or extensive). The major advantage of this classification, however, is that it encourages a physician to examine systematically the entire reproductive system and to document his findings by a drawing on the sketch of pelvic organs included in the classification form. Classification forms are available at a modest charge from the AFS. This standard AFS classification, in its present or perhaps a slightly modified form, will, one hopes, become generally accepted and encourage careful documentation of pelvic findings at the time of laparoscopy or laparotomy. This, in turn, may allow a better understanding of the natural course of endometriosis and a more precise

AMERICAN FERTILITY SOCIETY CLASSIFICATION OF ENDOMETRIOSIS

Patient's name _____

Stage I	(Mild)	1–5
Stage II	(Moderate)	6–15
Stage III	(Severe)	16–30
Stage IV	(Extensive)	31–54

Total _____

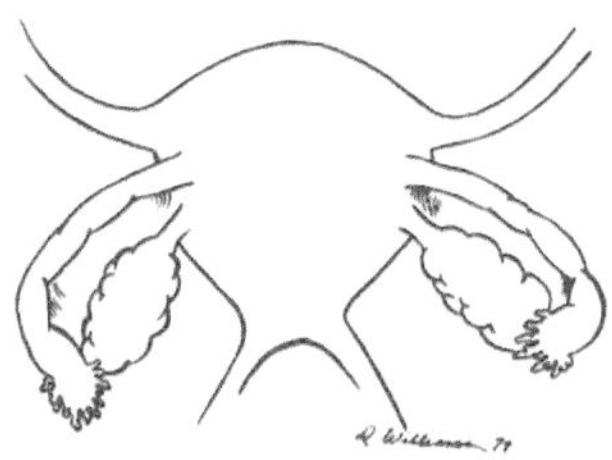

	ENDOMETRIOSIS	<1 cm	1–3 cm	>3 cm
PERITONEUM		1	2	3
	ADHESIONS	Filmy	Dense with partial cul-de-sac obliteration	Dense with complete cul-de-sac obliteration
		1	2	3
OVARY	ENDOMETRIOSIS	<1 cm	1–3 cm	>3 cm or ruptured endometrioma
	R	2	4	6
	L	2	4	6
	ADHESIONS	Filmy	Dense with partial ovarian enclosure	Dense with complete ovarian enclosure
	R	2	4	6
	L	2	4	6
TUBE	ENDOMETRIOSIS	<1 cm	>1 cm	Tubal occlusion
	R	2	4	6
	L	2	4	6
	ADHESIONS	Filmy	Dense with tubal distortion	Dense with tubal enclosure
	R	2	4	6
	L	2	4	6

Associated pathology:

Figure 1. American Fertility Society endometriosis classification form.

comparison of the results of treatment with different therapeutic methods.

HORMONAL MANAGEMENT

The rationale for hormonal treatment of endometriosis is based on the clinical observation that symptoms and signs of this disease improve during the amenorrhea of pregnancy and menopause. The purpose of hormonal therapy is to stop cyclic endometrial stimulation by estrogen and progesterone, inhibit proliferative, secretory, and desquamative endometrial changes, and induce amenorrhea. The establishment of amenorrhea suppresses cyclic peritoneal bleeding from ectopic endometrial lesions. Atrophy of both uterine and ectopic endometrium results, and healing of endometriosis begins.

Currently, there are two acceptable and reasonably effective methods of hormonal treatment of endometriosis: pseudopregnancy and pseudomenopause. Just as pregnancy is less predictable in its beneficial effect on endometriosis than is menopause, pseudopregnancy is less consistent in this respect than pseudomenopause. Pseudomenopause is more beneficial, has fewer and better tolerated side effects, and requires less time to achieve a desirable improvement.

Effect of Pregnancy

If a young woman suffering from endometriosis is capable and willing to conceive, pregnancy will be the most common recommendation that she will receive from her gynecologist. It is a common belief that repeated gestations in some way prevent development of endometriosis and that the disease undergoes involution during gestation. A review of the literature, however, indicates that the beneficial effects of pregnancy on symptoms and signs of endometriosis have been variable and inconsistent.[19] Symptomatic improvement and decrease in the size of endometriotic lesions appear to be associated with the third trimester of pregnancy and the postpartum lactation period. A worsening of the symptoms and increase in the size of endometriotic lesions are generally observed during early pregnancy. Histological changes in the ectopic endometrium during pregnancy correspond to those occurring in the uterine endometrium and reflect the hormonal status of pregnancy, specifically the increased activity of estrogens and progesterone. Endometrial hypertrophy, increased vascularity, edema, and decidualization are observed early in pregnancy. As pregnancy advances, atrophic changes in the ectopic endometrium begin to take place.[20] This sequence of histological changes explains variable clinical effects of pregnancy on endometriosis.

Effect of Menopause

The effect of menopause on endometriosis is probably more consistent. In the absence of estrogenic and progestational stimulation of the ectopic endometrium, the disease regresses, and symptomatic improvement immediately begins. This is particularly evident following surgical menopause when abrupt and complete withdrawal of all ovarian hormonal secretion results in a prompt and complete atrophy of the ectopic and uterine endometrium. Physiological menopause is characterized by much less complete and much less abrupt withdrawal of hormonal support to the endometrium. Estrogen production, although not cyclic and without additional progestational effect, may continue in many patients well past menopause. Active endometriosis may remain in such patients.

PSEUDOMENOPAUSE

Induction of amenorrhea, of the so-called "pseudomenopause," is a relatively recent approach to the treatment of endometriosis. Danazol, a synthetic steroid with potent antigonadotropic properties, induces pseudomenopause characterized by complete ovarian suppression and hypoestrogenic amenorrhea.

Biological Properties of Danazol

Chemically, danazol (Fig. 2) is an isoxazol derivative of 17α-ethinyl testosterone (ethisterone). The antigonadotropic properties of danazol have been demonstrated in various animal species and in humans by different investigators using both bioassay and radioimmunoassay techniques.[21] The compound inhibits pituitary secretion of both FSH and LH, and the effect is dose dependent. The results of LHRH testing to determine the mechanism of danazol action at the hypothalamo-pituitary level have been inconsistent. It is still unclear whether danazol inhibits the response of the pituitary to LHRH or acts through suppression of hypothalamic LHRH secretion. The FSH- and LH-suppressing properties of danazol are comparable to those of other sex steroids such as estradiol, testosterone, and dihydrotestosterone. The antigonadotropic effect of danazol is demonstrable at a dose that does not produce peripheral endocrine effects, whereas a similar antigonadotropic effect of the other steroids mentioned only occurs at doses that are either strongly androgenic or estrogenic.[22] Danazol, as could be anticipated from its chemical structure which is related to that of testosterone, displays some androgenic and anabolic properties. The androgenic effect of danazol is statistically significant at a higher dose level than its an-

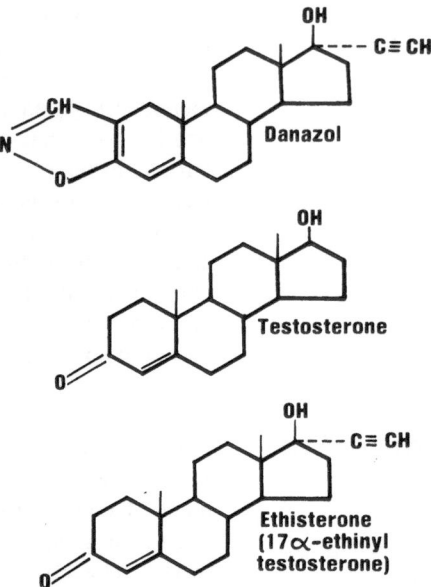

Figure 2. Chemical structures of danazol, testosterone, and ethisterone.

tigonadotropic effect (12 mg/kg vs. 4mg/kg), leaving a relatively wide therapeutic safety margin between desirable antigonadotropic and undesirable androgenic properties. In a bioassay system, the androgenic effect of danazol was about 200 times lower and the anabolic effect about 24 times lower than that of testosterone.[23] Thus, danazol appears to be relatively more anabolic than androgenic.

The suppressive effect of danazol on basal plasma FSH and LH levels has been somewhat more difficult to demonstrate in human than in animal studies, particularly when the drug was administered on a short-term basis. Even with short-term administration, however, the midcycle FSH and LH surges have usually been well suppressed.[24] During chronic administration of the drug, absence of FSH and LH peaks and decreased plasma FSH levels have been noted.[25] The effect of danazol on elevated postmenopausal FSH and LH titers is not entirely clear. In one study, danazol did not modify elevated FSH and LH in two women a few days after oophorectomy,[26] whereas in another study, a significant suppression of gonadotropins was observed in five postmenopausal women.[27]

In clinical studies on both men and women, danazol initiates characteristic changes related to gonadotropin suppression.[21] When administered to women with normal menstrual cycles, danazol brings about the multitude of endocrine and clinical changes listed in Table I. The midcycle FSH and LH surges are suppressed from the beginning of treatment and are followed by a decrease in the basal levels of both gonadotropins. Plasma estradiol levels are either undetectable or lie in the early follicular range, and the preovulatory rise of this hormone is not observed. Plasma progesterone is low, and ovulation detection tests indicate an anovulatory state. Amenorrhea develops, usually within the first 4–6 weeks of treatment, although occasionally irregular spotting throughout the course of therapy may be observed. Gross and microscopic examination of the endometrium indicates marked thinning of the endometrial layer and atrophic changes in the endometrial glands and stroma. Vaginal cytology is hypoestrogenic. Some women report hot flashes, night sweats, and other vasomotor disturbances characteristic of menopause. Androgenic and anabolic effects of danazol have also been observed in clinical studies. They are usually mild and can readily be con-

Table I
Endocrine and Clinical Effects
of Danazol in Normal Women

Endocrine effects
    Inhibition of midcycle FSH and LH surge
    Lowering of basal FSH and LH titers
    Persistently low plasma estradiol
    Persistently low plasma progesterone
Clinical effects
    Anovulation
    Amenorrhea
    Hypoestrogenic vaginal cytology
    Atrophic endometrium
    Monophasic basal body temperature
Side effects in some women
    Hot flashes, sweats, and other vasomotor disturbances
    Androgenic effects
    Anabolic effects

trolled by a decrease in the daily dose. Those most commonly noted include increased skin oiliness, acne, and weight gain. Deepening of the voice and increased hair growth have been observed only occasionally, and true virilization has not been reported.

Danazol is well absorbed from the gastrointestinal system and is rapidly metabolized. After administration of a single oral dose of 400 mg, plasma levels of danazol in ten female volunteers reached a mean maximum value of 80 ng/ml within 2 hr.[28] Although individual variability was observed, none of the subjects had measurable plasma danazol levels after 8 hr, and the average half-life of the compound was about 4.5 hr. Experimental studies with radiolabeled danazol in rhesus monkeys indicate that the drug is eliminated in about equal portions in urine and feces, and its total recovery exceeds 80% after 48 hr and 90% after 4 days.[28] The major metabolite of danazol in plasma, urine, and feces is 2-hydroxymethylethisterone. Other identified metabolites include Δ^1-hydroxymethylethisterone and 2-ketoethisterone.

Although danazol is rapidly and extensively metabolized with resulting cleavage of the isoxazol ring, several studies seem to indicate that the biological effect is caused by danazol itself and not by its metabolites. None of the five metabolites of danazol had significant androgenic or antigonadotropic activities as compared with the parental molecule.[29] Furthermore, concurrent administration of danazol and its metabolic blockers to rats resulted in an increase of the antigonadotropic function of this compound.[30]

Treatment of Endometriosis with Danazol

To exert its effect, danazol, as do natural steroids, binds competitively, and probably at various levels in the reproductive system, to the cytoplasmic receptor proteins specific for these steroids.[31] In addition to the central, antigonadotropic effect, danazol may be directly inhibiting ovarian steroidogenesis[32] and, as postulated by some, may also have a direct effect at the endometrial level.[33] However, the mechanism of danazol's beneficial effect on endometriosis can be explained solely through its antigonadotropic function.

A schematic outline in Fig. 3B illustrates the effect of danazol on the reproductive function in the female as compared to normal relationships demonstrated in Fig. 3A. Acting at the hypothalamus and/or the pituitary, danazol either inhibits the pituitary response to LHRH or suppresses hypothalamic secretion of LHRH. The net result of this effect is suppression of FSH and LH release from the pituitary, the antigonadotropic effect. Suppression of FSH and LH results in anovulation and inhibition of ovarian steroidogenesis. The ovary becomes small, without gross evidence of follicular or luteal activity, resembling an inactive menopausal ovary. Histologically, most of the follicles are in the early preantral stage of development, and no corpora lutea are present. Endocrine assays demonstrate persistently low plasma FSH and LH titers, comparable to those of the midfollicular range. Plasma progesterone is persistently below 2 ng/ml, indicating anovulation. Uterine endometrium grossly is markedly atrophic and microscopically resembles the inactive endometrium of menopause, with small atrophic glands and dense inactive stroma.

Ectopic endometrium demonstrates atrophic changes histologically similar to those observed in the uterine endometrium.[24] Small and medium-sized thin-walled endometriomas regress completely. Large endometriomas, and especially those with thick walls surrounded by dense connective tissue, may only decrease in size. In many areas where active endometriosis was present prior to treatment, adhesive disease may develop, and hemosiderin-laden macrophages may be seen histologically.[15] Along with atrophy of endometriotic lesions, pelvic congestion and vascularity related to endometriosis and estrogenic stimulation decrease. Uterus, ovaries, and Fallopian tubes may also undergo atrophy similar to that observed during menopause.

Amenorrhea usually begins with the onset of treatment. Hypoestrogenic changes in the vaginal epithelium are observed in most patients and in some may lead to a predisposition to vaginal infections. Hot flashes, sweats, and other symptoms of vasomotor instability are observed in some patients. These symptoms and findings, in some ways resembling menopause, prompted the term "pseudomenopause" for the state induced by danazol therapy.[34] How-

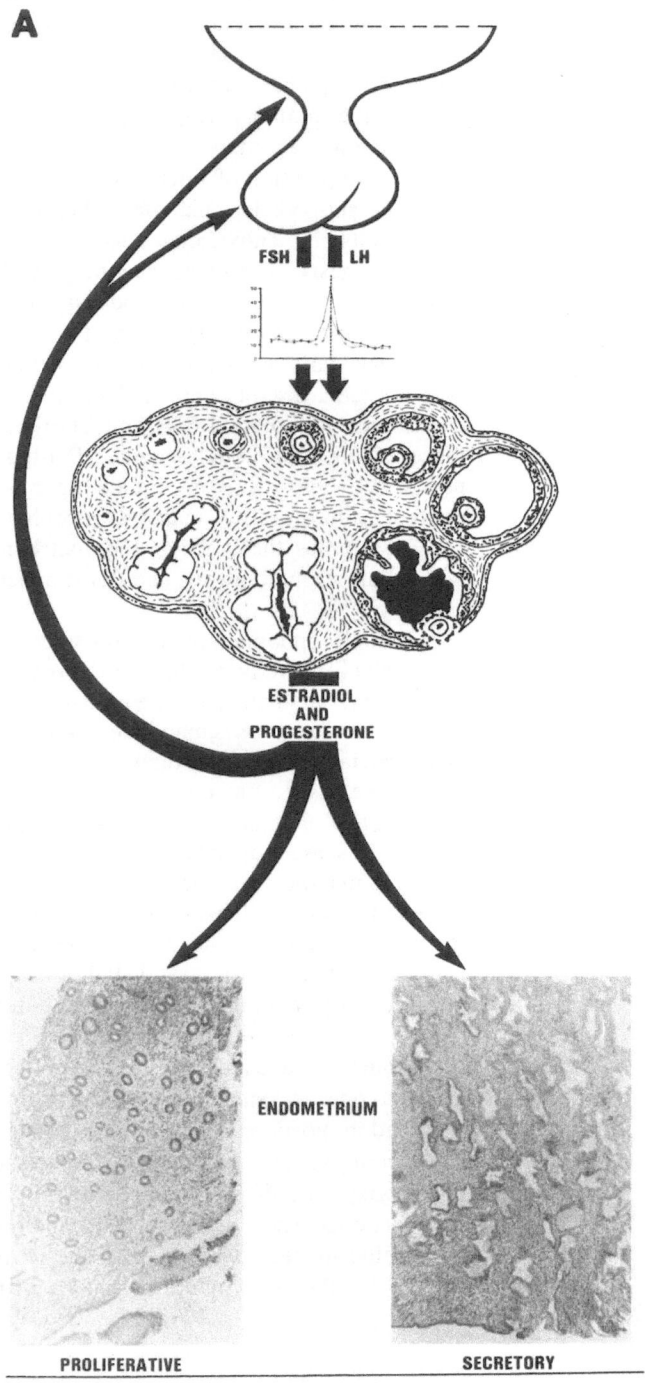

Figure 3. Hypothalamo–pituitary–gonadal–endometrial relationships in (A) normally cycling women; (B) women treated with danazol; (C) women treated with estrogen plus progestogen.

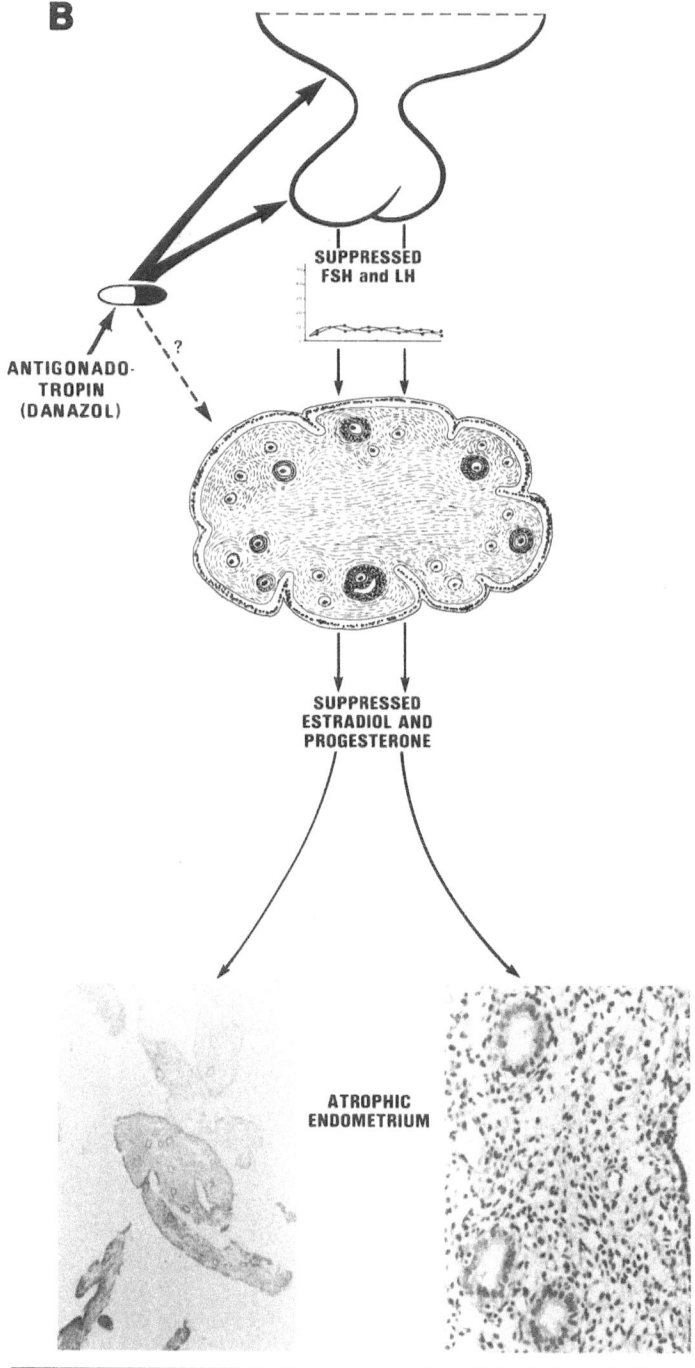

B

ANTIGONADO-
TROPIN
(DANAZOL)

SUPPRESSED
FSH and LH

SUPPRESSED
ESTRADIOL AND
PROGESTERONE

ATROPHIC
ENDOMETRIUM

Figure 3.   (*continued*)

MANAGEMENT OF PELVIC ENDOMETRIOSIS | **247**

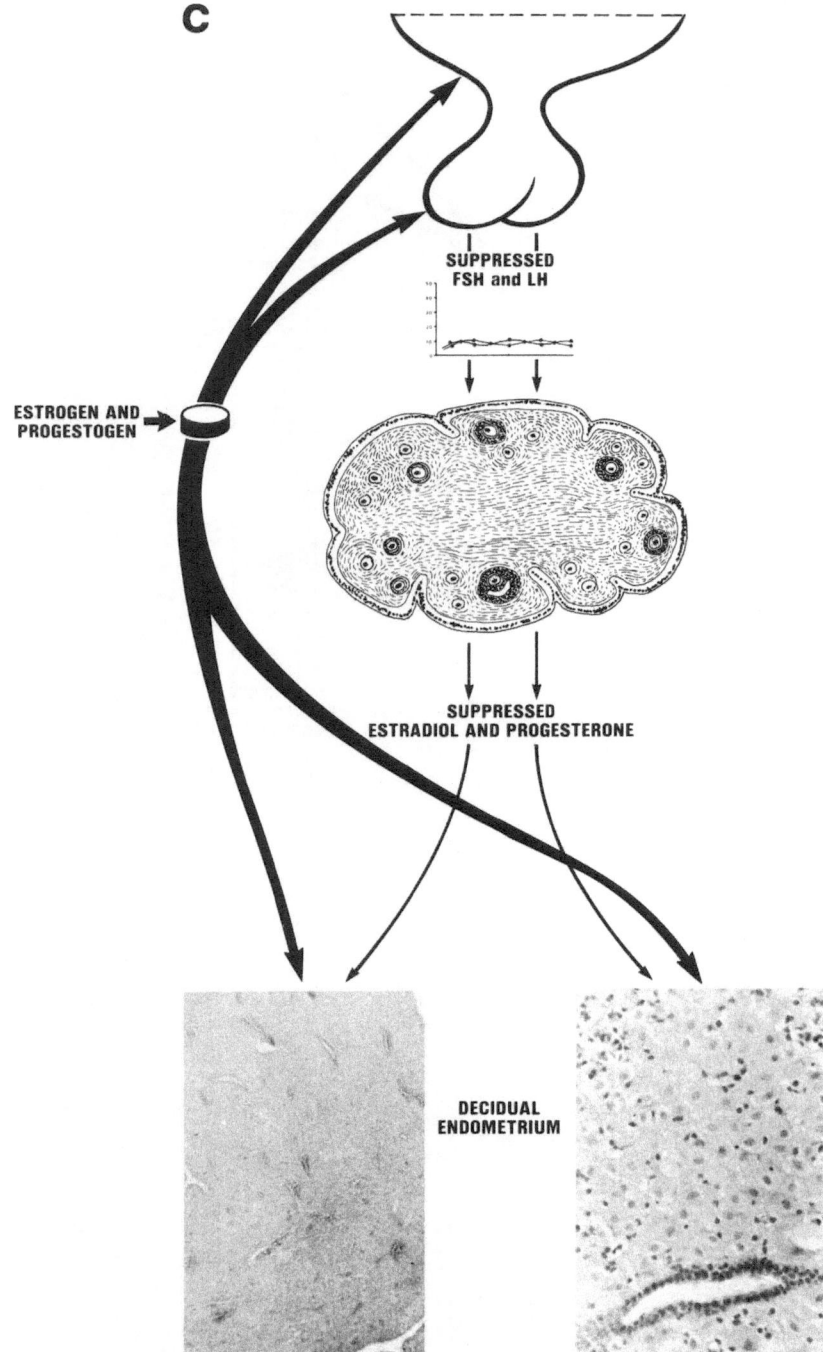

C

SUPPRESSED
FSH and LH

ESTROGEN AND
PROGESTOGEN

SUPPRESSED
ESTRADIOL AND PROGESTERONE

DECIDUAL
ENDOMETRIUM

Figure 3. *(continued)*

ever, in contradistinction to physiological menopause, plasma gonadotropin levels are suppressed, not elevated during pseudomenopause. Pseudomenopause terminates with the end of danazol treatment.

The beneficial effect of danazol in endometriosis was first reported by Greenblatt and co-workers.[24] In their group of 40 patients, the authors noted symptomatic improvement in over 90% and clinically evident regression of the disease in over 50%. Laparotomy demonstrated regression of endometriotic lesions and atrophic changes in the ectopic endometrium. Subsequent studies by other investigators have confirmed these findings. Symptomatic improvement was reported in up to 94% of patients and objective improvement in up to 87%.[15,35-41] Along with symptomatic and clinical improvement, an increased incidence of posttreatment pregnancies has been reported.

Essentially any patient with confirmed diagnosis of endometriosis can be a candidate for danazol therapy. Induction of pseudomenopause is probably the best currently available medical treatment of endometriosis. Even those patients in whom surgery is considered the treatment of choice may benefit if pretreated with danazol. The best candidates for danazol therapy, however, are infertile women with mild or moderate endometriosis.

Pseudomenopause is induced with danazol administered in a dose of 200 mg q.i.d. for a period of 3–9 months. In many patients, the effective daily dose of danazol may be lower than 800 mg. Recent experience of several investigators indicates that although a lower dose may be beneficial in some patients, it is associated with a higher incidence of the residual disease.[42,43] From the practical standpoint, it seems advantageous to begin the patient on a full 800 mg/day dose. This could be subsequently decreased to 600 and 400 mg/day if the patient responds well in terms of symptomatic and clinical improvement and in the appearance of amenorrhea. Underweight patients can probably begin with the lower initial dose of 600 mg/day. Selection of the lowest optimal dose for a particular patient should decrease the incidence of androgenic side effects, which are dose related. A dose lower than 200 mg/day will probably be only minimally effective.

Administration of danazol on a twice-a-day schedule as recommended in the package insert may be inadequate in some patients. Studies on animals and on human volunteers indicate that the half-life of danazol administered orally is about $4\frac{1}{2}$ hr.[28,44] An interval of 12–16 hr between doses may result in a significant fluctuation of plasma danazol levels and may be the cause of persistent bleeding. Administration of the drug according to a four-times-a-day schedule corrects the problem.

The treatment with danazol should begin on the first day of the menstrual cycle. Beginning therapy later on in the cycle may delay the onset of amenorrhea and may be associated with irregular bleeding during the first few weeks of therapy. Furthermore, unless treatment coincides with the beginning of the cycle, early conception cannot be excluded. The drug should not be used during pregnancy because virilization of the female fetus may occur.

The length of danazol therapy should be adjusted individually on the basis of the initial extent of the disease and the clinical response of the patient. In patients with mild disease, a 3- to 4-month course of treatment is adequate. Patients with moderate endometriosis and endometriomas up to 3 cm in diameter will require a longer course of 6–8 months. Those with severe endometriosis and large pelvic endometriomas, especially if associated with pelvic adhesive disease, may take longer, and regression of endometriosis may never be complete. In such patients, conservative surgery should be considered on discontinuation of danazol therapy.

Repeated second-look laparoscopy may be indicated after termination of pseudomenopause. In patients with moderate or severe disease in whom pelvic adhesions have been observed or suspected, second-look laparoscopy should probably be done immediately after discontinuation of danazol and should be followed by lysis of adhesions. In patients with mild or moderate disease without adhesions who improved well clinically during the course of treatment, second-look laparoscopy is probably not necessary immediately after discontinuation of therapy. It should be considered, however, if pregnancy does not follow within 6–12 months.

Following pseudomenopause, as after other methods of treatment, endometriosis demonstrates tendencies to recur. In some patients it may be a *de novo* process; in others it may be a reactivation of residual endometriotic lesions. The incidence of posttreatment recurrence was 39% after an average of 37 months from the completion of danazol treatment.[38] This consisted of the annual recurrence rate of 23% during the first year, 5% during the second, and 9% during the third year. The recurrence rate was lower, and the average interval between the end of treatment and the onset of recurrence was longer, in those patients who conceived after treatment. There are no contraindications to repeated danazol treatment in patients with recurring disease. If, however, there is evidence of incomplete clinical response, or if recurrence is observed early, alternative approaches such as conservative surgery should be considered.

Following treatment of endometriosis with pseudomenopause, spontaneous conceptions occur in many patients with previously longstanding infertility. Most conceptions are observed immediately after completion of treatment, and the cause-and-effect relationship between treatment of endometriosis and improved fertility can be readily established. In two separate studies, the corrected pregnancy rates after danazol treatment were 72% and 76%.[35,38] Dmowski and Cohen,[38] who reported a 72.2% overall occurrence of pregnancy within 37 months after pseudomenopause, had 83% conceptions among patients with mild endometriosis, 73% in those with moderate, and 38% in patients with severe disease. Twenty-three of 39 conceptions in that study occurred within 6 months from discontinuation of danazol, and a total of 30 within the first year after completion of treatment.

PSEUDOPREGNANCY

A beneficial effect of pregnancy on some patients with endometriosis has been repeatedly observed by clinicians and was discussed earlier in this chapter. Unfortunately, pregnancy as a treatment for endometriosis may be applied only seldom, since a significant proportion of patients afflicted by this disease are infertile. A hormonal status similar to that of pregnancy, however, may be achieved by continuous administration of estrogens and progestogens in high doses. A state of hyperhormonal amenorrhea is induced, and along with it a multitude of symptoms and findings resembling changes that occur during normal pregnancy. During the course of treatment, functional endometriotic tissue undergoes decidual transformation and subsequently necrobiosis and absorption.

This method of treatment for endometriosis, introduced by Kistner[45] in 1958, has been aptly called "pseudopregnancy." Kistner, in several publications, has probably reported on the largest group to date of patients treated with various pseudopregnancy regimens.[8,45–48] The symptomatic response in his series varied between the lowest of 72.7% and the highest of 87.3%. Kistner[49] recommends pseudopregnancy "only for those patients who are infertile and in whom moderate degrees of surface ovarian endometriosis are demonstrated at endoscopy." In the experience of other investigators whose patient selection criteria were different, the results of pseudopregnancy have been more variable. The symptomatic response rate was reported as low as 60%[50] and as high as 94%.[51]

The mode of action of estrogen–progestogen preparations in endometriosis is demonstrated in Fig. 3C. The exogenous steroids, and especially the estrogenic component, suppress hypothalamic LHRH and, therefore, FSH and LH secretion from the pituitary. Without FSH and LH stimulation, ovaries become atrophic with deeply corrugated cortex and without evidence of follicular or luteal activity. Microscopically, ovarian follicles are in the early preantral stage, and there are no active corpora lutea. As a result, ovarian secretion of estrogen and progesterone is suppressed. Cyclic endometrial stimulation by endogenous steroids is replaced by the continuous effect of exogenously supplied hormones. The uterine and ectopic endometrium undergoes initial stimulation, hypertrophy, vascular congestion and edema, and decidual transformation induced by progestogen. Later during the course of treatment, necrobiosis and resorption of the endometriotic tissue begin to take place.[8]

Exogenous estrogen–progestogen preparations, in contrast to endogenous steroids, are capable of suppressing ectopic and uterine endometrium for two reasons: (1) their effect is continuous and not cyclic; and (2) progestogen is administered simultaneously with estrogen so that the overall effect of the medication is strongly progestational. It should be emphasized, however, that to induce and maintain amenorrhea of pseudopregnancy, estrogen–progestogen preparations should be used continuously and not cyclically, and that the dose should be increased at every episode of breakthrough bleeding.

A variety of preparations have been recommended to induce pseudopregnancy. The doses and regimens used are illustrated in Table II. Those found most effective have been oral contraceptives with strong progestational properties such as norethynodrel, 10 mg, plus mestranol, 100 μg; norethindrone, 10 mg, plus mestranol, 60 μg; and norgestrel, 0.5 mg plus ethinyl estradiol, 50 μg. The usual therapeutic regimen consists of one tablet daily, continuously for 6–9 months, with an increase of one tablet for

Table II
Therapeutic Regimens for Induction of Pseudopregnancy
with Currently Available Preparations

Drugs	Regimen	References
Norethynodrel + mestranol (Enovid)	2.5 mg for 1 week, then 5 mg for 1 week, then 10 mg for 2 weeks, then 15 mg for 2 weeks, then 20 mg daily; increase by 10 mg for BTB^a	53
	20 mg daily; increase by 10 mg for BTB	54
	30 mg daily; increase by 10 mg for BTB	69,51,52
Norethindrone + mestranol (OrthoNovum, Norinyl)	10 mg for 2 weeks, then 20 mg for 2 weeks, then 30 mg daily; increase by 10 mg for BTB	53
Ethynodiol diacetate + mestranol (Ovulen)	2 mg daily; increase by 2 mg for BTB	69,47
Norethindrone acetate + ethinyl estradiol (Norlestrin)	5 mg daily; increase by 2.5 mg for BTB	48
Mesgestrol acetate + ethinyl estradiol	5 mg daily; increase by 5 mg for BTB	47
Norgestrel + ethinyl estradiol (Ovral)	0.5 mg daily; increase by 0.5 mg for BTB	
Medroxyprogesterone acetate (Provera)	30 mg daily	70
Depo-medroxyprogesterone acetate (Depo-Provera)	100 mg IM every 2 weeks for 4 doses; then 100 mg every 4 weeks; add oral or parenteral estrogen for BTB	53
	100 mg IM every 2 weeks with or without oral estrogens	71

^{a} BTB: breakthrough bleeding.

each episode of breakthrough bleeding. In this way, the lowest effective dose is determined individually for each patient.

The use of progestational preparations alone has been associated with a much higher incidence of breakthrough bleeding, and generally, addition of an estrogenic component is recommended. The results of treatment with progestogens alone probably do not differ significantly from those obtained with estrogen–progestogen preparations. In specific circumstances, however, long-acting parenteral progestogens such as depo-medroxyprogesterone acetate may be of benefit. They seem to be of special advantage in an older patient not interested in fertility, who has moderately extensive, symptomatic endometriosis and who, for one reason or another, cannot be treated surgically. It has been demonstrated that depo-medroxyprogesterone acetate may remain in the body for several months, and sometimes years, exerting a prolonged effect on the hypothalamo–pituitary-gonadal axis. For this reason, it should not be used in infertile patients who would like to conceive after completion of therapy.

During the early phase of treatment with pseudopregnancy, exacerbation of symptoms and findings related to endometriosis may be observed in many patients. Some women may have breakthrough bleeding and may pass a thick, decidual cast of the uterine cavity. As previously mentioned, a similar exacerbation of symptoms may be observed during early pregnancy in those patients with endometriosis who conceive. It is related to hypertrophy, increased vascularity, and edema taking place during that time in the uterine as well as the ectopic endometrium.

Side effects of pseudopregnancy are numerous, and continuation rates of treatment have not been high in the experience of many investigators. The most common side effects include nausea, breast soreness, vaginal discharge, and fluid retention. Some patients note insomnia, restlessness, and irritability, whereas others complain of excessive lethargy and tiredness. Occasionally, severe and persistent headaches have been reported. Uterine leiomyomata increase in size during pseudopregnancy, and probably an alternative treatment method should be chosen for patients with these tumors. Uterine breakthrough bleeding occurs frequently before pseudopregnancy is established and may be associated with severe cramping and abdominal pains. Contraindications and potential complications of pseudopregnancy are the same as those associated with the use of oral contraceptives.

The recurrence rate of endometriosis after pseudopregnancy is variable and related to the time of follow-up. It is higher during the first year following treatment, which may indicate that it is related more to the residual disease than to the *de novo* process. Riva et al.[52] reported a 17.8% recurrence after an average of 10.9 months, and Kistner[53] a 16.6% recurrence after a similar period of time. During subsequent years, recurrence rates vary between 5% and 10% annually.

Posttreatment pregnancy rates after pseudopregnancy have been reported as low as 5%[50] and as high as 73%.[54] Kistner, who had an overall pregnancy rate of 50.8% in 186 patients, states that "a pregnancy rate of approximately 50% may be expected following pseudopregnancy in patients whose only abnormality is surface ovarian endometriosis without endometriomas or tubo-ovarian adhesions."[49]

OTHER HORMONAL METHODS

Androgens

Androgens such as testosterone and methyltestosterone have been employed for many years in the treatment of endometriosis, although there is no exact explanation as to the mechanism of their effect. Several reports are on record indicating their beneficial effect on endometriosis and specifically on amelioration of symptoms such as pelvic pain, dyspareunia, and dysmenorrhea.[55-59] The dose of androgen is not high enough to suppress ovarian function, at least not consistently. Ovulations and conceptions have been reported to occur during therapy. A direct effect of androgen on the endometrium has been suggested, but histological studies of the endometriotic tissue in monkeys on androgen treatment do not reveal microscopic changes that could be attributable to the therapy.[60]

The most common therapeutic regimen consists of methyltestosterone linquettes administered continuously for a period of about 6 months in a daily dose of 5–10 mg. The therapy should be discontinued immediately if conception occurs. Thus, the use of basal body temperature charts as well as other means to diagnose early pregnancy are necessary. Symptomatic improvement in the severity of dysmenorrhea, dyspareunia, and pelvic pain has been observed in about 75% of patients treated.[59] In most patients, however, the relief is only partial and temporary, and the symptoms tend to recur within a few cycles after discontinuation of treatment.

The pregnancy rate within a year after discontinuation of treatment is variable and has been reported in the range of 11% to 19%.[58,59] The major advantage of androgen therapy for endometriosis as opposed to other therapeutic regimens is its apparent lack of the inhibitory effect on ovulation. However, the clinical results and posttreatment pregnancy rates are not as good with androgens as those achieved with other methods of treatment.

Side effects of androgen therapy may be significant and are related to their inherent endocrine properties. Hirsutism, acne, deepening of the voice, and clitoral enlargement have been observed. If conception occurs during treatment, virilization of the female fetus may occur. Large doses of androgens may occasionally inhibit or delay ovulation.

Estrogens

Continuous administration of large doses of estrogens to induce "hyperhormonal amenorrhea" has been advocated for treatment of endometriosis by few investigators.[61,62] Although symptomatic improvement has been observed in some patients on this regimen, atrophic changes in the ectopic endometrium could not be demonstrated histologically.[49] On the contrary, endometrium, as expected, responds with the development of cystic and adenomatous hyperplasia.[63] The risks of such therapy, especially those associated with development of hyperplastic endometrial changes and thromboembolic disease along with multiple side effects such as peripheral edema, nausea, mastodynia, and heavy vaginal bleeding make this regimen currently not acceptable.

SURGICAL MANAGEMENT

Surgery is the traditional, time-sanctioned approach to the treatment of endometriosis. It allows direct visualization of the lesions and provides surgical specimens for histological evaluation and affirmative diagnosis. Resection of endometriosis and especially of large endometriomas is the quickest way to eradicate the disease and is of specific appeal to most surgically oriented gynecologists. Furthermore, if endometriosis is associated with pelvic adhesions immobilizing the ovaries and distorting Fallopian tubes, surgical excision of both endometriosis and adhesions is considered necessary to restore patient's fertility.

There are two major disadvantages, however, of the surgical approach: (1) surgery itself may frequently be followed by development of postoperative adhesions that further compromise the patient's chances for conception; and (2) surgical resection of endometriosis is often incomplete since not all endometriotic foci can be identified grossly and removed surgically, and especially not those involving vital intraperitoneal structures.

Surgical procedures employed in the treatment of endometriosis may be divided into two broad categories: conservative and definitive. Conservative surgery aims at resection of endometriosis as well as preservation and improvement of fertility, whereas definitive surgery involves hysterectomy, bilateral salpingo-oophorectomy, and excision or destruction of all visible areas of endometriosis.

Laparoscopy and Operative Laparoscopy

Endometriosis may frequently be confused with other diseases of inflammatory or neoplastic origin if symptoms and findings of pelvic examination are the only diagnostic information available. Such presumptive diagnoses should be confirmed through direct visualization and, in questionable cases, through histological examination of the lesions. This is especially important if hormonal treatment is contemplated. Laparoscopy is the most common technique utilized for visualization of the pelvic organs and hence is of special importance in the diagnosis of endometriosis.

The laparoscopic appearance of endometriosis and especially that of mild and moderate disease is characteristic. The laparoscopist should look for bluish-brown implants in the cul-de-sac and on the utero-sacral ligaments, posterior wall of the uterus, and ovaries. A thick brownish liquid material is frequently released when lesions are touched with the probe or biopsy forceps. Small endometriotic lesions may appear at times as fleshy irregular implants on the peritoneal surface and may be scooped up easily with biopsy forceps. At times, however, such implants may be a part of a larger lesion extending beneath the surface of the peritoneum. The surgeon should look for telltale signs of endometriosis on the peritoneal surface such as "powder burn" ecchymotic areas, "puckered" nodules, or "mulberry spots." Advanced endometriosis with massive adhesions between the reproductive system and neighboring organs may at times be difficult to evaluate and diagnose through the laparoscope. Careful exploration of such lesions with the laparoscopic probe may reveal typical endometriotic implants or suspicious lesions that can be biopsied for histological diagnosis.

Laparoscopy permits the affirmative diagnosis of endometriosis and allows an evaluation of the extent and location of both endometriosis and pelvic adhesions. On the basis of such evaluation, the duration of medical therapy or the need for surgical resection may be determined. Repeat "second-look" laparoscopy has been recommended to evaluate the results of treatment, to identify the need for additional therapy, and to detect pelvic adhesions that frequently are the sequelae of therapy. It is especially recommended if the infertile patient with endometriosis does not conceive within 6 months to a year after termination of medical therapy.

Some authors consider operative laparoscopy as the accepted and, at times, the preferred surgical technique for the treatment of mild endometriosis.[64,65] Minor surgical procedures may be performed with accessory instruments inserted through one or more puncture wounds in the abdominal wall. These include lysis of adhesions, cautery of endometriotic implants, transsection of utero-sacral ligaments, and even uterine suspension. It should be stressed, however, that such procedures may be technically difficult and should be attempted only by experienced laparoscopists. The risk of serious injury to vital organs such as bowels, bladder, ureters, and blood vessels is high.[66]

Meticulous hemostasis at the conclusion of the procedure is essential in preventing reappearance of pelvic adhesions. Therefore, irrigation and aspiration of the irrigating solution are used routinely at the conclusion of the operative laparoscopy.

Conservative Surgery

Conservative surgery for endometriosis consists of resection of endometriomas and small endometriotic lesions, lysis of pelvic adhesions, and reconstruction of pelvic anatomy. At the end of the procedure, at least one ovary with the corresponding Fallopian tube should be free of endometriosis and adhesions so that the patient's fertility is preserved and enhanced. Conservative surgery for endometriosis may be performed in the infertile patient with the primary purpose of improving her fertility. It is also performed to relieve symptoms and to resect the disease in the patient who wants to retain her reproductive function but at the time is not currently concerned with conception.

Conservative surgery for endometriosis is usually performed through a transverse suprapubic incision, although a midline incision may be necessary if endometriosis is severe. The decision as to the type and extent of surgery should be made following a thorough exploration of the pelvic organs and evaluation of the extent of destruction of each adnexa. Unilateral salpingo-oophorectomy may be the procedure of choice if one ovary is severely destroyed by the disease, especially if the corresponding Fallopian tube is compromised, and the contralateral adnexa are relatively free from endometriosis. Buttram,[67] in a recent report, indicates that such an approach may be more effective in terms of posttreatment incidence of conception than attempts to resect the disease and preserve both adnexae.

Once the decision has been made as to the type and extent of surgery, all endometriomas and endometriotic implants accessible to resection should be removed. Some surgeons advocate a point cautery if endometriotic implants are multiple. If this approach is selected, maximal care should be taken to avoid thermal injury to vital structures and to prevent formation of adhesions by complete removal of all necrotic tissue. Every effort should be made to excise ovarian endometriosis as completely as possible. Following resection, the ovaries should be reconstructed using fine, nonreactive suture material. All periovarian adhesions should be lysed so that ovarian mobility is restored. Endometriotic implants and adhesions involving the corresponding Fallopian tube should then be resected, and tubal mobility and patency restored. If contralateral adnexa are to be preserved, the same procedure is repeated on the other side.

Buttram[67] suggested recently that complete resection of endometriotic implants may not necessarily improve prognosis and chances for conception but, on the contrary, may increase the incidence of postsurgical adhesions. Many of his patients with incompletely resected disease conceived readily after surgery. This concept, however, is contrary to the opinion of other surgeons who advocate complete resection of endometriosis and postsurgical hormonal treatment if the resection was incomplete.[8]

Following resection of endometriosis, care should be taken to secure complete hemostasis and to reperitonealize any raw areas in order to prevent postoperative adhesions. Techniques advocated for tuboplasty—such as the use of optical loupes or operative microscope, constant irrigation and suction, dissection with the aid of an electrocautery needle, and use of fine, nonreactive suture material—help to insure the success of the procedure.

Ancillary surgical procedures such as anterior uterine suspension, presacral neurectomy, plication of utero-sacral ligaments, and free omental or peritoneal grafts to cover any raw surface have also been recommended. The intended purpose of these procedures has been to prevent development of postoperative adhesions and to keep the uterus and adnexae away from the cul-de-sac. Various pharmacological approaches for the same purpose have also been suggested. Use of corticosteroids and antihistamines administered systemically before and after surgery and intraperitoneally during the procedure as well as the use of intraperitoneal dextran have been recommended. The value, if any, of such treatment modalities has not been conclusively demonstrated.

Definitive Surgery   Endometriosis, regardless of the method of treatment, tends to recur posttreatment. Return of cyclic ovarian function after hormonal suppression or following surgery may stimulate residual endometriotic foci or may lead to reappearance of the disease through activitation of mechanisms not yet completely understood. Definitive surgery is the only mode of treatment for endometriosis that prevents subsequent recurrence.

The surgery involves abdominal hysterectomy, bilateral salpingo-oophorectomy, and resection of the endometriosis. The procedure should be reserved only for patients with extensive endometriosis, who have completed their families, and who suffer from severe symptoms, especially if involvement of neighboring structures is present. Although ideally, only older patients should be subjected to the definitive surgery, it may have to be performed at times in a younger infertile woman who has recurring extensive disease and severe symptoms. Residual foci of endometriosis that might have been left behind undetected or that could not be resected because of technical difficulties undergo rapid regression following castration.

Although preservation of ovaries has been advocated in younger women, the possibility of recurrence makes such a procedure undesirable. It has been demonstrated that preservation of an ovary or its fragment in a patient undergoing hysterectomy for severe endometriosis is associated with repeated surgery in as many as 85% of patients.[68] It does not have to be emphasized that hysterectomy for severe endometriosis effectively terminates the reproductive function of the patient. Preservation of the ovaries in such patients exclusively for their hormonal function does not justify the risk of recurrence of endometriosis. Controlled amounts of estrogen or estrogen and androgen combined, beginning 3–6 months after surgery when residual disease has regressed, can be used for the relief or prevention of symptoms and changes resulting from estrogen deficiency. If recurrence of endometriosis is stimulated by such a regimen, the medication can be stopped or the dose decreased.

COMBINED HORMONAL AND SURGICAL MANAGEMENT

Both hormonal and surgical management of endometriosis have specific advantages as well as specific limitations. A full understanding of these advantages and limitations may result in a choice of a combined approach for the management of many cases. In patients with moderate to severe endometriosis, especially if associated with pelvic adhesions, hormonal management may be only partially effective and most likely will not restore fertility. In such patients, conservative surgery at the end of hormonal therapy should offer better clinical results and a higher chance for pregnancy. Similarly, a conservative surgery may not remove all endometriotic lesions, and a follow-up hormonal treatment may be required.

A combination of pseudomenopause and surgery has been found advantageous by several investigators. Induction of pseudomenopause for 3–6 months prior to conservative surgery is probably more desirable than treatment with danazol of the residual disease. If surgery follows pseudomenopause, its extent is limited, and there is less vasocongestion and edema resulting in easier dissection and a more complete hemostasis. There is no increased risk of thromboembolic disease since danazol has no effect on the clotting mechanisms. Surgical resection of endometriosis following a course of pseudomenopause should be associated with resection of pelvic adhesions to further improve the patient's chances for conception.

A combination of conservative surgery and pseudopregnancy or androgen therapy has been evaluated by several investigators and generally found to be without particular advantage.[59,68,69] If used prior to conservative surgery, pseudopregnancy increases pelvic vascularity and edema and usually makes dissection and hemostasis more difficult. Furthermore, changes in the clotting mechanism induced by pseudopregnancy may increase the risk of thromboembolic complications following surgery.

INDIVIDUALIZED APPROACH TO TREATMENT

Clinical diagnosis of suspected endometriosis should be confirmed by laparoscopy or laparotomy. Patients should not be subjected to a lengthy and expensive hormonal therapy on the basis of clinical diagnosis alone. There is no disagreement on this matter. A controversy exists, however, as to when endometriosis should or should not be treated, what is the most advantageous therapeutic approach, should oophorectomy be a part of a definitive surgery, as well as in other areas.

Asymptomatic, mild endometriosis not associated with infertility probably does not require specific treatment. The patient, however, should be advised of the implications of this diagnosis in terms of future fertility and progression of the disease. She may be placed on a strongly progestational contraceptive pill administered cyclically to prevent excessive endometrial proliferation and, as suggested by some, to slow down the spread of endometriosis.

Various therapeutic modalities are available for the patient with more extensive or symptomatic disease. A specific therapeutic approach is chosen on the basis of the patient's age, family status, desire for conception, severity of symptoms, extent of disease, and the personal preference as well as the expertise of the physician. A suggested therapeutic approach to four typical clinical situations is discussed in the following sections.

Management of Endometriosis in a Young, Symptomatic Patient with Untested Fertility

The patient is seen initially because of symptoms such as secondary, progressive dysmenorrhea, pelvic pain, or dyspareunia. Pelvic examination may reveal tender cul-de-sac nodularities or unilateral or bilateral adnexal enlargement, or may be entirely negative. The patient is frequently unmarried or married but not planning to conceive in the immediate future. Clinical diagnosis of suspected endometriosis is confirmed by laparoscopy (Fig. 4). If the disease is mild and the patient is willing to begin her family, conception should be advised. Unmarried patients or those not interested in pregnancy can be treated symptomatically with prostaglandin inhibitors and placed on strongly progestational oral contraceptives such as norgestrel, 0.5 mg, plus ethinyl estradiol, 0.05 mg. If symptoms are severe and no improvement occurs on this treatment, pseudomenopause may be induced for 3–4 months.

In patients with moderate endometriosis, 3–6 months of pseudomenopause is recommended. Following treatment, conception should be advised, or the patient should be placed on strongly progestational oral contraceptives. In patients with severe endometriosis, pseudomenopause for 6–8 months or, when pelvic adhesions are present, pseudomenopause combined with conservative surgery are recommended. Following treatment, conception should be

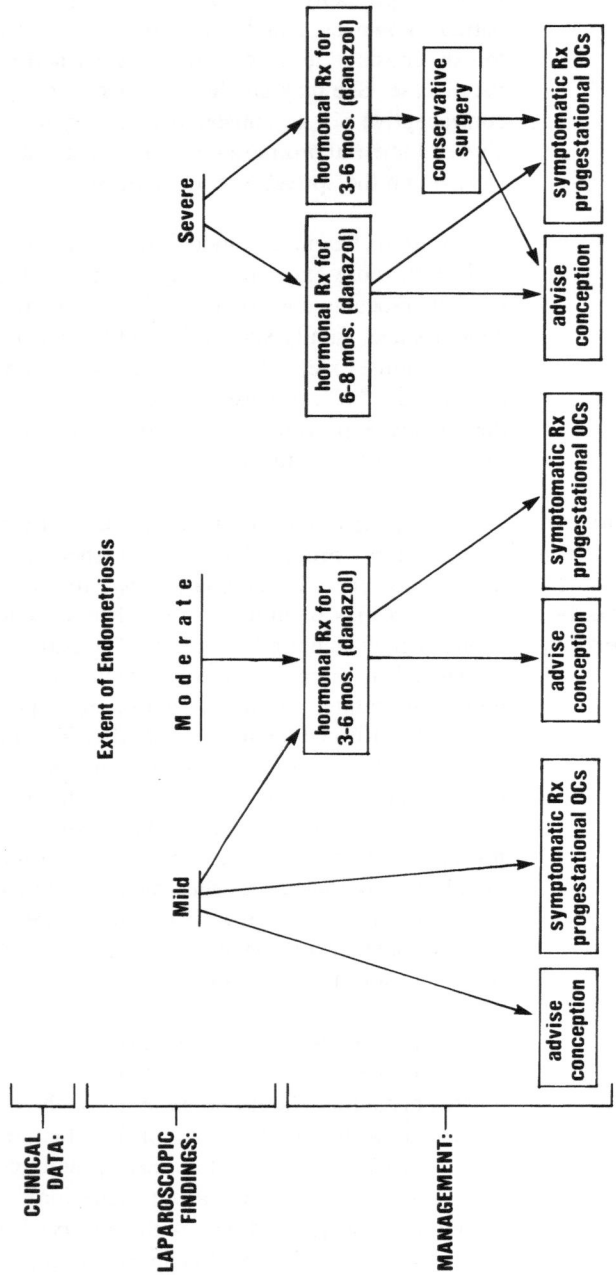

Figure 4. Management of endometriosis in a young, symptomatic patient with untested fertility.

attempted, or the patient should be placed on progestational oral contraceptives to prevent undue endometrial proliferation and recurrence of the disease.

Management of Endometriosis in a Young, Infertile Patient with no Other Causes of Infertility

The patient typically has been investigated for infertility by one or more specialists without identification of its cause. Infertility in such patients may be the only symptom, and pelvic findings may be entirely within normal limits. If laparoscopy reveals mild or moderate endometriosis without pelvic adhesions, the recommended treatment is pseudomenopause for a period of 3–6 months (Fig. 5). If conception does not follow within 6–12 months of treatment, a second-look laparoscopy may be indicated. In patients with moderate or severe endometriosis complicated by pelvic adhesions, 3–6 months of danazol treatment followed by resection of residual endometriosis and lysis of adhesions are recommended.

Management of Endometriosis in a Symptomatic Patient with Completed Family

The patient is usually in her late 30s or 40s and gives a history of one or more normal pregnancies at a relatively young age. At the time of the initial visit, she may be using some form of birth control or she might have undergone sterilization. The symptoms, usually dysmenorrhea or pelvic pain, began after the last pregnancy and are progressively getting worse. Pelvic findings may confirm the diagnosis of suspected endometriosis, and laparoscopy may reveal varying extent of the disease (Fig. 6). If the extent of endometriosis is mild, symptomatic treatment may be attempted. However, induction of pseudomenopause for 3–6 months will be more beneficial, especially in patients with severe symptoms. If endometriosis is moderate, either conservative surgery or hormonal treatment with danazol may be used. If endometriosis is severe, but the patient is relatively young, conservative surgery should be the treatment of choice. In older patients, definitive surgery should be considered.

Management of Endometriosis in a Patient with Recurrent Disease

The patient usually gives a history of endometriosis treated by a prior medical or surgical approach. The symptoms and pelvic findings are variable and depend on the extent of endometriosis and severity as well as location of adhesions. Infertility is frequently one of the major complaints. A second-look laparoscopy is indicated and strongly recommended. It should reveal the extent and location of

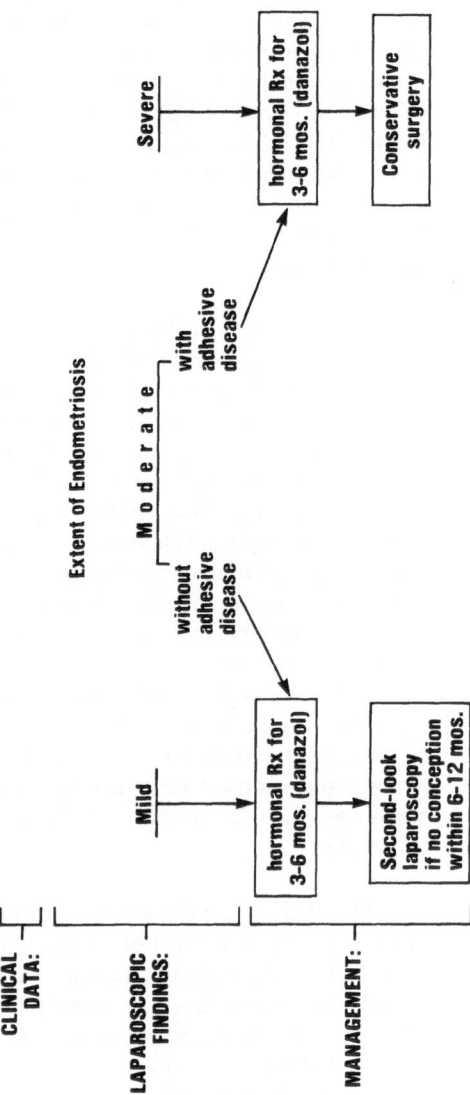

Figure 5. Management of endometriosis in a young, infertile patient with no other causes of infertility.

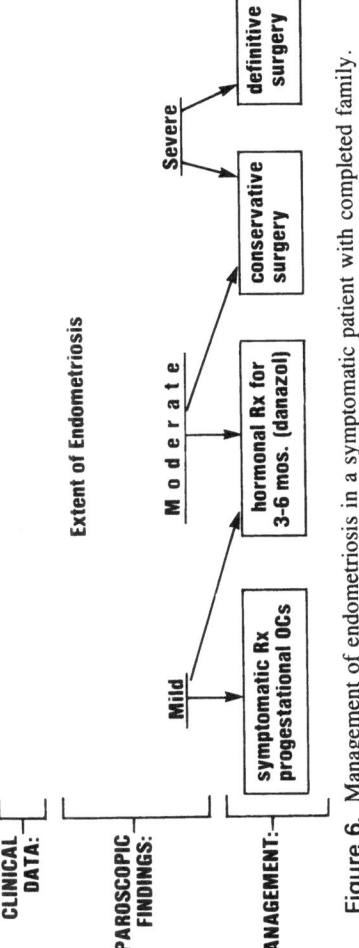

Figure 6. Management of endometriosis in a symptomatic patient with completed family.

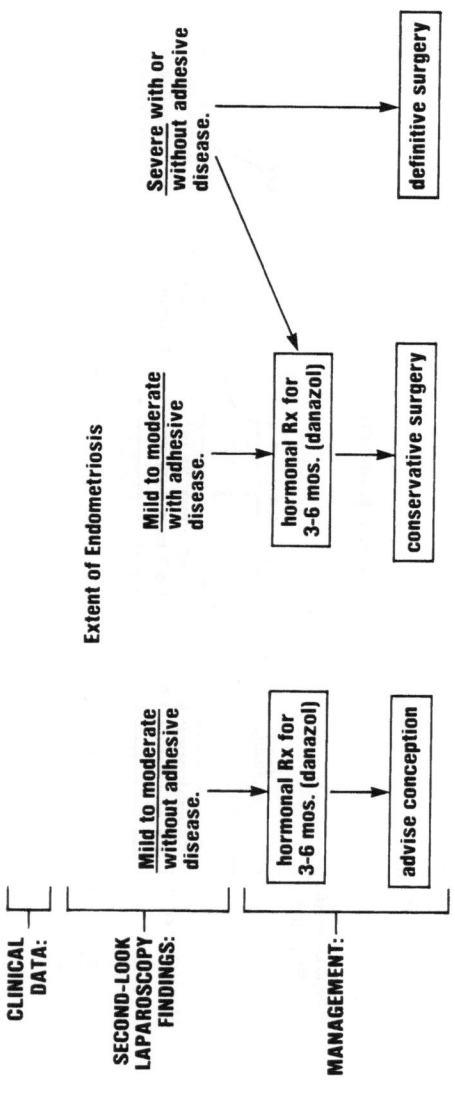

Figure 7. Management of endometriosis in a patient with recurrent disease.

the endometriosis as well as the extent and location of pelvic adhesions (Fig. 7). If mild to moderate endometriosis without adhesive disease is diagnosed, a 3- to 6-month course of treatment with pseudomenopause should be adequate. In patients with the same extent of endometriosis who have adhesions interfering with fertility, a 3- to 6-month course of danazol treatment followed by conservative surgery is recommended. If severe recurrent endometriosis is diagnosed, conservative surgery after treatment with danazol may be attempted. But if the patient has had previous surgery, and if overall chances for pregnancy are considered minimal, definitive surgery should be strongly considered.

REFERENCES

1. MacKenzie WF, Splitter GA, Valerio MG: Endometriosis in primates. *Med Primatol* 1:288, 1972.
2. Oliker AJ, Harris AE: Endometriosis of the bladder in a male patient. *J Urol* 106:858, 1971.
3. Pinkert TC, Catlow CE, Straus R: Endometriosis of the urinary bladder in a man with prostatic carcinoma. *Cancer* 43:1562, 1979.
4. Ebers G: *The Papyrus Ebers,* as quoted in Ridley JH: The histogenesis of endometriosis: A review of facts and fancies. *Obstet Gynecol Surv* 23:1, 1968.
5. Von Rokitansky C: 1860, as quoted in Ridley JH: The histogenesis of endometriosis: A review of facts and fancies. *Obstet Gynecol Surv* 23:1, 1968.
6. Sampson JA: Peritoneal endometriosis, due to menstrual dissemination of endometrial tissue into peritoneal cavity. *Am J Obstet Gynecol* 14:422, 1927.
7. Kistner RW: Endometriosis and infertility, in Behrman SJ, Kistner RW (eds): *Progress in Infertility,* ed 2. Boston, Little, Brown, 1975, p 345.
8. Kistner RW: Endometriosis, in Sciarra J (ed): *Gynecology and Obstetrics.* New York, Harper & Row, 1977, vol 1, p 1.
9. Meldrum DR, Shamonki I, Clark KE, et al: Prostaglandin content of ascitic fluid in endometriosis: A preliminary report. Presented at the 25th Annual Meeting of the Pacific Coast Fertility Society, Palm Springs, California, October, 1977.
10. Marik J, Hulka J: Luteinized unruptured follicle syndrome: A subtle cause of infertility. *Fertil Steril* 29:270, 1978.
11. Brosens IA, Koninckx PR, Corvelyn PA: A study of plasma progesterone, oestradiol-17β, prolactin and LH levels and of the luteal phase appearance of the ovaries in patients with endometriosis and infertility. *Br J Obstet Gynaecol* 85:246, 1978.
12. Dmowski WP, Rao R, Scommegna A: The luteinized unruptured follicle syndrome and endometriosis. *Fertil Steril* 33:30, 1980.
13. Weed JC, Arquembourg PC, Schneider GT: Autoimmunity in endometriosis: A preliminary study. Presented at the Central Association of Obstetricians and Gynecologists, Minneapolis, Minnesota, September 25, 1980.

14. Acosta AA, Buttram VC Jr, Besch PK, et al: A proposed classification of pelvic endometriosis. *Obstet Gynecol* 42:19, 1973.
15. Dmowski WP, Cohen MR: Treatment of endometriosis with an antigonadotropin, danazol: A laparoscopic and histologic evaluation. *Obstet Gynecol* 46:147, 1975.
16. Kistner RW, Siegler AM, Behrman SJ: Suggested classification for endometriosis: Relationship to infertility. *Fertil Steril* 28:1008, 1977.
17. Buttram VC Jr: An expanded classification of endometriosis. *Fertil Steril* 30:240, 1978.
18. The American Fertility Society: Classification of endometriosis. *Fertil Steril* 32:633, 1979.
19. McArthur JW, Ulfelder H: The effect of pregnancy upon endometriosis. *Obstet Gynecol Surv* 20:709, 1965.
20. Mocquot P, Musset R: Remarques sur la physiologie pathologique des endometrioses a propos de trois observations d'endometriose du cul-de-sac posterieur du vagin. *Gynecol Obstet* 48:135, 1949.
21. Dmowski WP: Endocrine properties and clinical application of danazol. *Fertil Steril* 31:237, 1979.
22. Eldridge JC, Dmowski WP, Mahesh VB: Effects of castration of immature rats on serum FSH and LH, and of various steroid treatments after castration. *Biol Reprod* 10:438, 1974.
23. Dmowski WP, Scholer HFL, Mahesh VB, et al: Danazol—a synthetic steroid derivative with interesting physiologic properties. *Fertil Steril* 22:9, 1971.
24. Greenblatt RB, Dmowski WP, Mahesh VB, et al: Clinical studies with an antigonadotropin—danazol. *Fertil Steril* 22:111, 1971.
25. Wood GP, Wu CH, Flickinger GL, et al: Hormonal changes associated with danazol therapy. *Obstet Gynecol* 45:302, 1975.
26. Andrews MC, Wentz AC: The effects of danazol on gonadotropins and steroid blood levels in normal and anovulatory women. *Am J Obstet Gynecol* 121:817, 1975.
27. Franchimont P, Cramilion C: The effect of danazol on anterior pituitary function. *Fertil Steril* 28:814, 1977.
28. Davison C, Banks W, Fritz A: The absorption, distribution and metabolic fate of danazol in rats, monkeys, and human volunteers. *Arch Int Pharmacodyn Ther* 221:294, 1976.
29. Rosi D, Neumann HC, Christiansen RG, et al: Isolation, synthesis, and biological activity of 5 metabolites of danazol. *J Med Chem* 20:349, 1977.
30. Potts GO: Pharmacology of danazol. *J Int Med Res* 5:1, 1977.
31. Chamness GC, Asch RH, Pauerstein CJ: Danazol binding and translocation of steroid receptors. *Am J Obstet Gynecol* 136:426, 1980.
32. Barbieri RL, Canick JA, Makris A, et al: Danazol inhibits steroidogenesis. *Fertil Steril* 28:809, 1977.
33. Asch RH, Fernandez EO, Siler-Khodr TM, et al: Mechanism of induction of luteal phase defects by danazol. *Am J Obstet Gynecol* 136:932, 1980.
34. Dmowski WP, Scommegna A: The rationale for treatment of endometriosis with danazol, in Greenblatt RB (ed): *Recent Advances in Endometriosis, Proceedings of a Symposium.* Amsterdam, Excerpta Medica, 1976, p 99.
35. Friedlander RL: The treatment of endometriosis with danazol. *J Reprod Med* 10:197, 1973.

36. Ansbacher R: Treatment of endometriosis with danazol. *Am J Obstet Gynecol* 121:283, 1975.
37. Chalmers JA, Shervington PC: Danazol treatment and follow-up of patients with endometriosis. *J Int Med Res* 5:72, 1977.
38. Dmowski WP, Cohen MR: Antigonadotropin (danazol) in the treatment of endometriosis. Evaluation of post-treatment fertility and three year follow-up data. *Am J Obstet Gynecol* 130:41, 1978.
39. Ingerslev M: Danazol: An antigonadotropic agent in the treatment of recurrent pelvic and intestinal endometriosis. *Acta Obstet Gynecol Scand* 56:343, 1977.
40. Lauersen NH, Wilson KH, Birnbaum S: Danazol: An antigonadotropic agent in the treatment of pelvic endometriosis. *Am J Obstet Gynecol* 123:742, 1975.
41. Young MD, Blackmore WP: The use of danazol in the management of endometriosis. *J Int Med Res* 5:86, 1977.
42. Moore EE, Archer DF, Harger JH: Treatment of pelvic endometriosis with low dose danazol. Presented at the American Fertility Society 36th Annual Meeting, Houston, Texas, March, 1980.
43. Dmowski WP, Kapetanakis M, Scommegna A: Variable effects on endometriosis of danazol at different low-dose levels: Laparscopic and histologic evaluation. In preparation.
44. Williams TA, Edelson J, Ross R Jr: A radioimmunoassay for danazol (17α-pregna-2,4,-dien-20-yno-[2,3-D]-isoxazole-17-ol). *Steroids* 31: 205, 1978.
45. Kistner RW: The use of newer progestins in the treatment of endometriosis. *Am J Obstet Gynecol* 75:264, 1958.
46. Kistner RW: The treatment of endometriosis by inducing pseudopregnancy with ovarian hormones: A report of 58 cases. *Fertil Steril* 10:539, 1959.
47. Kistner RW: Observations on the effects of a new synthetic progestogens on endometriosis in the human female. *Fertil Steril* 16:61, 1965.
48. Kourides IA, Kistner RW: Three synthetic progestins in the treatment of endometriosis. *Obstet Gynecol* 31:821, 1968.
49. Kistner RW: Management of endometriosis in the infertile patient. *Fertil Steril* 26:1151, 1975.
50. Timonen S, Johansson CJ: Endometriosis treated with lynestrenol. *Ann Chir Gynaecol Fenn* 57:144, 1968.
51. Andrews MC, Andrews WC, Strauss AF: Effects of progestin induced pseudopregnancy on endometriosis: Clinical and microscopic studies. *Am J Obstet Gynecol* 78:776, 1959.
52. Riva HL, Wilson JH, Kawaski DM: Effect of norethynodrel on endometriosis. *Am J Obstet Gynecol* 82:109, 1961.
53. Kistner RW: Infertility with endometriosis. A plan of therapy. *Fertil Steril* 13:237, 1962.
54. Williams BFP: Conservative management of endometriosis: Follow-up observations of progestin therapy. *Obstet Gynecol* 30:76, 1967.
55. Hirst JC: Conservative treatment and therapeutic test for endometriosis by androgens. *Am J Obstet Gynecol* 53:483, 1947.
56. Creadick RN: The non-surgical treatment of endometriosis. *NC Med J* 11:576, 1950.
57. Preston SN, Campbell HB: Pelvic endometriosis: Treatment with methyltestosterone. *Obstet Gynecol* 2:152, 1953.
58. Katayama KP, Manuel M, Jones HW, et al: Methyltestosterone treat-

ment of infertility associated with pelvic endometriosis. *Fertil Steril* 27:83, 1976.

59. Hammond MG, Hammond CB, Parker RT: Conservative treatment of endometriosis externa: The effects of methyltestosterone therapy. *Fertil Steril* 29:651, 1978.

60. Scott RB, Wharton LR: The effect of testosterone on experimental endometriosis in rhesus monkeys. *Am J Obstet Gynecol* 78:1020, 1959.

61. Karnaky KJ: The use of stilbestrol for endometriosis. *South Med J* 41:1109, 1948.

62. Hoskins AL, Woolf RB: Stilbestrol-induced hyperhormonal amenorrhea for the treatment of pelvic endometriosis. *Obstet Gynecol* 5:113, 1955.

63. Douglas CF, Weed JC: Endometriosis treated with prolonged administration of diethylstilbestrol: A report of a case. *Obstet Gynecol* 13:744, 1959.

64. Hasson HM: Electrocoagulation of pelvic endometriotic lesions with laparoscopic control. *Am J Obstet Gynecol* 135:115, 1979.

65. Sulewski JM, Curcio FD, Bronitsky C, et al: The treatment of endometriosis at laparoscopy for infertility. *Am J Obstet Gynecol* 138:128, 1980.

66. Cheng YS: Ureteral injury resulting from laparoscopic fulguration of endometriotic implant. *Am J Obstet Gynecol* 126:1045, 1976.

67. Buttram VC: Surgical treatment of endometriosis in the infertile female: A modified approach. *Fertil Steril* 32:635, 1979.

68. Hammond CB, Rock JA, Parker RT: Conservative treatment of endometriosis: The effects of limited surgery and hormonal pseudopregnancy. *Fertil Steril* 27:756, 1976.

69. Andrews WC, Larsen GD: Endometriosis: Treatment with hormonal pseudopregnancy and/or operation. *Am J Obstet Gynecol* 118:643, 1974.

70. Moghissi KS, Boyce CR: Management of endometriosis with oral medroxyprogesterone acetate. *Obstet Gynecol* 47:265, 1976.

71. Gunning JE, Moyer D: The effect of medroxypreogesterone acetate on endometriosis in the human female. *Fertil Steril* 18:759, 1967.

13 Magnified Surgery of the Vas Deferens

Lawrence Dubin and Richard D. Amelar

Department of Urology
New York University School of Medicine
New York, New York 10016

Careful surgery is a must in dealing with the vas deferens. The use of magnification in this surgery has certainly increased the success rate when compared to series performed only 10 years ago.[1] The type and degree of magnification necessary will vary from surgeon to surgeon depending on that surgeon's visual acuity and microsurgical ability.

We find both the microscope and high- and low-power loupes extremely helpful but recommend that surgeons practice with these optical aids prior to actually performing surgery with them. Belker et al.[2] have devised an excellent method of doing this using preserved vasectomy specimens. A novice using the microscope or high-powered loupes is doomed to frustration and failure.

We suggest that surgeons try working with loupes and the microscope. Later, they can decide which is better in their hands. Recently an expanded-field loupe telescope has been developed (Designs for Vision, New York) that makes magnified surgery much easier. These loupes, which are available from $\times 2$ to $\times 8$, are shown in Fig. 2 of Chapter 4.

Microsurgery requires "micro" instruments. Many instruments already used by ophthalmologists and plastic surgeons will be useful for this surgery. Many companies are manufacturing special instruments for microsurgery as well. The individual surgeon must choose those instruments with which he works best.

VASOVASOSTOMY

There has been a marked increase in the number of requests for vasectomy reversal in the past decade. The publicized fact that reversal operations can often be successful has led many men to consider this option.

The reason for desiring vas reanastomosis and restored fertility are various: (1) a subsequent marriage (usually to a younger woman) with a desire to have children in this new union, (2) death or severe injury of children, (3) change of heart in a patient who thought as a young man that sterilization would aid society and zero population growth, (4) improvement in the economic situation of a couple, making children more desirable, and (5) psychological inability to tolerate the concept of being sterile.

We recently have seen several patients who requested vasectomy reversal because they had exhausted the supply of their own semen, which had been frozen and stored in a commercial bank for fertility insurance before vasectomy. Their wives had failed to conceive by repeated inseminations with the stored frozen semen.[3]

Alexander and Clarkson have reported an increase in diet-induced atherosclerosis in a small series of monkeys after vasectomy.[4] Extensive studies in a large series of monkeys are now in progress. If this preliminary study is confirmed in man, the demand for vasectomy reversal would certainly increase markedly.

ANATOMIC AND PHYSIOLOGICAL CONSIDERATIONS

The vas deferens is easily palpable in the scrotum as a portion of the spermatic cord. It is about 35 cm in length and 3 mm in diameter. The vas has a thick muscular wall, and the vas lumen has a mean diameter of 1.0 mm.[5] The vas extends from the cauda epididymis, where it originates as a convoluted structure, and, after its proximal 2 cm, it becomes straight and courses upward through the scrotum, the inguinal canal, retroperitoneum, and pelvis, over the ureter, and behind the bladder. The terminal portion enlarges to form an ampullary portion that joins the duct of the seminal vesicle, forming the ejaculatory duct. Histologically, the vas deferens is lined by mucosa and is surrounded by a wall composed of three layers of smooth muscle: longitudinal muscle in the outer and inner layers and circular muscle in the middle. This thick muscular wall affords powerful peristaltic motion. Exterior to this muscle layer there is a sheath of connective tissue. The epithelial lining of the lumen varies along the length of the vas deferens. Near the epididymis, the mucosa resembles the epithelium in the cauda epididymidis and is characterized by large columnar cells with regularly placed pairs of cilia that are actually sterocilia or microvilli that may have an absorptive function. These sterocilia do not move as do the cilia of the rete testis and the efferent ductules. Distally, the epithelial cells lining the lumen of the vas deferens become nonciliated and smaller in size.

Anatomically, the portion of the vas deferens of clinical interest for performing vasectomy is generally in the midscrotal portion.

The blood supply to the vas deferens is derived from the deferential artery, a branch of the inferior vesical artery, which provides an important collateral blood supply to the testis. At the time of vasectomy, if the deferential artery is not carefully ligated or coagulated, it may be a potential site of hemorrhage. The sheath of the vas deferens contains nerve fibers for pain and sympathetic fibers that release norepinephrine. These fibers may be responsible for the presence of the spontaneous motility of the human vas deferens that has been demonstrated *in vitro*. The presence of spontaneous motility *in vitro* leads to the working hypothesis that there is spontaneous motility of the human vas deferens *in vivo*.

Tone in the sympathetic fibers innervating the vas deferens probably is dependent on the integrity of the spinal center. It is believed that the intrinsic rhythmicity of the vas deferens depends on the local concentration of norepinephrine. However, the powerful and coordinated series of contractions that propel sperm from the epididymis to the urethra during ejaculation are initiated and controlled by the release of substantial amounts of norepinephrine from the sympathetic nerve endings. It is well known that spermatozoa are expelled from the cauda epididymidis and vas deferens at the time of ejaculation.

Vasectomy results in the division of the inferior spermatic nerve that runs parallel to the vas deferens and innervates it. Attempts at vasectomy reversal may fail to restore fertility because, although the sympathetic fibers are strongly regenerative and, consequently, if divided would probably grow from the vas deferens to reinnervate the lower vas and epididymis, iatrogenic surgical factors may prevent regeneration and restoration of the sympathetic nerve supply. These factors include (1) the removal of a large segment of the vas, (2) the placement of a suture or clip too close to the sheath around the stump of the vas, and (3) an inflammatory reaction in scar tissue in response to the trauma of the operation. An intact sympathetic nerve supply probably is essential for the transport of sperm from the epididymis at the time of ejaculation. Without such a supply to the vas deferens and epididymis, complete recovery of sperm output is unlikely to be achieved after a functional vasovasostomy.

After vasectomy, the lumen of the testicular side of the vas increases 70% in mean diameter because of the obstruction.[6] Silber believes that this dilatation on the testicular side can be reduced by intentionally allowing sperm leakage from the testicular end of the vas at the time of vasectomy,[7] but this suggestion has precipitated a great deal of criticism,[8] and Silber has since retracted this suggestion for use as a routine in performance of vasectomy until further experimental evidence is accumulated.

The difference in the relative size of the two vas lumina requires that the anastomosis unite lumina of different diameters, and efforts should be made to avoid subsequent leakage of sperm at the site of the anastomosis, which can lead to the formation of granulomas with subsequent antibody formation.[9]

RESULTS   The reported experience with vasectomy reversal operations is shown in Table I.

Table I
Selected World Experience with Vasectomy Reversal

Author	Number of cases	% With sperm	% Pregnancies
O'Connor (Survey) (1948)[10]	420	45%	Not reported
Phadke and Phadke (1967)[12]	76	83%	55%
Hulka and Davis (1972)[11]	705	60%	Not reported
Lee (1975)[13]	156	81%	35%
Owen (1977)[15]	50	98%	72%
Silber (1978)[7]	400	94%	71%
Schmidt (1975, 1978)[14]	45	80–90%	42%
Middleton and Henderson (1978)[16]	110	74%	39%
Amelar and Dubin (before 1976)[17]	93	84%	33%
Amelar and Dubin (1976–1978)	69	87%	55%

O'Connor reported a survey of American urologists in 1948 with a success rate of 45% for 420 vasovasostomies accomplished by many different splinted and nonsplinted techniques.[10] However, it must be remembered that there is a difference between sperm appearing in the ejaculate and the occurrence of pregnancy.

Hulka and Davis compiled the results from 705 vasovasostomies from the world literature.[11] In 60% of these cases, reappearance of sperm was reported. Phadke and Phadke had 83% of 76 cases with sperm and 55% pregnancy rate.[12] Lee reported 156 cases of vas reanastomosis: 81% of these patients had viable sperm in the ejaculates, but there was a pregnancy rate of only 35%.[13] Schmidt has reported 80–90% sperm appearance with 42% pregnancy rates.[14] Owen achieved 98% sperm appearance and 72% pregnancy rate with unilateral vasovasostomy using a two-layer microsurgical technique.[15]

Silber, using the operating microscope and a two-layer anastomosis in a series of 400 patients, reported excellent results[5] with at least some sperm present in 94% of patients and a 71% pregnancy rate in the first 42 patients followed for $1\frac{1}{2}$ years.

Middleton and Henderson used a simple nonmagnified technique with a 6-0 Prolene® and reported the reappearance of sperm in 74% and a pregnancy rate of 39% in 110 vasectomy reversals in the last $6\frac{1}{2}$ years.[16]

In our own series of 93 vasovasostomies, which were performed before 1976 and followed for at least 2 years, sperm were present in 78 men (84%). Thirty-one couples had children (a pregnancy rate of 33%).[16] In 69 vasectomy reversals that we have performed using magnification during the years 1976 through December 1978, sperm were found in 60 cases (87%), and pregnancies have occurred so far in 38 cases (55%).

It is of interest that spontaneous recanalization of the vas does occur in 1–2% of the cases after vasectomy.[18-21] Semen analysis should be performed before vas reanastomosis lest the operation not be necessary at all. It is amazing that even after a highly tortuous and scarified spontaneous reanastomosis, semen qualities of significant fertility potential may be present.

SURGICAL TECHNIQUE OF VASOVASOSTOMY

We are now using a nonsplinted technique with surgical ocular lenses of 6-power magnification (Fig. 1) and eight 6-0 Prolene® sutures. The increased magnification afforded by the expanded-field surgical telescope has contributed, we believe, to our recent better results as compared to our results in the operation we performed prior to 1976.

The scrotum is well prepared with antiseptic and draped appropriately. The scrotum is then palpated to identify the scarred area or granuloma secondary to the vasectomy and the ends of the vas if possible. An incision of 2–3 in. is then made in the scrotum over this area, and the testis and spermatic cord are delivered from the scrotum. The fascia is incised to expose the scarred ends of the vas, which must be excised. The distal vas is incised, cannulated with a blunt needle, and tested for patency by injection of hydrogen peroxide dyed with methylene blue. Spatulation of the distal end may be necessary, since the proximal end usually is dilated and has a greater diameter. The proximal vas is then incised, and fluid from the vas is placed on a microscope slide and examined by an assistant for the presence of sperm. Efforts should be made to prevent spillage of vasal fluid containing sperm into the tissues to prevent granuloma or antibody formation.

Vasoepididymal anastomosis should be considered if no sperm are found in the proximal vas.

Using 6-power ocular loupe magnification, eight through-and-through 6-0 Prolene® sutures are placed with the knots on the outside of the lumen of the vas. The first four sutures are placed at each quadrant, and the remaining four are placed between the quadrant sutures (Fig. 1). This procedure gives a closure that aligns mucosa to mucosa and serosa to serosa. The closure is watertight and should not be under tension. Freeing the distal vas will often relieve any possible tension.

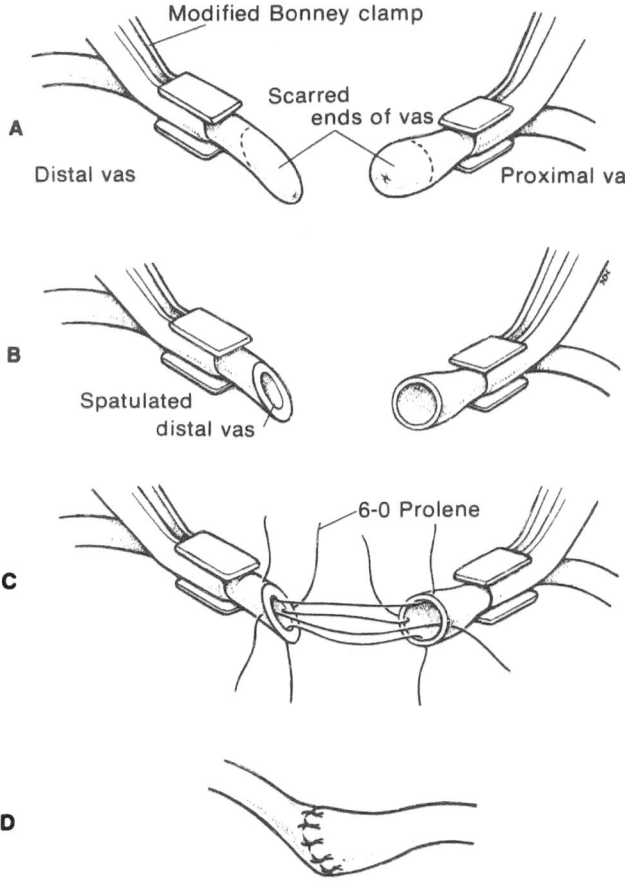

Figure 1. Vasovasostomy. (A) Ends of vas deferens are exposed, and scarred ends are excised. (B) After patency has been tested, distal vas deferens may require spatulation. (C) Vasovasostomy with interrupted 6-0 prolene atraumatic sutures. (D) completed anastomosis. (From Amelar et al.,[22] reprinted with permission.)

The fascia is then closed above the anastomosis. Small indwelling Penrose drains are left, depending on the extent of the operation, and the skin is closed with catgut sutures. A pressure dressing or scrotal support is then applied.

Schmidt uses a similar nonsplinted one-layer anastomosis, but he uses an operating microscope for the placement of 7-0 to 9-0 nylon sutures. Silber uses the delicate two-layer anastomosis with the operating microscope and emphasizes the importance of a precise watertight anastomosis. Magnification of $\times 16$ or $\times 25$ is used with 9-0 nylon suture material.[7]

The reasons for the marked discrepancy between the presence of sperm after vasovasostomy and the pregnancy rates remain obscure. Certainly, there may be a relationship between fertility and the presence of sperm-agglutinating and -immobilizing antibodies in as many as 62% of men tested after vasectomy.[23-28] Significantly high titers (1 : 32 or greater) of antibodies also were found in 18 of 29 men (62.1%) with congenital bilateral absence of the vasa deferentia.[29] Such titers may be related to epididymal obstruction.

High antibody titers per se are not a contraindication to an operation, although they may be a poor prognostic sign. We have seen these titers return to normal in some patients after successful vasovasostomy. In others, the levels remained elevated, and sperm motility was poor.

Semen analysis after vasovasostomy may show sperm as early as 1 month postoperatively, but sperm may not appear in some cases until 6 months later. Poor sperm motility is likely to be noted in the early ejaculates, but motility should be at an adequate level by 6 months. If the semen qualities are poor, further investigation of the patient for other causes of infertility (for example, varicocele or hormonal imbalance) and appropriate therapy are indicated.

The improved results with vas reanastomosis recently reported by urologists using various techniques may be related to the elimination of the use of exteriorized intravasal splints that generally were removed several days or even weeks postoperatively. Such stents would often lead to sperm leakage and granuloma formation at the point of exit from the vas with subsequent obstructions and an increased incidence of antisperm antibody formation.[28] These exteriorized splints also could be a pathway for infection.

The consensus after a panel discussion on the various current techniques for vasectomy reversal by vasovasostomy (nonmagnified single layer, ocular loupe-magnified single layer, microsurgical single layer, and microsurgical double layer) is that, at the present time, long-term comparative results are simply not available.[30] There were present a number of urologic surgeons who have acquired considerable experience with vas reconstruction, and they are having fair success in terms of subsequent pregnancies using a variety of surgical techniques with or without the operating microscope. Certainly, the more experience with a particular technique the surgeon has acquired, the better will be the results. This definitely is not an operation to be performed casually by the urologist who does not have a special interest and expertise in treating infertility problems.

The interval between vasectomy and vas reanastomosis usually does not appear to influence the rate of success in vasectomy reversal, but this interval may be critical in the individual patient who has suffered irreversible obstructive damage to the testes or epididymides after vasectomy. Schmidt has reported successful reanastomosis as long as 21 years after vasectomy.[6] Phadke and Phadke also have reported success regardless of the time between vasectomy and reanastomosis.[12] Silber reported that he obtained poor results in patients who had vasectomies performed more than 10 years before reanastomosis and excellent results when the vasectomy was performed within 2 years of the reversal operation.[7] However, most patients who request vasectomy reversal within 2 years probably should never have been sterilized in the first place. Silber believes that a prolonged duration of vas obstruction has a deleterious effect on the successful return of fertility after reconstruction of the vas deferens and that any series of vasovasostomies weighted toward patients whose vasectomies were performed more recently, no matter which surgical technique is used, will have a higher success rate than a series weighted toward patients whose vasectomies were performed more than 10 years previously. The data that would allow conclusions with respect to a critical interval beyond which reconstruction of the vas should not be attempted are still not available.

EPIDIDYMO-VASOSTOMY

When the seminal ejaculate is azoospermic but contains fructose, and the testicular biopsy has demonstrated normal spermatogenesis, epididymal obstruction is highly probable. Multiple cystic anomalies of microscopic size and other congenital defects are presently far more common causes of such obstruction than are postinflammatory obstructive lesions resulting from untreated gonorrhea. The fructose test serves to differentiate congenital absence of the ductal system form occlusions of the duct. Complete azoospermia resulting from tuberculosis is generally not amenable to surgical correction because of the extensive involvement of the epididymides, vasa, and seminal vesicles.

Robert Schoysman of Belgium suggests that there is no necessity for preliminary biopsy of the testis. He feels that the presence of an epididymis distended with sperm as seen under a microscope at the time of exploration is sufficient evidence of active spermatogenesis in the testis and obstruction of the epididymis (R. Schoysman, personal communication, 1974).

Postinflammatory lesions of the tail of the epididymis offer the best chance for cure. Among patients successfully undergoing this operation, about 20% have been able to achieve pregnancy, and these patients deserve the champagne. Sperm may appear in the ejaculate of a much higher percentage of the patients, however.

Only rare success has been reported in those cases in which azoospermia results from congenital anomalies rather than from postinflammatory obstruction.

Hanley[31] reported only one pregnancy after 83 vaso-epididymal anastomoses. In these patients, sperm were found in the head of the epididymis, and the vas was patent, but a congenital anomaly of the epididymis was present.

In our own series of 69 cases of azoospermia secondary to epididymal obstruction, all performed more than 1 year ago, there were 24 patients with a definite history of epididymitis, and the other 45 patients had congenital epididymal obstructions. Bilateral side-to-side epididymo-vasostomy on the 24 patients with epididymitis resulted in 14 patients able to produce sperm in their ejaculates (55%), but only six (20%) had good semen quality. Seven men caused pregnancies that resulted in six normal children, and there was one early miscarriage.

The procedure we have used in these cases is a modification of techniques first described by Hagner, Humphreys, and Hotchkiss.[22] The principle of this operation is the anastomosis of a minute elliptical opening in the vas to a similar opening in the epididymis where live sperm have been recovered.

In our operative technique, the testes, epididymides, and spermatic cords are exposed through bilateral scrotal incisions. The straight portions of the vasa are identified and are freed from the other cord structures, taking care to avoid devascularization of the vasa. A sufficient length of vas is mobilized so that it can be easily approximated to the epididymis without tension.

Using a number 11 blade, an incision is made into the epididymis at the level of the globus minor on the border opposite its testicular attachment. Any fluid that escapes from the epididymal incision is collected on a sterile glass slide, mixed with a drop of saline, and handed to an assistant outside the sterile field, who places it under the microscope. In favorable cases, many motile sperm will be identified. If sperm are few or absent, another incision is made into the more proximal parts of the epididymis, and the procedure is repeated until a satisfactory site is found for anastomosis.

By making the first exploratory epididymal incision at a point some distance from its proximal portion, part of the epididymis can be preserved for whatever function it affords the sperm. If the operation fails, a second attempt can be made at a later date, using the remaining proximal areas for a new anastomosis.

Once a favorable site in the epididymis has been selected on each side, the vas is brought adjacent to it, and

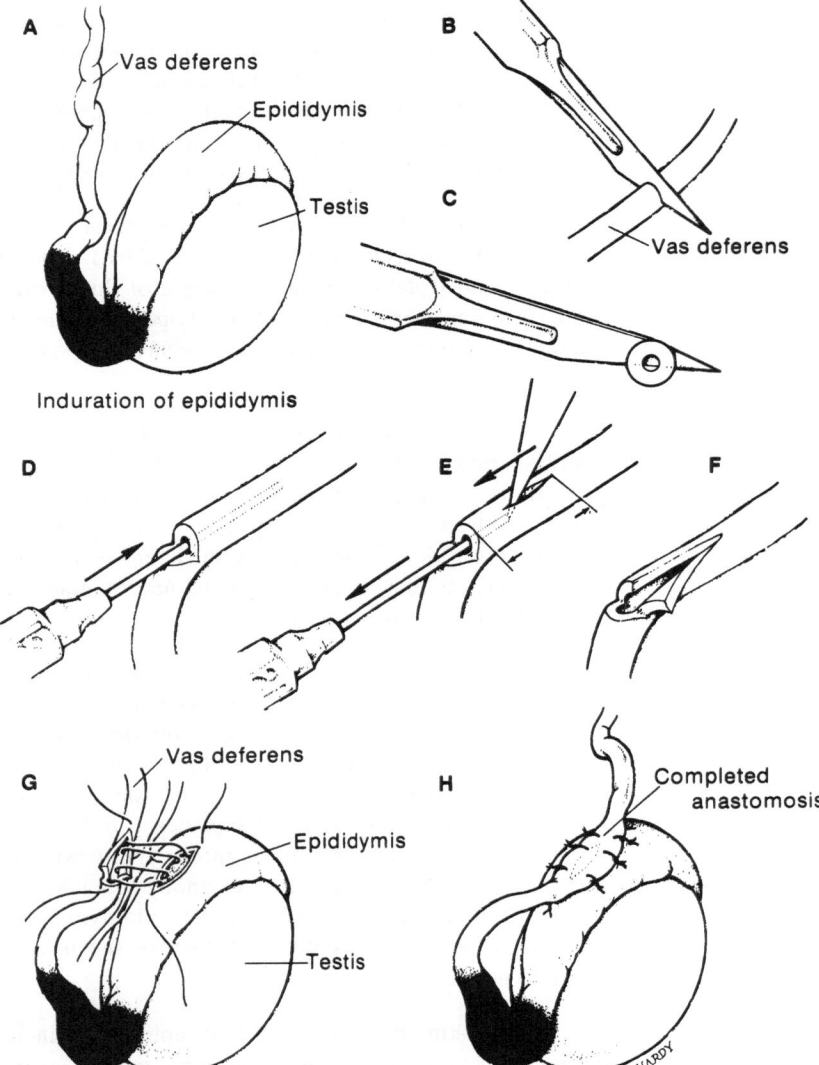

Figure 2. Method of epididymovasostomy. (A) Exposure of anatomy and area of induration and obstruction. (B–F) Method of incision of vas deferens and preparation of the vas for epididymovasostomy. (G) Vasoepididymal anastomosis using interrupted 6-0 Prolene® sutures. (H) Completed anastomosis. (From Amelar et al.,[22] reprinted with permission.)

an incision is made into the vas. An invaluable surgical maneuver for making a clean and adequate incision is to support the vas on the index finger of the left hand while making the transverse incision through the upper portion of the tubular vas with the right hand. The incision should be just deep enough to expose the lumen, and care must be taken not to cut entirely through the vas (see Fig. 2).

A 21-gauge hypodermic needle, the tip of which has been honed to blunt its sharp edge, is inserted into the lumen of the distal segment of the vas. A few milliliters of hydrogen peroxide that has been colored blue with a few drops of indigo carmine is injected to insure that the vas is patent. The tip of the needle is then withdrawn to a point 0.5 cm above the transverse incision. The point of the #11 blade is inserted into the wall of the vas so that it engages the lumen of the blunted end of the needle. Then, as the needle is pulled downward with gentle traction, the knife engaged in the tip of the needle cuts the desired uniform opening through the wall of the vas.

If the blue peroxide solution does not flow easily into the vas, or if there is any doubt about patency, a catheter can be passed into the bladder. If the vas is patent, the urine will be blue. If it is necessary to perform this procedure with the other vas, the bladder will have to be irrigated until the return fluids are clear.

If no solution can be injected into the vas, #1 nylon suture can be passed into the vas as a probe to locate the site of the obstruction. If the obstruction is in an accessible area of the vas, it may be possible to reenter the vas above the point of obstruction and make another test of patency. Occasionally, multiple points of obstruction may be encountered, and if it is not feasible to detour around them, the vasoepididymal anastomosis will have to be eliminated on that side.

Atraumatic 6-0 Prolene® sutures are used for the anastomosis. The sutures are placed through each wall of the incised vas and then deeply into the epididymis in such a manner that all knots are outside the anastomosis. We have found it helpful to use an ocular loupe with 6-power magnification during the placing of these sutures.

At the conclusion of the anastomosis, the scrotal contents are replaced, and the scrotum is closed in two layers with interrupted 3-0 chromic catgut sutures. Penrose drains are used and are left in place for 24 hr. Sterile dressings and a scrotal suspensory or pressure drainage are applied. The patient may be discharged from the hospital on the third or fourth postoperative day.

The procedure of epididymovasostomy is performed on both sides unless the preliminary biopsy has revealed a hopeless condition in one of the testes. On occasion, when the testicle is normal on one side but its vas is occluded, and the opposite testicle is deficient but has a patent vas, a crossed anastomosis has been done successfully. In one such case, the patient had unilateral testicular atrophy on the right side and an injured left vas incidental to a difficult low ureterolithotomy, resulting in sterility. At operation, the proximal left vas from the healthy testicle was anastomosed by crossover to the patent distal vas on the right side. He subsequently was found to have good semen quality and has since had two children.

In one case in which the point of obstruction on the right side appeared to be at the ejaculatory duct itself, an attempt was made to release the obstruction by forcible irrigation. All that we succeeded in accomplishing on this side was to blow up the seminal vesicle to enormous proportions, but the blue tinted radiographic fluid still would not enter the bladder. The temporary seminal vesicle distention was confirmed by radiographic and rectal examinations immediately after the operative procedures. On the left side, however, there was congenital atresia of the epididymis and the convoluted lowermost segment of the vas; the remainder of the vas was patent. A crossed anastomosis was performed in this instance, and sperm were subsequently found in the ejaculum, but so far a pregnancy has not occurred.

When the anastomosis is successful, sperm may be found in the ejaculum within 3–6 months; but occasionally, it may require up to a year before sperm appear. Periodic follow-up with semen analysis should be performed for at least 1 year before it is determined that the procedure has not been successful.

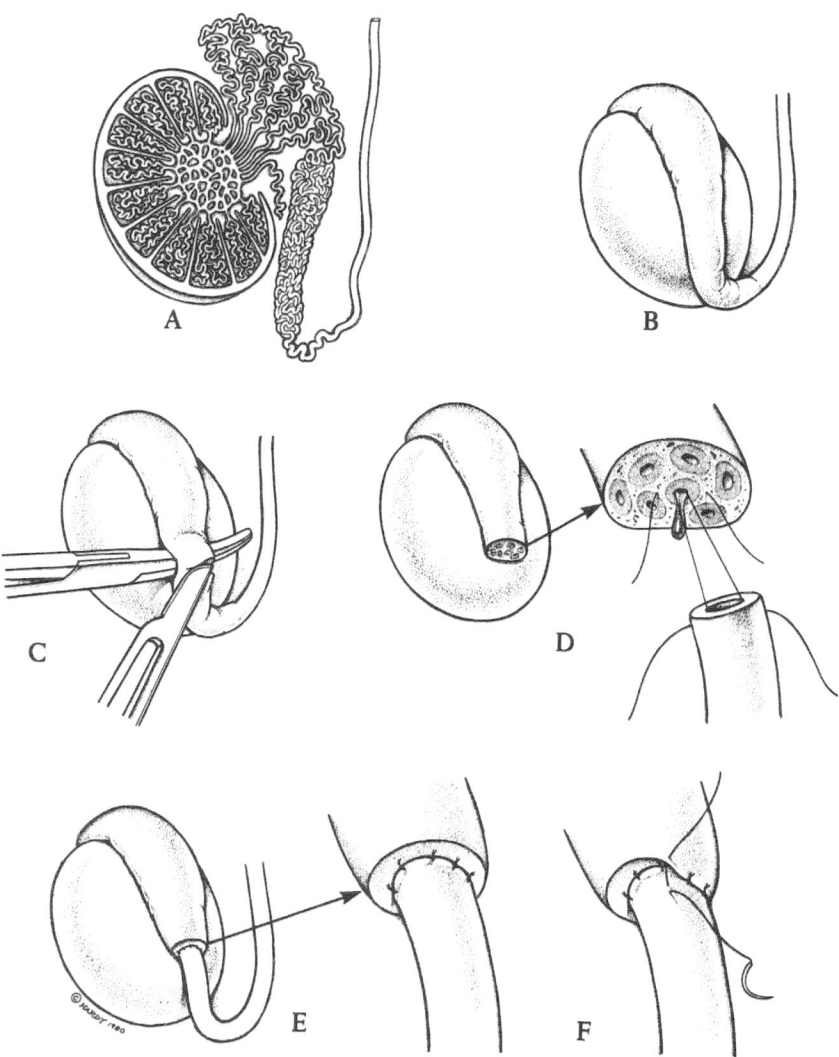

Figure 3. Dubin and Amelar modification of epididymovasostomy. (A and B) Anatomy. (C) Epididymis is transected. (D) Tubule with sperm-rich fluid is identified. (E and F) Anastomosis.

In 1978, Silber proposed a new surgical approach to the problem of epididymal obstruction that may offer a much better prognosis than we have been able to achieve so far using the conventional technique we have just described.[32] The epididymis is one long tube, 22 ft long, coiled into a space $1\frac{1}{2}$ in. long. After an incision is made into the epididymis, any sperm leaking out are indeed leaking out from only one of the many convolutions of that tube that has been cut. Careful inspection using magnification will reveal the specific epididymal tubule that is leaking sperm. Silber now employs a delicate microsurgical technique to create an end-to-end anastomosis between the inner lumen of the vas and the one specific epididymal tubule after he has completely transected the vas and the epididymis; he reports success in a small number of patients.[33]

We have modified Silber's technique of epididymovasostomy in our own practice, but it is too soon to cite our results with this technique. The concept of end-to-end anastomosis between the single leaking epididymal tubule and the vas seems to be an excellent one, and at least it offers hope for improved results.

Our method is shown in Fig. 3.

The testis is delivered as previously described. The distal vas is mobilized and cannulated. Dye or hydrogen peroxide is injected to prove distal patency. The epididymis is then transected. Observation with 6-power loupe or the microscope is now necessary to locate the tubule from which the sperm-containing fluid is flowing. The fluid should be checked for the presence of sperm with the light microscope if available. It is quite difficult to find the exact tubule, but one can locate the area of the epididymis from which the fluid is arising. Using magnification, an end-to-end anastomosis is performed using 6-0 Prolene® sutures. A second layer from the edge of the epididymis to the serosa of the vas can also then be performed. The testis is returned to the scrotum, and a Penrose drain is brought out through a stab wound. A pressure dressing is applied.

REFERENCES

1. Belker AM: Urologic microsurgery. Current perspectives: I: Vasovasostomy. *Urology* 14:325, 1979.

2. Belker AM, Acland RD, Sexter MS, et al: Microsurgical two-layer vasovasostomy: Laboratory use of vasectomized segments. *Fertil Steril* 29:48, 1978.

3. Amelar RD, Dubin L: Frozen semen—a poor form of fertility insurance. *Urology* 14:53, 1979.

4. Alexander NJ, Clarkson TB: Vasectomy increases the severity of diet induced atherosclerosis in *Macaca fascicularis. Science* 201:538, 1978.

5. Brueschke EE, Burns M, Maness JH, et al: Development of a reversible vas deferens occlusive device. I. Anatomical size of the human and dog vas deferens. *Fertil Steril* 25:659, 1974.

6. Schmidt SS: Anastomosis of the vas deferens: An experimental study, II. Success and failures in experimental anastomosis. *J Urol* 81:203, 1959.

7. Silber SJ: Vasectomy and vasectomy reversal. *Fertil Steril* 29:125, 1978.

8. Stewart BH: Letter to the editor. *Fertil Steril* 29:472, 1978.

9. Alexander NJ, Schmidt SS: Incidence of antisperm antibody levels and granulomas in men. *Fertil Steril* 28:655, 1977.

10. O'Connor VJ: Anastomosis of the vas deferens after purposeful division for sterility. *J Urol* 59:229, 1948.

11. Hulka JF, Davis JE: Vasectomy and reversible vasocclusion. *Fertil Steril* 23:683, 1972.

12. Phadke AM, Phadke AG: Experience in the reanastomosis of the vas deferens. *J Urol* 97:888, 1967.

13. Lee H: Technique and results of vasectomy in Korea, in Sciarra JJ (ed): *Control of Male Fertility.* New York, Harper & Row, 1975, p 76.

14. Schmidt SS: Principles of vasovasostomy. *Contemp Surg* 7:13, 1975.

15. Owen ER: Microsurgical vasovasostomy: A reliable vasectomy reversal. *Aust NZ J Surg* 47:305, 1977.

16. Middleton RG, Henderson D: Vas deferens reanastomosis without splints and without magnification. *J Urol* 119:763, 1978.

17. Amelar RD, Dubin L: Review article. Vasectomy reversal. *J Urol* 121:547, 1979.

18. Bunge RG: Bilateral spontaneous reanastomosis of the ductus deferens. *J Urol* 100:762, 1968.

19. Blandy J: Vasectomy. *Br J Hosp Med* 9:319, 1973.

20. Marshall S, Lyon RP: Transient reappearance of sperm after vasectomy. *JAMA* 219:1753, 1972.

21. Schmidt SS: Techniques and complications of elective vasectomy. The role of spermatic granuloma in spontaneous recanalization. *Fertil Steril* 17:467, 1966.

22. Amelar RD, Dubin L, Walsh PC: *Male Infertility.* Philadelphia, W. B. Saunders, 1977.

23. Phadke AM, Padukone K: Presence and significance of autoantibodies against spermatozoa in the blood of men with obstructed vas deferens. *J Reprod Fertil* 7:162, 1964.

24. Rumke P: Sperm-agglutinating autoantibodies in relation to male infertility. *Proc R Soc Med* 61:275, 1968.

25. Shulman S, Zappi E, Ahmed U, et al: Immunologic consequences of vasectomy. *Contraception* 5:269, 1972.

26. Ansbacher R: Vasectomy: Sperm antibodies. *Fertil Steril* 24:788, 1973.
27. Alexander NJ, Wilson BJ, Patterson GD: Vasectomy: Immunologic effects in rhesus monkeys and men. *Fertil Steril* 25:149, 1974.
28. Alexander NS, Schmidt SS: Incidence of antisperm antibody levels and granulomas in men. *Fertil Steril* 28:655, 1977.
29. Amelar RD, Dubin L, Schoenfeld C: Circulating sperm-agglutinating antibodies in azoospermic men with congenital bilateral absence of the vasa deferentia. *Fertil Steril* 26:228, 1975.
30. Amelar RD, Alexander N, O'Connor VJ Jr, et al: Vasectomy reversal. Panel discussion presented at the Annual Meeting of the American Urological Association, Washington, D.C., May 21–25, 1978.
31. Hanley HG: The surgery of male subfertility. *Ann R Coll Surg* 17:159, 1955.
32. Silber SJ: Microscopic vasoepididymostomy. *Fertil Steril* 30:565, 1978.
33. Silber SJ: Vasoepididymostomy to the head of the epididymis: Recovery of normal spermatozoal mobility. *Fertil Steril* 34:149, 1980.

Index